Marine Chitin 2019

Marine Chitin 2019

Special Issue Editors

Hitoshi Sashiwa

Hironori Izawa

MDPI • Basel • Beijing • Wuhan • Barcelona • Belgrade • Manchester • Tokyo • Cluj • Tianjin

Special Issue Editors
Hitoshi Sashiwa
Kaneka Co., Ltd.
Japan

Hironori Izawa
Tottori University
Japan

Editorial Office
MDPI
St. Alban-Anlage 66
4052 Basel, Switzerland

This is a reprint of articles from the Special Issue published online in the open access journal *Marine Drugs* (ISSN 1660-3397) (available at: https://www.mdpi.com/journal/marinedrugs/special_issues/Marine_Chitin_2019).

For citation purposes, cite each article independently as indicated on the article page online and as indicated below:

LastName, A.A.; LastName, B.B.; LastName, C.C. Article Title. *Journal Name* **Year**, *Article Number*, Page Range.

ISBN 978-3-03936-072-7 (Pbk)
ISBN 978-3-03936-073-4 (PDF)

Contents

About the Special Issue Editors vii

Preface to "Marine Chitin 2019" ix

Deeb Abu Fara, Linda Al-Hmoud, Iyad Rashid, Babur Z. Chowdhry and Adnan Badwan
Understanding the Performance of a Novel Direct Compression Excipient Comprising Roller Compacted Chitin
Reprinted from: *Mar. Drugs* **2020**, *18*, 115, doi:10.3390/md18020115 1

May Wenche Jøraholmen, Abhilasha Bhargava, Kjersti Julin, Mona Johannessen and Nataša Škalko-Basnet
The Antimicrobial Properties of Chitosan Can Be Tailored by Formulation
Reprinted from: *Mar. Drugs* **2020**, *18*, 96, doi:10.3390/md18020096 23

Shun-Hsien Chang, Ching-Hung Chen and Guo-Jane Tsai
Effects of Chitosan on *Clostridium perfringens* and Application in the Preservation of Pork Sausage
Reprinted from: *Mar. Drugs* **2020**, *18*, 70, doi:10.3390/md18020070 39

Raúl Cazorla-Luna, Araceli Martín-Illana, Fernando Notario-Pérez, Luis Miguel Bedoya, Aitana Tamayo, Roberto Ruiz-Caro, Juan Rubio and María-Dolores Veiga
Vaginal Polyelectrolyte Layer-by-Layer Films Based on Chitosan Derivatives and Eudragit® S100 for pH Responsive Release of Tenofovir
Reprinted from: *Mar. Drugs* **2020**, *18*, 44, doi:10.3390/md18010044 55

Hyunwoo Moon, Seunghwan Choy, Yeonju Park, Young Mee Jung, Jun Mo Koo and Dong Soo Hwang
Different Molecular Interaction between Collagen and α- or β-Chitin in Mechanically Improved Electrospun Composite
Reprinted from: *Mar. Drugs* **2019**, *17*, 318, doi:10.3390/md17060318 77

Francisco Avelelas, André Horta, Luís F.V. Pinto, Sónia Cotrim Marques, Paulo Marques Nunes, Rui Pedrosa and Sérgio Miguel Leandro
Antifungal and Antioxidant Properties of Chitosan Polymers Obtained from Nontraditional *Polybius henslowii* Sources
Reprinted from: *Mar. Drugs* **2019**, *17*, 239, doi:10.3390/md17040239 89

Chien Thang Doan, Thi Ngoc Tran, Van Bon Nguyen, Anh Dzung Nguyen and San-Lang Wang
Production of a Thermostable Chitosanase from Shrimp Heads via *Paenibacillus mucilaginosus* TKU032 Conversion and its Application in the Preparation of Bioactive Chitosan Oligosaccharides
Reprinted from: *Mar. Drugs* **2019**, *17*, 217, doi:10.3390/md17040217 105

Christine Klinger, Sonia Żółtowska-Aksamitowska, Marcin Wysokowski, Mikhail V. Tsurkan, Roberta Galli, Iaroslav Petrenko, Tomasz Machałowski, Alexander Ereskovsky, Rajko Martinović, Lyubov Muzychka, Oleg B. Smolii, Nicole Bechmann, Viatcheslav Ivanenko, Peter J. Schupp, Teofil Jesionowski, Marco Giovine, Yvonne Joseph, Stefan R. Bornstein, Alona Voronkina and Hermann Ehrlich
Express Method for Isolation of Ready-to-Use 3D Chitin Scaffolds from *Aplysina archeri* (Aplysineidae: Verongiida) Demosponge
Reprinted from: *Mar. Drugs* **2019**, *17*, 131, doi:10.3390/md17020131 119

Ruilian Li, Xianghua Yuan, Jinhua Wei, Xiafei Zhang, Gong Cheng, Zhuo A. Wang and Yuguang Du
Synthesis and Evaluation of a Chitosan Oligosaccharide-Streptomycin Conjugate against *Pseudomonas aeruginosa* Biofilms
Reprinted from: *Mar. Drugs* **2019**, *17*, 43, doi:10.3390/md17010043 . . . . **143**

Yue Yang, Ronge Xing, Song Liu, Yukun Qin, Kecheng Li, Huahua Yu and Pengcheng Li
Immunostimulatory Effects of Chitooligosaccharides on RAW 264.7 Mouse Macrophages via Regulation of the MAPK and PI3K/Akt Signaling Pathways
Reprinted from: *Mar. Drugs* **2019**, *17*, 36, doi:10.3390/md17010036 . . . . **155**

Dalila Miele, Silvia Rossi, Giuseppina Sandri, Barbara Vigani, Milena Sorrenti, Paolo Giunchedi, Franca Ferrari and Maria Cristina Bonferoni
Chitosan Oleate Salt as an Amphiphilic Polymer for the Surface Modification of Poly-Lactic-Glycolic Acid (PLGA) Nanoparticles. Preliminary Studies of Mucoadhesion and Cell Interaction Properties
Reprinted from: *Mar. Drugs* **2018**, *16*, 447, doi:10.3390/md16110447 . . . . **167**

Ángela Sánchez, María Mengíbar, Margarita Fernández, Susana Alemany, Angeles Heras and Niuris Acosta
Influence of Preparation Methods of Chitooligosaccharides on Their Physicochemical Properties and Their Anti-Inflammatory Effects in Mice and in RAW264.7 Macrophages
Reprinted from: *Mar. Drugs* **2018**, *16*, 430, doi:10.3390/md16110430 . . . . **185**

Chien Thang Doan, Thi Ngoc Tran, Van Bon Nguyen, Anh Dzung Nguyen and San-Lang Wang
Reclamation of Marine Chitinous Materials for Chitosanase Production via Microbial Conversion by *Paenibacillus macerans*
Reprinted from: *Mar. Drugs* **2018**, *16*, 429, doi:10.3390/md16110429 . . . . **199**

Jianying Qian, Xiaomeng Wang, Jie Shu, Chang Su, Jinsong Gong, Zhenghong Xu, Jian Jin and Jinsong Shi
A Novel Complex of Chitosan–Sodium Carbonate and Its Properties
Reprinted from: *Mar. Drugs* **2018**, *16*, 416, doi:10.3390/md16110416 . . . . **213**

Nathanael D. Arnold, Wolfram M. Brück, Daniel Garbe and Thomas B. Brück
Enzymatic Modification of Native Chitin and Conversion to Specialty Chemical Products
Reprinted from: *Mar. Drugs* **2020**, *18*, 93, doi:10.3390/md18020093 . . . . **225**

Mitchell Jones, Marina Kujundzic, Sabu John and Alexander Bismarck
Crab vs. Mushroom: A Review of Crustacean and Fungal Chitin in Wound Treatment
Reprinted from: *Mar. Drugs* **2020**, *18*, 64, doi:10.3390/md18010064 . . . . **253**

About the Special Issue Editors

Hitoshi Sashiwa was born in Osaka, Japan, in 1963. He received his Ph.D. degree from Hokkaido University (Japan) under the supervision of Professor S. Tokura in 1991. He then served as Assistant Associate Professor at Tottori University (Japan) from 1988 to 2000 before moving to University of Ottawa (Canada), where he worked with Professor R. Roy during 1998–2000. He served as a postdoctoral scholar at AIST Kansai (Japan) during 2000–2004. He has been affiliated with Kaneka Co., Ltd. (Japan) since April 2004. His research interests include chemical modification of chitin and chitosan and their biomedical applications. He is the sole author of 70 publications and co-author of 30 publications. He has served as Guest Editor of Special Issues of the MDPI journals *Marine Drugs* and *IJMS*.

Hironori Izawa received his PhD in 2010 from Kagoshima University under the supervision of Prof. Jun-ichi Kadokawa. He spent a postdoctoral research stay at the National Institute for Materials Science (NIMS) under the supervision of Prof. Katsuhiko Ariga (2010–2012). In 2012, he moved to Tottori University as Assistant Professor. In 2020, he was promoted to Associate Professor. His major interests are in the preparation of functional polymeric materials, including gel and film materials, through enzymatic or chemical processes.

Preface to "Marine Chitin 2019"

Biomass-based polymers from renewable resources have recently been receiving increasing attention due to the depletion of petroleum resources. Natural polysaccharides derived from natural resources, including cellulose, hemicellulose, and starch, are among the candidates for use in biomass polysaccharide products such as bioplastics. Although numerous kinds of anionic polysaccharides such as alginic acid, hyaluronic acid, heparin, and chondroitin sulfate exist in nature, examples of natural cationic polysaccharides are relatively rare. Chitin is second only to cellulose as the most natural abundant polysaccharide in the world. Chitosan, the product derived from the *N*-deacetylation of chitin, appears to be the only example of a natural cationic polysaccharide. Therefore, due to their unique properties, chitin and chitosan are expected to continue to offer a vast number of possible applications not only for chemical or industrial use but also biomedical treatments. The research history on chitin, one of the most abundant natural polysaccharides on earth, started around 1970. Since the 1980s, chitin and chitosan research (including D-glucosamine, *N*-acetyl-D-glucosamine, and their oligomers) has progressed significantly in several stages covering both fundamental research and industrial fields.

In launching this book, our idea was to present an authoritative and exciting issue that will encompass breakthroughs in the scientific and industrial research conducted in this field. A large volume of chitin and chitosan research involves biomedical objectives, in particular, controlled drug release. Nevertheless, this book covers recent trends in all aspects of basic and applied scientific research on chitin and chitosan as well as their derivatives.

Hitoshi Sashiwa, Hironori Izawa
Special Issue Editors

marine drugs

MDPI

Article

Understanding the Performance of a Novel Direct Compression Excipient Comprising Roller Compacted Chitin

Deeb Abu Fara [1,*], Linda Al-Hmoud [1], Iyad Rashid [2], Babur Z. Chowdhry [3] and Adnan Badwan [2]

1 Chemical Engineering Department, School of Engineering, University of Jordan, Amman 11942, Jordan; l.alhmoud@ju.edu.jo
2 Research and Innovation Centre, The Jordanian Pharmaceutical Manufacturing Company (JPM), P.O. Box 94, Naor 11710, Jordan; irashid@jpm.com.jo (I.R.); adnanbadwan@gmail.com (A.B.)
3 School of Science, Faculty of Engineering & Science, University of Greenwich, Medway Campus, Chatham Maritime, Kent ME4 4TB, UK; b.z.chowdhry@greenwich.ac.uk
* Correspondence: abufara@ju.edu.jo; Tel.: +962-799182424

Received: 7 January 2020; Accepted: 12 February 2020; Published: 17 February 2020

Abstract: Chitin has been investigated in the context of finding new excipients suitable for direct compression, when subjected to roller compaction. Ball milling was concurrently carried out to compare effects from different energy or stress-inducing techniques. Samples of chitin powders (raw, processed, dried and humidified) were compared for variations in morphology, X-ray diffraction patterns, densities, FT-IR, flowability, compressibility and compactibility. Results confirmed the suitability of roller compaction to convert the fluffy powder of raw chitin to a bulky material with improved flow. X-ray powder diffraction studies showed that, in contrast to the high decrease in crystallinity upon ball milling, roller compaction manifested a slight deformation in the crystal lattice. Moreover, the new excipient showed high resistance to compression, due to the high compactibility of the granules formed. This was correlated to the significant extent of plastic deformation compared to the raw and ball milled forms of chitin. On the other hand, drying and humidification of raw and processed materials presented no added value to the compressibility and compactibility of the directly compressed excipient. Finally, compacted chitin showed direct compression similarity with microcrystalline cellulose when formulated with metronidazole (200 mg) without affecting the immediate drug release action of the drug.

Keywords: chitin; roller compaction; ball milling; direct compression; compression work; crushing strength; Hausner ratio; Kawakita analysis; bulk density; dissolution

1. Introduction

Pharmaceutical excipients for direct compression (DC) applications are mostly favored in relation to saving time, cost and labour for solid dosage form preparations and tableting [1,2]. The foregoing advantages are due to their ability to provide the three main requirements associated with excipients for DC processing, i.e., compressibility, compactibility, and flowability [3,4]. Many DC excipients are manufactured from natural sources (e.g., cellulose and starch), from existing excipients of synthetic origin or from binary mixtures of non-DC excipients [5,6]. The necessity for structural modification and industrial manufacture is attributed to the detrimental physical properties of most pharmaceutical excipients before being processed. These properties include poor compactibility, compressibility, and flowability.

Industrially, different processes have been used in the scale-up production of DC excipients. Spray-drying and spray-granulation represent the most two common processes in DC excipient production [7–9]. However, apart from the high cost and investment of time, these techniques commonly impose complexity in terms of operational procedures, as well as process control [10]. Moreover, prior to spray drying, most excipients are subjected to physical and chemical treatment in order to provide specific functionalities for in vivo drug delivery purposes [11,12]. Such pre-treatment steps add to the complexity of product manufacture.

Dry granulation represents a preferred industrial alternative in order to minimize time and cost for a myriad of pharmaceutical applications. This is due to the fact that neither liquids nor heat is involved in the dry processing of powders. Arguably, the most promising dry granulation technique, to date, is roller compaction, since it has proved to be effective in replacing powders that are conventionally processed using wet granulation [13,14]. However, most applications of roller compactors are confined to the improvement of powder flow of pharmaceutical preparations comprising mixtures of API(s) and excipient(s) [15]. Nevertheless, there have been attempts to employ roller compaction technology for the conversion of poorly compressible/compactable starch and α-lactose monohydrate into DC excipients [16,17]. In this regard, specific intensive compaction pressures were able to produce DC excipients via the mechanism of gelatinization and reduction in crystallinity for starch and α-lactose monohydrate, respectively.

Recently, there has been a significant interest in the development of chitin for pharmaceutical use, especially in direct compression processing. The basic asset of chitin that renders such a development to be advantageous lies in its ability to provide vital multi-functionalities in tablet processing. In this regard, chitin showed good tabletability, fast disintegration properties, in addition to improved flowability, compressibility, and compactibility when processed with other common excipients, such as calcium carbonate and magnesium silicate [18–23]. Despite the foregoing comments, chitin lacks essential manufacturing requirements for the processing of DC excipients. In this regard, the low bulk density and poor powder flowability represent the two major inherent shortcomings of chitin. Nevertheless, numerous attempts have been made to convert chitin into a pharmaceutical DC excipient. Most of these attempts have adopted co-processing techniques, whereby another excipient has been involved in, e.g., wet granulation methodologies for product manufacturing [20,23]. However, the manufacturing procedures and processing time and cost of such methodologies are, relatively, complex. This necessitates searching for new technical alternatives for the processing of chitin in order for it to be used as an excipient with DC functionality.

The research reported herein attempts to extend the usefulness and opportunities that roller compaction may provide in obtaining a new DC excipient using chitin. Because roller compaction is a pressure inducing technique, it was concurrently compared with ball milling in order to further support an understanding of the performance of modified chitin, as an excipient, when subjected to pressure.

2. Results

2.1. SEM

SEM of raw, ball milled, and compacted chitin particles display the morphology presented in Figure 1. Originally, the raw chitin particles are thin, and most of their surfaces are flat with some degree of folding. The shape did not change dramatically upon ball milling; however, the surface of the particles became more flattened with some degree of surface damage and tearing. In contrast, compacted chitin particles were thick and displayed a high degree of surface irregularities.

2.2. XRPD Analysis

The XRPD spectra of raw chitin, and that subjected to roller compaction and ball milling for 36 h, is presented in Figure 2. Initially, the pattern for the raw chitin shows two main sharp peaks indicative of α-chitin at 2θ = 9° and 19°, whereby the intensity of the peak at 19° is higher than that at 9° [24]. It is obvious that ball milling decreased the intensities of these much more than roller compaction indicating the sever action of the ball milling process. When the area under the diffraction peaks are considered for the two planes (010) and (020), the summation of the areas are 1984, 787, and 174 for raw, compacted, and ball milled chitin powders, respectively (Table 1).

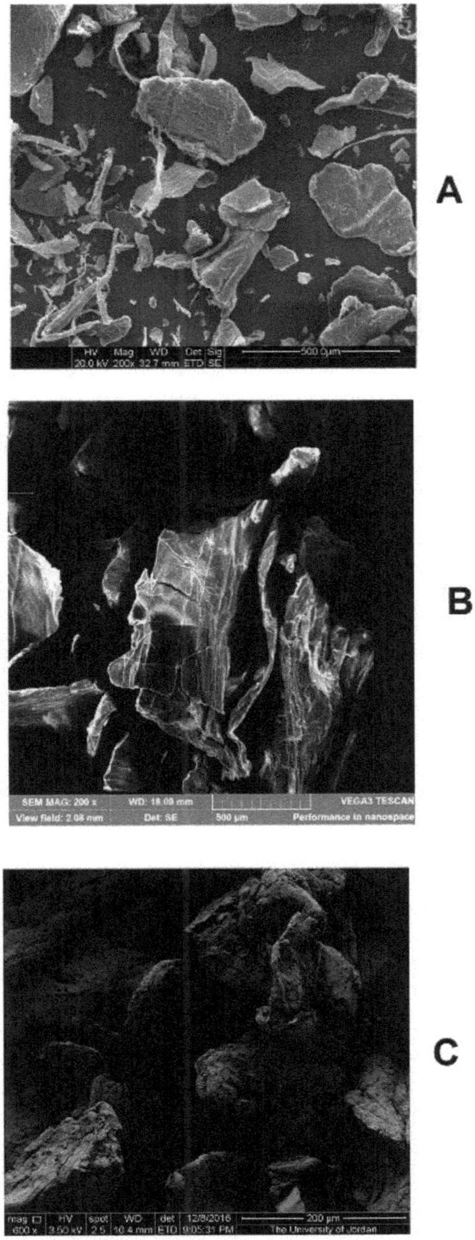

Figure 1. SEM images of raw chitin (**A**), ball milled chitin (**B**), and compacted chitin (**C**).

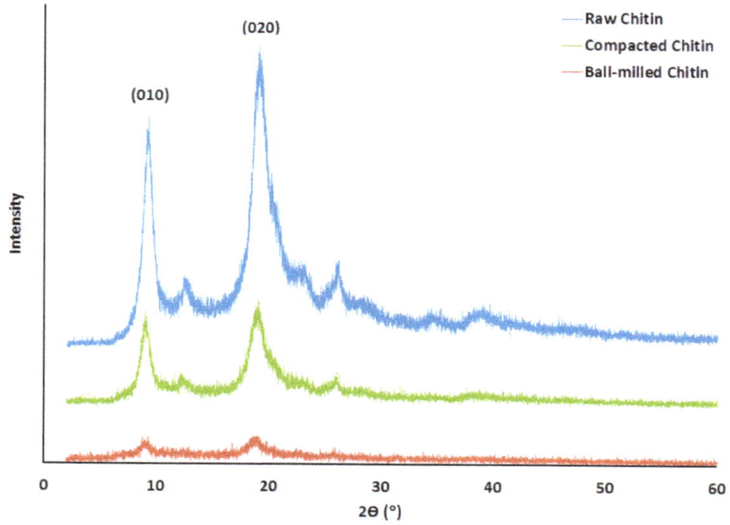

Figure 2. XRPD spectra of raw chitin (blue), and that subjected to roller compaction (green) and ball milling (red).

Table 1. Peak areas of XRPD spectrum of raw chitin, and that subjected to ball milling and roller compaction.

Chitin \ Area under the Peak	A9[1]	A19[2]	A9/A9R[3]	A19/A19R[4]
Raw	512	1472	1	1
Compacted	242	545	0.47	0.37
Ball milled	58	116	0.24	0.21

A9 = Area under the peak at 2θ = 9°; A19 = Area under the peak at 2θ = 19°; A9R = Area under the peak at 2θ = 9° of raw chitin; A19R = Area under the peak at 2θ = 19° of raw chitin.

2.3. FTIR Spectrophotometry

FTIR spectra of raw, ball milled, and compacted chitin samples are presented Figure 3A–C, respectively. The main characteristic bands of chitin (Figure 3A) were detected at 1620 and 1660 cm^{-1} for amide I and at 1560 cm^{-1} for amide II regions. These bands did not change when chitin was subjected to roller compaction (Figure 3B) and ball milling (Figure 3C). However, there was broadening and a decrease in band intensities for the identity bands of ball milled chitin.

2.4. Bulk, Tapped Density and True Density

The bulk and tapped densities of the light, fibrous raw chitin material increased with ball milling and compaction, whereby the later technique produced the densest powder (Table 2). Bulk and tapped densities were found to be affected by the number of water molecules within the chitin powder. In this regard, when the powder was subjected to humidification, under 93% RH for 30 days, the measured bulk density underwent a decrease for all three samples of chitin. In contrast, drying of the samples at 95 °C for four days caused an increase in bulk and tapped densities for all types of powders; raw-unprocessed, ball milled, and compacted.

The true density of chitin raw material underwent a decrease by 8% when the raw material was subjected to ball milling; the results are also illustrated in Table 2. In the same regard, roller compaction did not change the true density of chitin. Nevertheless, a further decrease in true density of the raw material was recorded when it was subjected to humidity conditions. However, true density values were the highest when the raw and processed materials were dried at 95 °C for four days.

Table 2. Bulk, tapped, and true densities of raw, ball milled, and compacted chitin, before and after humidification or drying.

Chitin. / Condition	Bulk Density			Tapped Density			True Density		
	Raw	Ball Milled	Compacted	Raw	Ball Milled	Compacted	Raw	Ball Milled	Compacted
BHD *	0.19 ± 0.01	0.28 ± 0.01	0.52 ± 0.01	0.29 ± 0.01	0.30 ± 0.01	0.64 ± 0.02	1.35 ± 0.01	1.24 ± 0.02	1.35 ± 0.01
Humidified	0.15 ± 0.02	0.20 ± 0.03	0.32 ± 0.02	0.19 ± 0.01	0.25 ± 0.02	0.52 ± 0.01	1.33 ± 0.02	1.22 ± 0.03	1.37 ± 0.01
Dried	0.33 ± 0.01	0.36 ± 0.01	0.69 ± 0.02	0.48 ± 0.02	0.56 ± 0.01	0.73 ± 0.02	1.37 ± 0.02	1.26 ± 0.01	1.32 ± 0.02

* BHD: before humidification or drying.

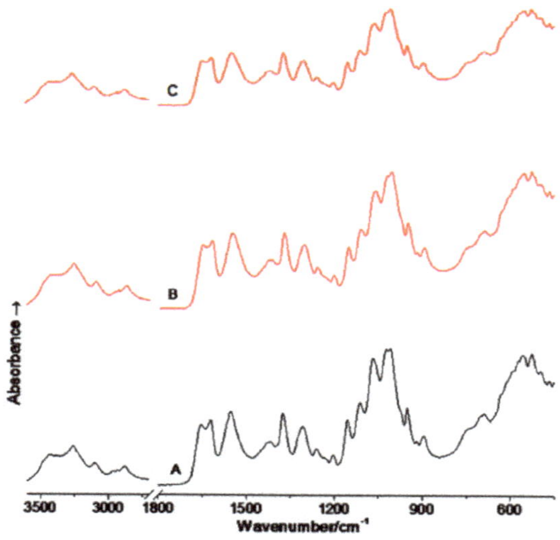

Figure 3. IR spectra of raw chitin (**A**), compacted chitin (stage 5) (**B**), and ball milled chitin (36 h) (**C**).

2.5. Particle Size Distribution

Results of the particle size analysis of raw, ball milled, and compacted chitin are illustrated in Table 3. Ball milling was able to reduce the particle size of the raw material of chitin ($d_{0.5}$ = 613 μm) to a value of $d_{0.5}$ = 384 μm, whereas, roller compaction increased the particle size to a value of $d_{0.5}$ = 877 μm. These values were the actual particle sizes resulting from roller compaction and ball milling. As such, the values are larger than the particle size distribution for common DC excipients, e.g., lactose DC and Avicel® 200 [25,26]. Therefore, all powders subjected to investigation, including processed and unprocessed chitin were passed over a mesh size 250 μm and collected on a 90 μm mesh. The new particle size distribution after sieving is presented in Table 3.

Table 3. Particle size based on 10%, 50% and 90% distribution of the total sample volume, before and after sieving the powders through a mesh size 250 μm and collected on a 90 μm mesh.

	Particle Size (μm) before Sieving			Particle Size (μm) after Sieving		
Material	$d_{0.1}$	$d_{0.5}$	$d_{0.9}$	$d_{0.1}$	$d_{0.5}$	$d_{0.9}$
Raw chitin	107	613	1179	98	178	223
Compacted chitin	156	877	1253	126	199	246
Ball milled chitin	58	384	902	93	121	141

2.6. Hauser Ratio

The Hausner ratios of all types of chitin powders (unprocessed, balled milled, and roller compacted), are presented in Table 4. Chitin, and to the same extent, ball milled chitin displayed poor flowability (HR > 1.45). However, roller compaction improved the powder flow to 'fair' criteria (HR; 1.19–1.25). Such an improvement was further noticed when chitin, as raw material, was subjected to humidity conditions. In this regard, a 'passable' flow criteria was recorded (HR: 1.26–1.34). In contrast, drying resulted in powders with poor flow property. A similar observation in flow behavior when the powder was humidified and dried was noticed for ball milled chitin, whereby the dried powders presented poor flow. However, the observation was the opposite for roller compacted chitin. In this regard, dried powders of this type showed the best improvement in powder flow where an 'excellent' flow criteria were recorded (HR < 1.11). In the same regard, a poor powder flow was recorded when the compacted powder was subjected to humidity conditions.

Table 4. Hausner ratios of raw, ball milled, and compacted chitin, before and after humidification or drying.

Condition \ Chitin	Raw	Ball Milled	Compacted
BHD *	1.55 ± 0.046	1.47 ± 0.041	1.23 ± 0.036
Humidified	1.26 ± 0.037	1.27 ± 0.038	1.59 ± 0.047
Dried	1.46 ± 0.043	1.54 ± 0.046	1.06 ± 0.032

* BHD: before humidification or drying.

2.7. Water Content

Results of the Karl Fischer water content for the chitin samples are presented in Table 5. The test clearly shows that humidification doubled the amount of water content from its initial value at room temperature for raw and processed chitin. In contrast, water content was reduced when the samples underwent drying. The decrease was more enhanced for processed chitin than for the raw material.

Table 5. Water content of raw chitin, ball milled chitin and roller compacted chitin in different conditions.

Condition	Chitin	Water Content (% *w/w*)
Room conditions	Raw	7.350 ± 0.049
	Ball milled	7.150 ± 0.057
	Roller compacted	7. 245 ± 0.014
Humidification at 93% RH at 25 °C	Raw	14.742 ± 0.106
	Ball milled	14.895 ± 0.099
	Roller compacted	14.5947 ± 0.014
Drying at 95 °C	Raw	4.705 ± 0.035
	Ball milled	2.080 ± 0.028
	Roller compacted	3.180 ± 0.014

2.8. Specific Surface Area

Specific surface area measurements give an indication in the difference between the two particle deformation techniques, ball milling and compaction. Results of these measurements are presented in Table 6 for the raw, ball milled, and compacted chitin powders. As expected, raw chitin showed a high specific surface area which underwent an increase or a decrease when the powder was subjected to ball milling or roller compaction, respectively.

Table 6. The specific surface area of raw chitin, ball milled chitin (36 h), and compacted chitin (stage 5).

Material	BET Surface Area, m^2/g
Non-compacted chitin	41.5
Chitin/ball milled	49.3
Chitin/compacted	0.84

2.9. Tablet Crushing Force

Results for the tablet crushing force when the different powders were compressed into 6 mm diameter tablets (75 ± 1 mg each) using the GTP at compression loads of 100 to 500 kg (34.67– 173.35 MPa pressure), are presented in Figure 4. At a compression force of 100 kg (34.67 Mpa), neither the raw nor the ball milled chitin powders (humidified and dried) were able to be compressed into tablets. The aforementioned materials started to form proper tablets at 200 kg of compression load (69.34 Mpa).

When the foregoing was increased, the crushing force, ultimately, underwent an increase. Within the same range of compression load, i.e., 100 to 500 kg (34.67–173.35 Mpa pressure), the crushing force of tablets made using roller compacted powder was significantly higher than tablets made of raw and ball milled chitin. These results indicate the high compactibility of chitin when subjected to roller compaction. On the other hand, the data in Figure 4 further indicates that all types of humidified powders (raw-unprocessed and processed) produce tablets with higher crushing force than raw and dried materials.

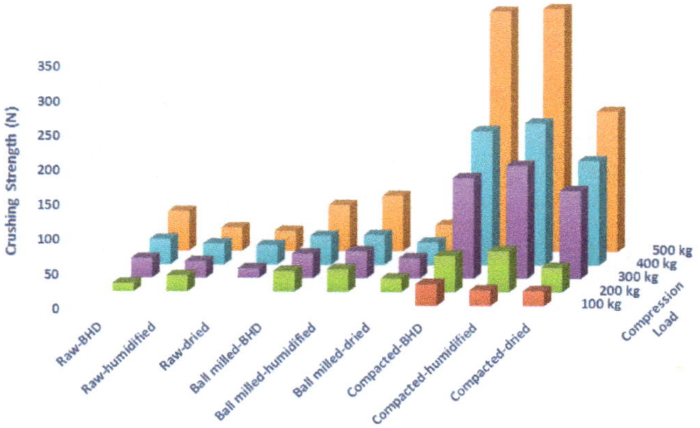

Figure 4. Crushing strength of tablet made of raw (unprocessed), ball milled, and compacted chitin, before and after humidification or drying [BHD: before humidification or drying].

2.10. Kawakita Compression Analysis

The three main parameters (a, P_k and ab) obtained via Kawakita analysis (explained in Section 4.2.5 of the method section) were analyzed in an attempt to interpret the compression behavior of the three samples of chitin. The values of each parameter for each powder type (raw and processed) under the two set conditions (humidified and dried) are presented in Figures 5–7.

The maximum volume reduction that can be attained (a) is presented in Figure 5 and illustrates that compacted chitin underwent the lowest volume reduction when a compression force was applied compared to raw and ball milled chitin. For the latter two materials, volume reduction of raw-unprocessed chitin was the highest followed by ball milled chitin. Furthermore, the two types of processed chitin—compared to their initial status (pre-drying and pre-humidification)—underwent either an increase in volume reduction when they were subjected to humidification, or a decrease upon drying.

P_k, which represents the pressure needed to reduce (a) into half its initial value, is the most important Kawakita parameter to be tested. This is due to the fact that it represents how hard the granules are, and therefore, their ability to be used in direct compression applications [27]. The data in Figure 6 shows that the P_k values of compacted raw chitin powder were the highest amongst all three types of samples. Ball milling causes a slight increase in the P_k value compared to the raw material. However, such an increase is not comparable to roll compacted powder. It is worth noting that although humidification improved the compressibility of all the powders, P_K values were dramatically reduced even for roller compacted chitin. With regard to dried powders, drying caused a small decrease in P_K values for all the powders when compared with non-dried samples.

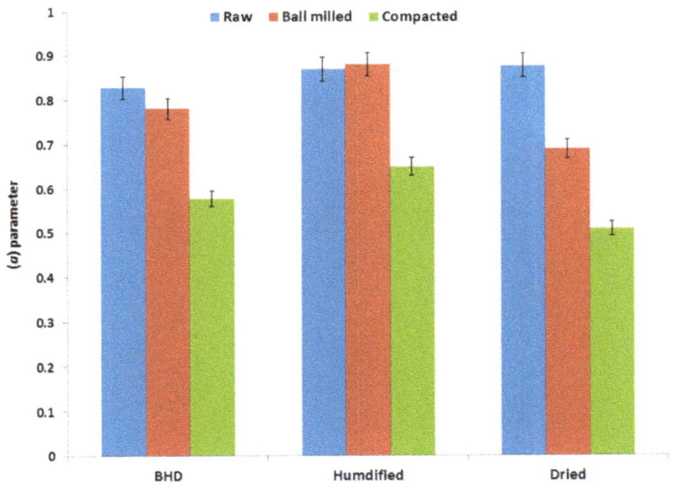

Figure 5. Kawakita parameter (*a*) of raw (unprocessed), ball milled, and compacted chitin, before and after humidification or drying [BHD: before humidification or drying].

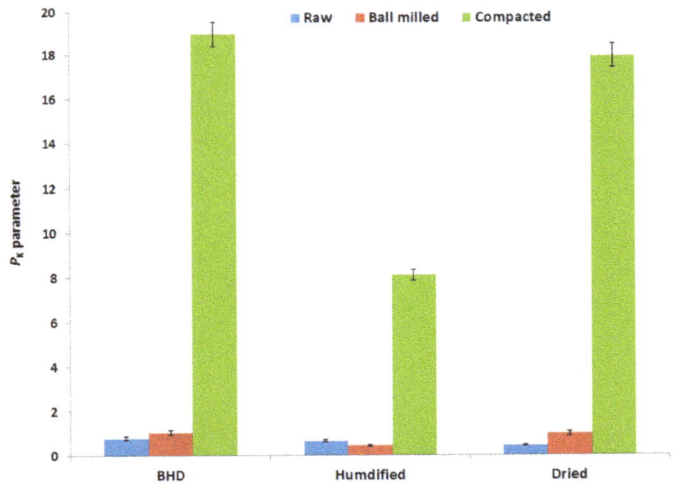

Figure 6. Kawakita parameter (p_k) of raw (unprocessed), ball milled, and compacted chitin, before and after humidification or drying [BHD: before humidification or drying].

The last Kawakita parameter that was used in this work to describe the compression behavior is *ab*. This parameter gives an indication of the degree of rearrangement of powder particles [28,29], Figure 7. Compared to the raw material, processing of chitin either by ball milling or by roller compaction reduced the extent of particle rearrangement (*ab*) upon compression. In the same regard, the value of *ab* was the lowest for the roller compacted powder. The data in Figure 7 also indicates that humidification increased the extent of particle rearrangement, especially for ball milled chitin, whereas, the values for *ab* for dried powders (ball milled and compacted) were almost similar to the values of the powders in the pre-dried state.

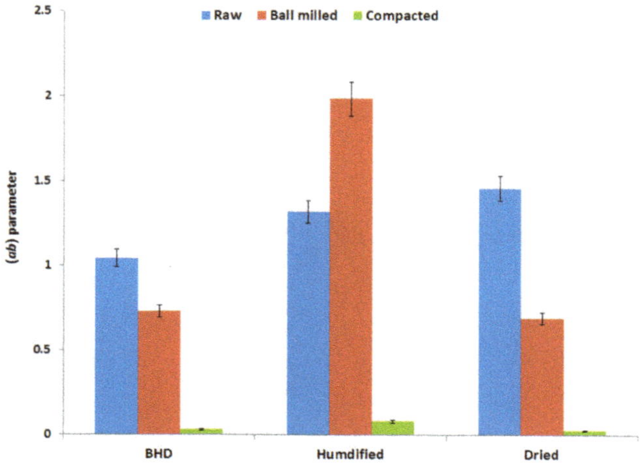

Figure 7. Kawakita parameter (*ab*) of raw (unprocessed), ball milled, and compacted chitin, before and after humidification or drying [BHD: before humidification or drying].

2.11. Heckel Compression Analysis

Compression analysis was further examined using the empirical Heckel model of compression analysis. In this model, the yield pressure, or P_Y, represents a critical parameter which reflects the type and extent of deformation, i.e., plastic/elastic or brittle-fracture. The data in Figure 8 illustrates the yield pressure values for all the powders tested. Results show that when the two stress-inducing techniques are compared with each other and with the raw material, the P_Y ranking followed the order: Raw chitin > ball milled chitin > roller compacted chitin. Humidification of each type of powder (raw and processed) further reduced the value of P_Y. Moreover, P_Y values of the three types of chitin (raw-unprocessed, ball milled, and compacted) underwent an increase upon drying.

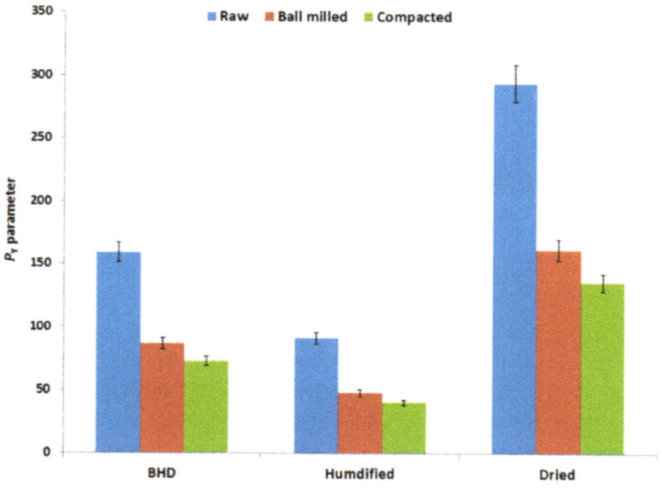

Figure 8. Heckel parameter (P_Y) of raw (unprocessed), ball milled, and compacted chitin, before and after humidification or drying [BHD: before humidification or drying].

2.12. Work of Compression

When powders of different types were compressed using the GTP, the instrument displays the force displacement curve during the descending/compression and decompression of the powders. The work of compression (W_c), which is represented by the area under the compression curves of the F-D profiles, is shown in Figure 9. W_c values were calculated at each compression force used. Results indicate that at all loads, W_c of raw-unprocessed chitin > W_c of roller compacted chitin > W_c of ball milled chitin. Moreover, above 300 kg of compression load (i.e., at 400 and 500 kg), drying of raw and processed materials rendered W_c higher than both humidified and un-dried powders.

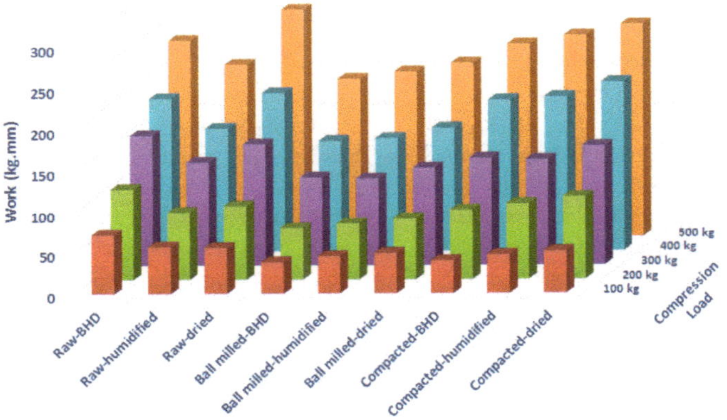

Figure 9. Compression work for raw (unprocessed), ball milled, and compacted chitin, before and after humidification or drying [BHD: before humidification or drying].

2.13. Characterization of Metronidazole Tablets Comprising Drug/Compacted-Chitin Matrix

Tablet properties and dissolution are illustrated in Table 7 and Figure 10. These results demonstrate that tablets comprising chitin are harder in terms of crushing force and faster in disintegration time than tablets made of MCC PH 200®. Moreover, full drug release of metronidazole/chitin matrix was achieved within 5 min of dissolution time. This was faster than tablets comprising metronidazole/MCC matrix, which resulted in full drug release within 20 min of dissolution time.

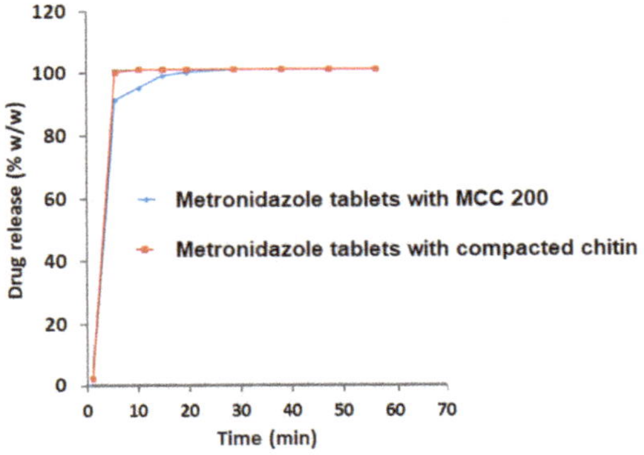

Figure 10. Dissolution profiles for metronidazole (200 mg) tablets comprising compacted chitin or MCC 200® excipients.

Table 7. Crushing strength, disintegration time, and time for full drug release for metronidazole (200 mg) tablets comprising compacted chitin or MCC PH 200® excipients.

Excipient Used in Metronidazole Preparation	Crushing Strength (N)	Disintegration Time (min)	Complete Dissolution Time (min)
Compacted chitin	110–120	<1	4–5
MCC PH 200®	100–105	<12	15–20

3. Discussion

The research presented herein is mainly focused on the assessment of the use of roller compaction technique for the development of DC pharmaceutical excipients from raw alpha chitin. Ball milling, as another stress-inducing technique, was tested for comparison and evaluation of changes in the physical properties and compression behavior of chitin powder. The main challenge in this work is to obtain workable chitin with suitable DC properties to facilitate compaction and compression in the industrial set up. FTIR test of ball milled, and compacted chitin indicates that no chemical change took place during these processes. This guarantees that the intended excipients are chemically stable when exposed to ball milling or compaction. Another objective was to reduce crystallinity to facilitate flow and compression. In this regard, materials are known to undergo plastic deformation with regular particle shape and consequently improved flowability once their amorphous character is increased [30]. Testing the raw chitin showed the necessity to alter the physical state of chitin, namely particle size and crystallinity. In this work, XRPD was used to assure that crystallinity raw chitin was modified, enabling treated chitin to be utilized in pharmaceutical processing.

XRPD results indicated that roller compaction and ball milling techniques affect the crystalline structure of chitin in different ways. A decrease in crystallinity of the semi-crystalline structure of raw chitin was generally the predominant change in the crystal lattice enhanced by both techniques (Figure 2). However, this decrease is more pronounced by ball milling when operated for 36 h. In fact, ball milling converts chitin into a material of a highly amorphous character. In this regard, the decrease in the two main crystalline planes of α-chitin represented by (010) and (020) at $2\theta = 9°$ and $19°$, respectively indicates a change in the crystalline nature of chitin. Ioelovich [31] suggests the use of integral intensities (areas) of the X-diffractions, especially for the (020) plane, instead of peak height as an indication of crystalline and amorphous contents for chitin. Based upon his finding, irrespective of which plane is more indicative of any crystallinity change, the summation of the peak areas of the two planes (010) and (020) follows the decreasing order: Raw, compacted, and ball milled. Such crystallinity change caused by roller compaction on chitin is similar to reported results on the effect of roller compaction on α-lactose monohydrate [17]. On the other hand, Alves et al. showed that ball milling of chitosan (de-acetylated chitin) caused a loss of the crystal plane (010); however, there was an increase in the intensity of the peak at the 020 plane [32]. The latter change further contradicts the finding by Ioelovich [31] who—as previously mentioned—states that crystallinity changes are associated with changes in the 020 crystal plane. In order to understand the foregoing contradiction, it is suggested that the dissimilarity with the findings of Alves et al., is more likely to be attributed to the fact that milling—in their work—was carried out for a maximum time of 3 h. The foregoing is too short to represent the extensive duration of the ball milling undertaken in the current work. Therefore, it is the intense stress applied to the powder that imparts a high reduction in its crystallinity. In fact, high stress induction applied to a structurally similar polysaccharide powder, e.g., cellulose, was reported to reduce crystallinity to 54.1% when using simple crushing, and down to 21.7% upon using ball milling [33]. Therefore, for the two techniques employed in this work, it is correct to assert that roller compaction—as a scalable process—can be regarded as a short time ball milling which, in the case of the latter method, is hard to scale-up.

At the molecular level, it has been reported that destruction of both planes at $2\theta = 9°$ and $19°$ causes a reduction in the hydrogen bond network which is responsible for imparting structural integrity and flexibility to the chitin chains [34]. Other studies (see Reference [33]) have reported that such a reduction causes a loss in the glycosidic linkages connecting acetylated glucosamine subunits which form the main structural backbone of chitin [33]. On the other hand, the increase in the amorphous character was further evident in the broadening and decrease in band intensities for the IR bands of ball milled chitin (Figure 3C) when the latter is compared with raw chitin (Figure 3A). However, changes in crystallinity for compacted chitin were not detectable using the same technique as the IR bands of roller compacted chitin did not undergo any changes (Figure 3B).

Moving from the molecular level to the particle behavior of the chitin powder, the first most crucial property to investigate was bulk density with respect to its impact on pharmaceutical processing of powders. In this regard, increasing the bulk density is advantageous in tablet manufacturing, whereby bulky materials enhance powder compression processing, and more specifically, in die filling procedures [35]. The increase in bulk density of chitin, due to ball milling is attributed to the size reduction of the particles, due to high energy impacts between the chitin particles during collision. In comparing the two different stress-inducing techniques, ball milling of chitin is not as good as a powder densification technique compared to roller compaction; the later methodology, imparted a greater increase in the powder bulk density.

The increase in bulk and tapped densities of chitin, due to humidification is attributed to the low optimal packing caused by strong cohesion -due to interparticle water bridging- between the molecules. Such behavior is generally anticipated when the water content of a material is increased, due to humidification as typically induced in the current case [36]. This further suggests an improvement in particle packing when the powders were subjected to drying for four days. In this regard, dried powder presented the highest recorded bulk and tapped densities in all cases.

The second most affected factor in dry granulation is particle size distribution. Ball milling is well known as a particle size reducing technique, due to the high energy of impact when the balls collide with chitin [37]. On the other hand, roller compaction is used for powder densification. Consequently, the two techniques are diametric to each other with respect to the changes, increasing or decreasing, they impart to particle size. Although all powders were passed and collected through sieves between 250 and 90 μm, roller compaction imparts high size distribution towards the upper limit of particle size between the aforementioned sieve ranges (Table 3). In contrast, ball milling imparts a high distribution towards the lower limit of particle size. These changes in particle size impart another opposing explanation to the bulk density increase caused by ball milling and roller compaction. In the former, reduction of particle size renders a fixed sample volume to be occupied by small chitin particles rather than large ones. Thus, a higher bulk density is attained upon milling compared to the raw material. On the other hand, despite the increase in particle size in case of roller compaction, the extent of densification is suggested to be high enough to overcome the effect of particle size towards variations in bulk density. It has to be emphasized herein that the aforementioned particle size and bulk density of compacted chitin were only possible after the powder was allowed to be compacted five times up to an applied pressure of 166 Mpa.

The two aforementioned properties; i.e., density and size of the granules, have a direct impact on powder flow, especially when the powders are subjected to humidification. In this regard, the improved flow for raw and ball milled chitin powders subjected to high humidification conditions is suggested to be attributed to the lubrication effect generally induced by water molecules [38,39]. Such a lubrication-flow theory is also aligned with the apparent poor powder flow when such an effect is reduced as the materials undergo drying (Table 4). However, the same theory does not align with the excellent powder flow when compacted chitin was dried. In this case, it is suggested that the effect of bulk density may have overcome the aforementioned concerns related to water content on powder flow. In other words, the significant increase in bulk density noticed for compacted chitin compared to the raw and ball milled chitin has rendered the compacted powders highly flowable. Drying further increases the bulk density value and bulk density difference of the compacted compared to the raw and ball milled chitin powders, and this may justify the excellent flowability of dried compacted chitin.

The same justification is valid when compacted chitin was subjected to humidification. In this regard, the sharp decrease in the bulk density of the humidified compacted powder is the main reason behind its poor flowability.

Measuring changes in true density for each stress-inducing technique was tested despite the fact that, theoretically, the true density value of chitin was expected not to be affected by means of pore volume reduction. This is based on the fact that the value is constant for solid matter and excludes any empty space considerations upon measurement. Such a perspective is valid for the material subjected to roller compaction. However, it has been reported that a reduction in the true density of a material can take place when the structure undergoes a polymorphic transformation [40,41]. In this regard, changes in the molecular arrangement of a powder can result in loose packing at the particulate level. Generally, amorphous materials have a lower density than their crystalline counterparts as the atoms of the former are located at further distances from each other than the latter. Therefore, a decrease in crystallinity results in an increase in lattice volume, and thereby, a decrease in density [42]. Thus, the decrease in crystallinity of chitin to a less ordered amorphous structure is suggested to be the main reason behind the decrease in true density of chitin upon ball milling. Water content, on the other hand, lowers the true density of raw chitin, since the measured value is the sum of the true densities of both water and chitin. When water is removed, the measurement will solely include the solid material and without the presence of other materials which disrupt the volume needed to be occupied by chitin for measurement [43]. Based upon the foregoing, the true densities of dried materials, unprocessed and processed, were the highest compared to the humidified ones.

The last property to be tested, and one which varies with pressure, is a specific surface area. Initially, the high specific surface area of raw chitin is attributed to its highly porous structure [44]. The increase in particle surface area, due to ball milling is typical behavior for a size reducing technique that principally imparts high energy upon collision of the falling balls with powder particles. In contrast, the decrease in particles surface area, due to roller compaction is more likely to be attributed to extensive folding and packing of the particles. Such densification is responsible for reducing the porous structure of raw chitin, and consequently, a decrease in the specific surface area is attained.

Although an increase in the surface area of granules is advantageous in providing new fresh particles surfaces and extra contact points for binding [45], the crushing force of compacted powders of lower surface area was the highest. In contrast, the increase in surface area upon ball milling had no significant effect on crushing force in comparison with roller compaction. Hence, the mechanism for strong binding between the granules is not directly related to the actual surface area of the granules. In fact, it is more likely to be attributed to the mode of deformation when a force is applied. In this regard, plastic deformation of chitin enables extensive folding, thereby providing new surfaces for bridging via new contact points. On the other hand, the presence of water, when the materials were humidified, is a typical action of a granulating medium. The foregoing is known to enforce greater adhesion between wet than dried surfaces [46]. This justifies the increase in crushing force for all the materials when they were humidified.

The hard granules produced by roller compaction showed high resistance to compression force rendering the granules with low maximum volume reduction or '*a*' values. Concurrently, the same hard granules manifested the highest compression force (P_k) needed for (a/2) volume reduction as well as minimal particle rearrangement compared to ball milled, and raw chitin. The closer crushing force values of ball milled to raw chitin further rendered similarly closer a, P_K and ab values. Accordingly, ball milled chitin particles do not provide any added value to the compressibility and compactibility of raw chitin.

When all the materials were humidified, the compressibility (represented by the '*a*' and to some extent the '*ab*' parameters), underwent an improvement. This is due to the fact that water acts as a plasticizer. The foregoing statement can be justified by the removal of water, as the compressibility of the dried materials decreased. On the other hand, high humidification levels (95% RH) weakened the inter-particulate bonding for all materials as the P_K required for (a/2) volume reduction underwent a decrease; thus, resulting in weak humidified granules and for the decrease in tablet hardness attained when the powders were compressed.

The high compactibility of roller compacted chitin powder was further confirmed using the P_Y parameter from the Heckel model. A lower P_Y value is preferable for plastically deforming materials, as it indicates a higher extent of deformation. The foregoing gives rise to a greater degree of folding, and thus, the appearance of fresh new particle surfaces for bridging with nearby surfaces [47]. Roller compacted powders manifested a high extent of plastic deformation compared to ball milled chitin which, in turn, displayed greater plasticity than the raw chitin. It is suggested that such high plasticity is attributed to the presence of denser chitin particles, due to roller compaction, and thus, new added surfaces are available for deformation. On the other hand, the high plastic deformation presented when the materials were subjected to humidification is, as stated previously, attributed to the plasticizing effect of water.

The compression force and the volume reduction can be combined together to describe the work of compression manifested by the area under the F-D curve. The fact that the work of compression is the product of force applied (f) $\times$ the displacement (d) of the compressed powder, means that this reflects how easy or hard the granules can be compressed, and/or reflects the extent of plastic/elastic or brittle deformation the particles are undergoing when pressure is applied. Because compressibility is a volume reduction parameter that has a physical displacement implication (d), it is suggested that the high W_c values for raw chitin- compared to ball milled- are attributed to its high a value. Thus, the impact of W_c was found to be valid at all compression pressures used. Similarly, using the fxd correlation to interpret W_c data, high W_c values of dried- compared to humidified- powders are more likely to be related to the increase in P_k values when the powders were dried. In this regard, P_K has a physical implication for f values in the F-D data.

Lastly, in metronidazole preparations comprising drug/compacted-chitin matrix, the highly compactible tablets did not hinder the disintegration time and metronidazole immediate drug release. Such unaffected disintegration is more likely, as previously suggested, attributed to the presence of a larger mass of chitin material in compacted granules. The properties and dissolution of such preparation were even more favorable than tablets made of drug/MCC matrix.

It is evident that compaction results in a better flow of chitin powder and harder compacts. This may facilitate the utilization of such a powder without any further processing. Such processed powder is less liable to absorb water, as is the case for the ball milled chitin. Keeping the chitin excipient in a dry form allows it to be more appropriate for use in hot and humid climates where the drugs can be more stable when formulated with similar excipients. This behavior is unique when compared with other polymers, such as cellulose, where a balance between crystalline and amorphous states needs to be attained.

4. Materials and Methods

4.1. Materials

Chitin with an average molecular mass of 300 kDa and a degree of acetylation about 0.96 was obtained from G.T.C. Bio Corporation (Qingdao, China), metronidazole (G.D. Searle and Company, Skokie, IL, USA), microcrystalline cellulose (MCC PH 200®, FMC BioPolymer, Philadelphia, PA, USA), pharmaceutical grade talcium (Hubei Aoks Bio-Tech CO., Wuhan, China).

4.2. Methods

4.2.1. Sample Preparation Using Roller Compaction

Chitin (3.0 kg) was compacted using a production scale roller compactor (TFC-520 Roller Compactor, capacity of 100 kg/h, Vector Corporation, Freund Group Company, Marion, IA, USA). Repetition of compaction of the same powder was carried out several times until the bulk density of a representative sample exceeded 0.5 g/mL. The foregoing was accomplished after repeating the compaction five times. Every time the chitin sheets were passed through a conical screen mill (Quadro Comil, Ytron-Quadro Ltd, Chesham Bucks, UK) fitted with a 2.4 mm sieve. Compaction parameters for the five stages of compression are summarized in Table 8. Importantly, the milling speed was adjusted to 15, 25, 30, 30 and 30 Hz for stages 1, 2, 3, 4, and 5, respectively.

Table 8. Roller compaction parameters of chitin performed for five successive times.

	Stage 1	Stage 2	Stage 3	Stage 4	Stage 5
Roller type	DPS	DPS	DPS	DPS	DPS
Roller speed. rpm	16 rpm	16 rpm	14 rpm	16 rpm	16 rpm
Screw speed, HZ	4 HZ	8 HZ	8 HZ	8 HZ	8 HZ
Pressure, MPa	83	83	97	140	166
Roll gape, mm	2.8	3.0	3.0	3.0	3.0

4.2.2. Sample Preparation Using Ball Milling

1 kg of chitin was ball milled (Erweka, Langen, Germany) using porcelain balls of diameters ranging from 30 to 50 mm. The material and the balls were inserted in a sealed drum. Milling was carried out for four days, whereby the running time was adjusted to 9 successive hours every day. A sample was taken at the end of each 9 h run. Accordingly, five samples were collected at 0, 9, 18, 27, 36 h of ball milling.

4.2.3. Preparation of Humidified and Dried Chitin Samples

Three samples from each chitin type (raw, ball milled and compacted) were placed in plastic petri dishes (5 g for each sample) then inserted in desiccators for 30 days. The desiccator was over-saturated with potassium nitrate salt (Acros Organics, New Jersey, NJ, USA) at a relative humidity of 93% at room temperature (25–30 °C); from each sample, known weights were taken for compression analysis.

Another three samples from each chitin type (5 g for each sample comprising either raw, ball milled and compacted) were dried using a Vacucell vacuum drying oven (MMM Medcenter Einrichtungen, Germany). The samples were placed in glass petri dishes then inserted in the oven to dry at a temperature of 95 °C for four days. From each sample, known weights were examined for compression analysis.

4.2.4. Characterization of Powder Properties

Scanning Electron Microscopy (SEM)

The morphology of samples was determined using a Quanta-200 3D (ThermoFisher Scientific, Bend, OR, USA) SEM operated at an accelerating voltage of 1200 V. Samples (≈0.5 mg) were mounted on to a 5 × 5 mm silicon wafer affixed via graphite tape to an aluminum stub. The powder was then sputter-coated for 105 s at a beam current of 20 mA/dm^3 with a 100 Å layer of gold/palladium alloy.

X-Ray Powder Diffraction (XRPD)

XRPD test was carried out using an X-ray powder diffractometer (Bruker, Karlsruhe, Germany) in 2-theta range of 2–40° 2θ in reflection mode. The X-ray compartment is a D2 Phaser comprising a copper tube, using Kα X-rays of 300 watts of power at 1.54184 Å wavelength. DIFFRAC.SUITE™ computer software was used to analyze the data obtained.

IR Spectrophotometry

IR spectrophotometry was carried out using Perkin Elmer Spectrum Two UATR FTIR spectrometer, Akron, OH, USA) with a resolution of 4 cm^{-1}, data interval of 2 cm^{-1} and a scan speed of 0.2 cm/s operating in the range of 450–4000 cm^{-1}. The ATR sample base plate was equipped with a Diamond ZnSe crystal where an infrared background is collected for all FTIR measurements. Samples (2–5 mg) were placed on the ATR crystal, and apressure was applied to compress the sample in order to obtain the spectra. The IR spectra of chitin samples (raw, ball milled, and roller compacted) were examined.

Particle Size Distribution

A laser diffraction Malvern particle size analyzer (Malvern Panalytical Ltd, Malvern, UK) was employed to measure particle size distribution ranging from 0.02 to 2000 microns at room temperature. The instrument is connected to a computer that uses the Mastersizer 2000 (version 5.6) software to display the results.

Bulk, Tapped and True Density Measurement and Flow Determination

The bulk density of chitin samples (raw, ball milled and compacted) in g/mL was measured by pouring the powder into a 25 mL volumetric cylinder. The bulk density of all samples was calculated as the ratio of the mass over the volume it occupied. Tapped density measurements were carried out by physical tapping of the cylinder for 100 mechanical taps then dividing the mass over the tapped volume.

The reduction in the bulk volume of the powders, due to tapping is considered to be an indication of powder flowability, which was evaluated by the Hausner's ratio (HR). As HR increase in value, the flowability is reduced.

HR is calculated using Equation (1).

$$HR = \rho_{Tapped}/\rho_{Bulk} \tag{1}$$

The criteria for flow interpretation based on HR is as follows [48]:

Excellent: 1.00 < HR < 1.11;
Good: 1.12 < HR < 1.18;
Fair: 1.19 < HR < 1.25;
Passable: 1.26 < HR < 1.34;
Poor: 1.35 < HR < 1.45;
Very poor: 1.46 < HR < 1.59.

The true density was determined using a Pycn-020 Gas Pycnometer (Vivid Separation and Filtration, Amman, Jordan). Each sample was weighed then placed in a vial in the second chamber, while air is allowed to pass through the second chamber from the first one. Pressure was recorded in both chambers by a pressure gauge, and the volume of the sample was calculated using the following equation:

$$P_1 \times V_1 = P_2 \times (V_1 + V_2 - \text{vs.}) \tag{2}$$

where P_1, V_1 and P_2, V_2 are the pressure and volume in the first and the second chamber, respectively, and vs. is the volume of the sample. The mass of the sample divided by its true volume yields the true density in g/cm^3. The average of three measurements was carried out for each sample and for each type of density.

Water Content Determination

Raw, ball milled, and compacted chitin samples were analyzed for water content using Karl Fischer volumetric titrator (Mettlor Toledo, Hamburg, Germany). Each sample was tested under the following conditions; room temperature (25 °C), humidified for 30 days at 93% relative humidity (RH), dried for four days at 95 °C. Three samples were considered for each analysis.

Specific Surface Area Determination

BET specific surface area was determined by physical adsorption of nitrogen gas using a Nova 2200 multi-speed high gas sorption analyzer (version 6.11, Quantachrome Co., Syosset, NY, USA). Samples were subjected to nitrogen gas for adsorption under isothermal conditions at 77 K. The samples were initially placed in a vacuum oven at 60 °C for 24 h. A reference empty cell (Sartorius, analytic, A120s, Göttingen, Germany) and the sample (~500 mg) were placed in the chambers. The amount of adsorbate gas was measured, then calculations based on a monomolecular layer assumption were applied. BET surface area analysis was calculated from the linear region of the BET plot.

4.2.5. Powder/Tablet Characterization

Chitin samples (raw, ball milled and compacted) were compressed into tablets using an instrumental single punch bench top tablet press (GTP-1, Gamlen Tablet Press Ltd, Nottingham, UK). Compression was carried out at a punch speed of 60 mm/min by applying five different loads; 100, 200, 300, 400, 500 kg. The samples poured into the die of the GTP had a common weight of 75 ± 1 mg. The diameter and height of the die were 6 and 18.1 mm, respectively. The machine was run by software to display the force-displacement (F-D) curve. Kawakita and Heckel models, Equations (3) and (4), respectively, were utilized to describe the compression analysis of the powders [49,50].

Kawakita analysis describes a linear relationship between the ratio of pressure (MPa) to volume reduction (C) and the pressure. From the slope and intercept of this relationship, constants *'a'* and *'b'* can be deduced; *'a'* represents the maximum volume reduction that can be attained by the powder. *'1/b'* or *'P_K'* is another parameter that represents the force required to reduce the powder bed volume to half its maximum value.

$$\frac{P}{C} = \frac{P}{a} + \frac{1}{ab} \tag{3}$$

Heckel analysis describes a relationship between the logarithm of the inverse of compact porosity (ε) and the pressure applied.

$$\ln\frac{1}{\varepsilon} = kP + A \tag{4}$$

Porosity is calculated using the following equation:

$$\varepsilon = 1 - \rho_r \tag{5}$$

where ρ_r is the relative density of the compact and is calculated using the following equation:

$$\rho_r = \rho_c/\rho_T \tag{6}$$

where ρ_c and ρ_T are compact and true densities (kg/m^3), respectively.

The inverse of the slope of the Heckel equation or *'1/K'* is an important parameter which assigns the type of deformation of materials, whether plastic/elastic or brittle-fracture. This parameter is called the yield pressure and is signified by the symbol *'P_Y'*.

4.2.6. Application of Compacted Chitin Excipient Using Metronidazole as a Model Drug

It was desired to test the dissolution profile of six tablets (500 mg weight each) comprising the weakly compressible/compactable metronidazole drug (200 mg) and compacted chitin. The matrix will be compared with a reference (6 tablets) made of the same drug and microcrystalline cellulose (MCC). The powder for compression (50 g) was prepared by physically mixing metronidazole (44.4% *w/W*) with compacted chitin/or MCC (50% *w/w*) and talc (5.6%). The mixtures were compressed using a single punch tablet press (Manesty F3 single stroke tablet press; West Pharma services Ltd, Dorset, UK) at an applied pressure of 35 kN. The fitted die was flat, round and 12 mm in diameter. Prior to dissolution testing, the average crushing force and disintegration time of 10 tablets produced were measured using a crushing force (Pharma Test PTB 311E. Hainburg, Germany) and disintegration (CALEVA, Dorest, UK) testers. The disintegration time of the tablets was determined according to the European Pharmacopoeia Supplement, whereby six tablets were inserted in a water-filled basket-rack apparatus set at 37 °C [46].

Dissolution testing was conducted according to USP 32, whereby apparatus II was used (Erweka DT6, Langen, Germany) with paddles rotating at 50 rpm. 900 mL of 0.1 N HCl was used as the dissolution medium. The amount of drug released was analyzed by measuring the absorbance using a UV spectrophotometer (LABINDIA UV/VIS, UV 3000, Maharashtra, India) at a wavelength of 277 nm for metronidazole [51].

5. Conclusions

Dry granulation via roller compaction has proved to be reliable in the conversion of raw chitin into an excipient suitable for direct compression. The data reported herein illustrates that this can be achieved by multiple compaction of the raw material under high pressure. Analysis of ball milled chitin showed that a decrease in powder crystallinity does not necessarily provide excipients with the required DC specifications. In the same vein, the improvement in raw chitin powder physical properties, i.e., bulk density, flowability, compressibility and compactibility, is attributed to the increase in the amorphous character of raw chitin. The obtained crystal form results in the highly packed arrangement of granules with lower true density and specific surface area than raw and ball milled chitin. On the other hand, such compacted granules were hard and showed resistance to displacement upon compression; however, they manifested high plastic deformation. The foregoing justifies the high crushing strength of tablets produced from compacted chitin. Drying and humidification of granules obtained from ball milling and roller compaction techniques did not provide added value that could serve excipient processing in the context of DC applications. Finally, compacted chitin provided tablets with DC and immediate drug release requirements when formulated with metronidazole (200 mg) as a non-compressible and-non compactible model drug.

Author Contributions: All authors contributed to the idea and design of the work, evaluating the results and writing the manuscript. All authors have read and agreed to the published version of the manuscript.

Funding: This research received no external funding.

Acknowledgments: The authors wish to thank the Jordanian Pharmaceutical Manufacturing Co. (JPM) for providing materials, lab and testing facilities. The authors would also like to thank The University of Jordan and The University of Greenwich for their ongoing support.

Conflicts of Interest: The authors declare no conflict of interest. The Jordanian Pharmaceutical Manufacturing Company (JPM) did not have any role in the design of the study; in the collection, analyses or interpretation of data; in the writing of the manuscript; or in the decision to publish the results.

References

1. Gohel, M.C.; Jogani, P.D. A review of co-processed directly compressible excipients. *J. Pharm. Pharm. Sci.* **2005**, *8*, 76–93. [PubMed]
2. Gangurde, A.; Patole, R.K.; Sav, A.K.; Amin, P.D. A Novel Directly Compressible Co-Processed Excipient for Sustained Release Formulation. *J. Appl. Pharm. Sci.* **2013**, *3*, 89–97.
3. Michoel, A.; Rombaut, P.; Verhoye, A. Comparative evaluation of co-processed lactose and microcrystalline cellulose with their physical mixtures in the formulation of folic acid tablets. *Pharm. Dev. Technol.* **2002**, *7*, 79–87. [CrossRef] [PubMed]
4. Mangal, S.; Meiser, F.; Morton, D.; Larson, I. Particle Engineering of Excipients for Direct Compression: Understanding the Role of Material Properties. *Curr. Pharm.* **2015**, *21*, 5877–5889. [CrossRef] [PubMed]
5. Ogaji, I.J.; Nep, E.I.; Audu-Peter, J.D. Advances in Natural Polymers as Pharmaceutical Excipients. *Pharm. Anal. Acta* **2012**, *3*, 146. [CrossRef]
6. Lachman, L.; Liebaerman, H.A.; Kang, J.L. *The Theory and Practice of Industrial Pharmacy*, 3rd ed.; Mumbai, H.A., Kanig, J.L., Eds.; Verghese Publication House: New York, NY, USA, 1990; pp. 171–342.

7. Gonnissen, Y.; Remon, J.P.; Vervaet, C. Development of directly compressible powders via co-spray drying. *Eur. J. Pharm. BioPharm.* **2007**, *67*, 220–226. [CrossRef]
8. Shanmugam, S. Granulation techniques and technologies: recent progresses. *BioImpacts* **2015**, *5*, 55–63. [CrossRef]
9. Rashid, I.; Al Omari, M.M.H.; Badwan, A.A. From native to multifunctional starch-based excipients designed for direct compression formulation. *Starch-Stärke* **2013**, *65*, 552–571. [CrossRef]
10. Badwan, A.A.; Rashid, I.; Omari, M.M.; Darras, F.H. Chitin and chitosan as direct compression excipients in pharmaceutical applications. *Mar. Drugs* **2015**, *13*, 1519–1547. [CrossRef]
11. Dokala, G.K.; Pallavi, C. Direct Compression—An Overview. *Int. J. Res. Pharm. Biomed. Sci.* **2013**, *4*, 155–158.
12. Agarwal, R.; Naveen, Y. Pharmaceutical Processing—A Review on Wet Granulation Technology. *Int. J. Pharm. Front. Res.* **2011**, *1*, 65–83.
13. Freeman, T.; Bey, H.V.; Hanish, M.; Brockbank, K.; Armstrong, B. The influence of roller compaction processing variables on the rheological properties of granules. *Asian J. Pharm. Sci.* **2016**, *11*, 516–527. [CrossRef]
14. Gereg, W.; Cappola, M.L. Roller Compaction Feasibility for New Drug Candidates: Laboratory to production scale. *Pharm. Tech. Suppl.* **2002**, 14–23.
15. Sonam, D.; Pa, K.; Vs, K.; Jitendra, B.; Manoj, T. A Review: Roller Compaction for Tablet Dosage Form Development. *Mater. Sci.* **2013**, *2*, 68–73.
16. Rashid, I.; Al-Remawi, M.; Leharne, S.A.; Chowdhry, B.Z.; Badwan, A. A novel multifunctional pharmaceutical excipient: modification of the permeability of starch by processing with magnesium silicate. *Int. J. Pharm.* **2011**, *2011 15*, 18–26. [CrossRef]
17. Abu Fara, D.; Rashid, I.; Alkhamis, K.; Al-Omari, M.; Chowdhry, B.Z.; Badwan, A. Modification of α-lactose monohydrate as a direct compression excipient using roller compaction. *Drug Dev. Ind. Pharm.* **2018**, *44*, 2038–2047. [CrossRef]
18. Rashid, I.; Al-Remawi, M.; Eftaiha, A.; Badwan, A.A. Chitin-silicon dioxide coprecipitate as a novel superdisintegrant. *J. Pharm. Sci.* **2008**, *97*, 4955–4969. [CrossRef]
19. El-Barghouthi, M.; Eftaiha, A.; Rashid, I.; Al-Remawi, M.; Badwan, A.A. A Novel Superdisintegrating Agent Made from Physically Modified Chitosan with Silicon Dioxide. *Drug Dev. Ind. Pharm.* **2008**, *34*, 373–383. [CrossRef]
20. Rashid, I.; Daraghmeh, N.; Al-Remawi, M.; Leharne, S.A.; Chowdhry, B.Z.; Badwan, A.A. Characterization of Chitin–Metal Silicates as Binding Superdisintegrants. *J. Pharm. Sci.* **2009**, *98*, 4887–4901. [CrossRef]
21. Chaheen, M.; Soulairol, I.; Bataille, B.; Yassine, A.; Belamie, E.; Sharkawi, T. Chitin's functionality as a novel disintegrant: benchmarking against commonly used disintegrants in different physico-chemical environments. *J. Pharm. Sci.* **2017**, *106*, 1839–1848. [CrossRef]
22. Chaheen, M.; Sanchez-Ballester, N.M.; Bataille, B.; Yassine, A.; Belamie, E.; Sharkawi, T. Development of co-processed chitin-calcium carbonate as multifunctional tablet excipient for direct compression. *J. Pharm. Sci.* **2018**, *107*, 2152–2159. [CrossRef] [PubMed]
23. Chaheen, M.; Bataille, B.; Yassine, A.; Belamie, E. Development of Co-processed Chitin-Calcium Carbonate as Multifunctional Tablet Excipient for Direct Compression, Part 2: Tableting Properties. *J. Pharm. Sci.* **2019**, *108*, 3319–3328. [CrossRef] [PubMed]
24. Kumirska, J.; Czerwicka, M.; Kaczyński, Z.; Bychowska, A.; Brzozowski, K.; Thöming, J.; Stepnowski, P. Application of spectroscopic methods for structural analysis of chitin and chitosan. *Mar. Drugs* **2010**, *29*, 1567–1636. [CrossRef]
25. Understanding the Differences between Lactose Grades in Terms of Powder Flow, Technical Document. Available online: www.dfepharma.com (accessed on 31 January 2020).
26. Soppela, I.; Airaksinen, S.; Murtoma, M.; Tenho, M.; Hatara, J.; Räikkönen, H.; Yliruusi, J.; Sandler, N. Investigation of the powder flow behaviour of binary mixtures of microcrystalline celluloses and paracetamol. *J. Excip. Food Chem.* **2010**, *1*, 55–67.
27. Abu Fara, D.; Dadou, S.M.; Rashid, I.; Al-Obeidi, R.; Antonijevic, M.D.; Chowdhry, B.Z.; Badwan, A.A. A Direct Compression Matrix Made from Xanthan Gum and Low Molecular Weight Chitosan Designed to Improve Compressibility in Controlled Release Tablets. *Pharmaceutics* **2019**, *11*, 603. [CrossRef]
28. Nordström, J.; Klevan, I.; Alderborn, G. A particle rearrangement index based on the Kawakita powder compression equation. *J. Pharm. Sci.* **2009**, *98*, 1053–1063. [CrossRef]

29. Nordström, J.; Welch, K.; Frenning, G.; Alderborn, G. On the physical interpretation of the Kawakita and Adams parameters derived from confined compression of granular solids. *Powder Technol.* **2008**, *182*, 424–435. [CrossRef]
30. Augsburger, L.L.; Hoag, S.W. *Pharmaceutical Dosage Forms—Tablets*, 3rd ed.; CRC Press: Florida, FL, USA, 2008; pp. 560–581.
31. Ioelovich, M. Crystallinity and Hydrophility of Chitin and Chitosan. *Res. Rev. J. Chem.* **2014**, *3*, 7–14.
32. Alves, H.J.; Furman, M.; Kugelmeier, C.L.; Oliveira, C.R.; Bach, V.R.; Lupatini, K.N.; Neves, A.C.; Arantes, M.K. Effect of shrimp shells milling on the molar mass of chitosan. *Polímeros* **2017**, *27*, 41–47. [CrossRef]
33. Yuan, X.; Liu, S.; Feng, G.; Liu, Y.; Li, Y.; Lu, H.; Liang, B. Effects of ball milling on structural changes and hydrolysis of lignocellulosic biomass in liquid hot-water compressed carbon dioxide. *Korean J. Chem. Eng.* **2016**, *33*, 21–34. [CrossRef]
34. Chen, X.; Gao, Y.; Wang, L.; Chen, H.; Yan, N. Effect of Treatment Methods on Chitin Structure and Its Transformation into Nitrogen-Containing Chemicals. *Chempluschem.* **2015**, *80*, 1565–1572. [CrossRef] [PubMed]
35. Shah, R.B.; Tawakkul, M.A.; Khan, M.A. Comparative evaluation of flow for pharmaceutical powders and granules. *AAPS PharmSciTech.* **2008**, *9*, 250–258. [CrossRef] [PubMed]
36. Armstrong, B.; Brockbank, K.; Clayton, J. Understand the Effects of Moisture on Powder Behavior. *Chem. Eng. Prog.* **2014**, *110*, 25–30.
37. Shekunov, B.Y.; Chattopadhyay, P.; Tong, H.H.; Chow, A.H. Particle size analysis in pharmaceutics: principles, methods and applications. *Pharm. Res.* **2007**, *24*, 203–227. [CrossRef]
38. Shi, L.; Feng, Y.; Sun, C.C. Initial moisture content in raw material can profoundly influence high shear wet granulation process. *Int. J. Pharm.* **2011**, *416*, 43–48. [CrossRef]
39. Crouter, A.; Briens, L. The Effect of Moisture on the Flowability of Pharmaceutical Excipients. *AAPS PharmSciTech.* **2014**, *15*, 65–74. [CrossRef]
40. Hancock, B.C.; Carlson, G.T.; Ladipo, D.D.; Langdon, B.A.; Mullarney, M.P. Comparison of the mechanical properties of the crystalline and amorphous forms of a drug substance. *Int. J. Pharm.* **2002**, *241*, 73–85. [CrossRef]
41. Feng, B.; Fang, X.; Wang, H.X.; Dong, W.; Li, Y.C. The Effect of Crystallinity on Compressive Properties of Al-PTFE. *Polymers* **2016**, *8*, 356. [CrossRef]
42. Einfal, T.; Planinšek, O.; Hrovat, K. Methods of amorphization and investigation of the amorphous state. *Acta Pharm.* **2013**, *63*, 305–334. [CrossRef]
43. Boukouvalas, C.J.; Krokida, M.K.; Maroulis, Z.B.; Marinos-Kouris, D. Effect of Material Moisture Content and Temperature on the True Density of Foods. *Int. J. Food Prop.* **2006**, *9*, 109–125. [CrossRef]
44. Silva, S.S.; Duarte, A.R.; Carvalho, A.P.; Mano, J.F.; Reis, R.L. Green processing of porous chitin structures for biomedical applications combining ionic liquids and supercritical fluid technology. *Acta Biomater.* **2011**, *7*, 1166–1172. [CrossRef]
45. Šantl, M.; Ilić, I.; Vrečer, F.; Baumgartner, S. A compressibility and compactibility study of real tableting mixtures: the effect of granule particle size. *Acta Pharm.* **2012**, *62*, 325–340. [CrossRef] [PubMed]
46. *European Pharmacopoeia Supplement*; Council of Europe: Strasbourg, France, 2007.
47. Alakayleh, F.; Rashid, I.; Al-Omari, M.M.H.; Al-Sou'od, K.; Chowdhry, B.Z.; Badwan, A.A. Compression profiles of different molecular weight chitosans. *Powder Technol.* **2016**, *299*, 107–118. [CrossRef]
48. Powder Flow. *The United States Pharmacopeia*; The United States Pharmacopeial Convention: Rockville, MD, USA, 2002.
49. Ilkka, J.; Paronen, P. Prediction of the compression behavior of powder mixtures by the Heckel equation. *Int. J. Pharm.* **1993**, *94*, 181–187. [CrossRef]
50. Choi, D.H.; Kim, N.A.; Chu, K.R.; Jung, Y.J.; Yoon, J.-H.; Jeong, S.H. Material Properties and Compressibility Using Heckel and Kawakita Equation with Commonly Used Pharmaceutical Excipients. *J. Pharm. Invest.* **2010**, *40*, 237–244.
51. *The United States Pharmacopeia and National Formulary USP 32–NF 27*; The United States Pharmacopeial Convention, Inc.: Rockville, MD, USA, 2009.

marine drugs

MDPI

Article

The Antimicrobial Properties of Chitosan Can Be Tailored by Formulation

May Wenche Jøraholmen [1], Abhilasha Bhargava [1], Kjersti Julin [2], Mona Johannessen [2] and Nataša Škalko-Basnet [1,*]

1 Drug Transport and Delivery Research Group, Department of Pharmacy, Faculty of Health Sciences, University of Tromsø The Arctic University of Norway, Universitetsveien 57, 9037 Tromsø, Norway; may.w.joraholmen@uit.no (M.W.J.); abhilasha.b-94@hotmail.com (A.B.)

2 Research group for Host-Microbe Interaction, Department of Medical Biology, Faculty of Health Sciences, University of Tromsø The Arctic University of Norway, Sykehusveien 44, 9037 Tromsø, Norway; kjersti.julin@uit.no (K.J.); mona.johannessen@uit.no (M.J.)

* Correspondence: natasa.skalko-basnet@uit.no; Tel.: +47-7764-6640

Received: 10 January 2020; Accepted: 30 January 2020; Published: 31 January 2020

Abstract: Topical administration of drugs into the vagina can provide local therapy of vaginal infections, preventing the possible systemic side effects of the drugs. The natural polysaccharide chitosan is known for its excellent mucoadhesive properties, safety profile, and antibacterial effects, and thus it can be utilized in improving localized vaginal therapy by prolonging the residence time of a drug at the vaginal site while acting as an antimicrobial in synergy. Therefore, we aimed to explore the potential of chitosan, namely chitosan-coated liposomes and chitosan hydrogel, as an excipient with intrinsic antimicrobial properties. Liposomes were prepared by the thin-film hydration method followed by vesicle size reduction by sonication to the desired size, approximately 200 nm, and coated with chitosan (0.01, 0.03, 0.1, and 0.3%, w/v, respectively). The mucoadhesive properties of chitosan-coated liposomes were determined through their binding efficiency to mucin compared to non-coated liposomes. Non-coated liposomal suspensions were incorporated in chitosan hydrogels forming the liposomes-in-hydrogel formulations, which were further assessed for their texture properties in the presence of biological fluid simulants. The antibacterial effect of chitosan-coated liposomes (0.03%, 0.1% and 0.3%, w/v) and chitosan hydrogels (0.1% and 0.3%, w/w) on *Staphylococcus epidermidis* and *Staphylococcus aureus* was successfully confirmed.

Keywords: chitosan-coated liposomes; chitosan hydrogel; mucoadhesion; vaginal infections; antibacterial activity; *Staphylococcus epidermidis*; *Staphylococcus aureus*

---

1. Introduction

Although the antibiotics era enabled treatment of previously fatal infections, microorganisms managed to "fight back" and develop resistance, leading to an era of antimicrobial resistance. As a consequence, the antimicrobial treatment options became limited and the need for better antimicrobials more evident. In a search for novel antimicrobials, materials of natural origin with intrinsic antimicrobial properties become highly attractive, especially for localized antimicrobial therapy. A material exhibiting intrinsic antimicrobial properties can be used either as a pharmaceutical excipient, for example, as a vehicle for the antimicrobial agent, or as an active agent itself [1]. The choice of excipients of natural origin with intrinsic antimicrobial properties will be dependent both on the targeted microorganism but also on the features of the administration site such as skin, vagina, etc. The choice will also be influenced by the other characteristics of the material such as its muco- and bio-adhesiveness, stability in biological environment, toxicity, etc. Considering the vagina as an administration site, chitosan is among the most promising materials. We have extensively studied chitosan-based delivery systems [2–5], both for skin and vaginal administration. To date, no consensus in the field has been reached considering the exact mechanisms of the antimicrobial actions of chitosan. The antimicrobial effects of chitosan are attributed to its ability to destabilize the outer membrane of Gram-negative bacteria [6,7] and permeate the microbial plasma membrane [8]. The interaction between positively charged chitosan molecules and negatively charged microbial cell membranes is expected to lead to a disruption of microbial membrane, followed by a leakage of intracellular constituents [9]. It was proposed that at a lower concentration (< 0.2 mg/mL), the cationic groups of chitosan bind to the negatively charged bacterial surface leading to agglutination, while, at higher concentrations, the larger number of chitosan cationic groups form a net positive charge onto the bacterial surfaces resulting in a suspension [6]. Considering the optimal properties of chitosan, it seems that its hydrophilicity is essential for its antimicrobial potential. In addition, its molecular weight, degree of acetylation and ionic strength and pH of the dissolving medium will also affect antimicrobial properties of chitosan. Therefore, by tailoring the formulation features, it is possible to optimize the antimicrobial potential of chitosan-based formulations [10].

Genital infections can be caused by a variety of microorganisms. However, bacterial vaginosis remains among the most recurrent infections of genital tract [5]. There are several factors responsible for failure to eradicate bacterial vaginosis completely and prevent recurrence. However, it seems that persistent bacterial biofilms could be among the most contributing factors. Antibiotics fail to fully penetrate the negatively charged polysaccharide matrix coating the bacteria in biofilm, enabling the survival of bacteria in the deeper quarters of the biofilm. Therefore, utilizing material able to act on disruption of biofilms, as well as deliver other antimicrobial of interest within the same formulation, may lead to successful antibacterial therapy. Chitosan was proposed as a potent antimicrobial material acting on biofilms; chitosan gels were reportedly able to eradicate *Pseudomonas aeruginosa* biofilms in a pH-independent manner. Moreover, the chitosan concentration required to eradicate biofilms was rather low (0.13%) [11].

Treating vaginal infections requires careful tailoring of the formulation features, since the vagina as an administration site bears specific challenges which should be addressed/overcome when optimizing the therapy. The first consideration is probably the need to assure that the formulation does not disturb the natural vaginal environment [12]. A further challenge is sufficient residence time within the vaginal cavity. Formulations such as liposomes-in-hydrogel formulations can assure the required mucoadhesive properties and vaginal residence time [13–15]. A liposomes-in-hydrogel formulation can exhibit a synergic effect; poorly soluble active substances/drugs will be incorporated in liposomes whereas the extend residence time within the vaginal site will be assured by hydrogel as a vehicle [16,17]. Moreover, these hydrogels are often based on natural mucoadhesive polymers such as chitosan, assuring the formulation's biocompatibility and biodegradability [18].

In order to achieve maximal clinical outcome of novel formulation based on hydrogels in terms of improving retention of a drug and spreading within the vaginal cavity, it is necessary to highlight the importance of texture characterization of hydrogels [19]. Utilizing chitosan as a hydrogel vehicle with intrinsic biological activity enables synergy between the drug and excipient chitosan [20].

The additional advantage of chitosan is its ability to closely interact with mucus, thus providing an efficient contact-time between the formulation and the vaginal mucosal epithelium [3]. Chitosan can be used to prepare different mucoadhesive delivery systems and dosage forms either as a coating material for liposomes and a building block for nanoparticles or as a mucoadhesive hydrogel [21,22].

We aimed to evaluate whether the formulation type and features have an impact on the antimicrobial performance of chitosan-based formulations. To avoid interference from the active ingredients, we focused on drug-free formulations. We prepared and fully characterized two main formulation types, namely chitosan-coated liposomes and liposomes-in-chitosan hydrogel. The formulations were fully characterized and tested against *Staphylococcus epidermidis* and *Staphylococcus aureus* and their antimicrobial activity compared.

2. Results and Discussion

An optimal localized treatment of vaginal infections depends not only on the potency of the active ingredient/drug, but also on the physiochemical properties of the formulation; an ideal formulation can protect and enhance as well as act in synergy with antimicrobial to assure successful therapy [23]. Chitosan-based delivery systems exhibit strong mucoadhesive properties, an excellent safety profile and intrinsic antimicrobial activity of chitosan, which add to their attractiveness as pharmaceutical formulations, including those destined for vaginal delivery [4,17,24,25]. However, relatively little is known about the effects of the type of formulation on the antimicrobial performance of the formulation. Since the most interesting chitosan-based formulations are coated liposomes and chitosan hydrogels, we developed, characterized and evaluated these two formulations.

2.1. Liposomal Characteristics

The vesicle size of liposomes depends on the preparation method, and the thin-film hydration method is known to generate rather large heterogeneous multilamellar vesicles (MLVs). [26]. When aiming at vaginal mucosal delivery, the vesicle size range is suggested to be approximately 200 nm [12]. We, therefore, reduced the MLVs' size to close to 200 nm (Table 1). The size reduction by probe sonication resulted in a bimodal size distribution expressed as two vesicle populations. However, the polydispersity index (PI) was found to be acceptable with values below 0.4 (Table 1). A lower PI value indicates a more homogenous liposomal distribution [27].

Table 1. The effect of chitosan coating on liposomal size distribution. The values are presented as the mean ± SD (n = 3).

	Vesicle size				PI*
	Peak 1 (nm)	Weight Intensity (%)	Peak 2 (nm)	Weight Intensity (%)	
Non-coated	226 ± 10.2	89.2	55 ± 4.6	10.8	0.35
0.01	217 ± 0.7	90.2	49 ± 0.2	10.2	0.32
0.03	228 ± 2.4	90.5	54 ± 0.0	10.2	0.31
0.1	288 ± 71.1	74.9	75 ± 19.2	24.6	0.33
0.3	358 ± 90.8	63.5	106 ± 29.4	34.1	0.33

* Polydispersity index.

An increase in liposomal size was seen for the chitosan-coated liposomes coated with the higher chitosan concentration (0.1% and 0.3%, w/v), indicating that coating was successful. Further, the vesicle size increased with the increasing polymer concentration, in agreement with the literature [3,28–31]. Although the chitosan concentrations commonly utilized for coating of vesicles range from 0.1% to 0.6%, we tried to use even lower concentrations (0.01% and 0.03%, respectively). However, the lowest concentration of chitosan did not lead to an increase in the original liposomal size (Table 1). Lack of the change in vesicle size after the coating may indicate that the coating was unsuccessful, assuming that original vesicle size of neutral liposomes was representative. The polydispersity index indicates a rather heterogenous population of neutral liposomes (Table 1). NICOMP distributions categorize the vesicles in subpopulations of vesicles of similar size [28]. Therefore, results are an estimate based on the intensity of subpopulations. In this case, the degree of significance would not be relevant and was not calculated.

An increased zeta potential for chitosan-coated liposomes is expected due to the cationic character of chitosan and can be used as an indicator of successful coating. The zeta potential of all liposomal formulations was determined (Figure 1), confirming that chitosan coating with the higher chitosan concentration (0.1% and 0.3% w/v) resulted in an increase in liposomal surface charge compared to the non-coated liposomes, in agreement with the literature [3,32]. The increase in potential was lower compared to our previous findings [28,29]. However, the use of different origin chitosan, lipid, and the medium liposomes were dispersed in, might be the contributing factors to the observed differences [33].

The changes in the liposomal size (Table 1) and increase in zeta potential (Figure 1) confirmed the successful coating when higher chitosan concentrations were applied.

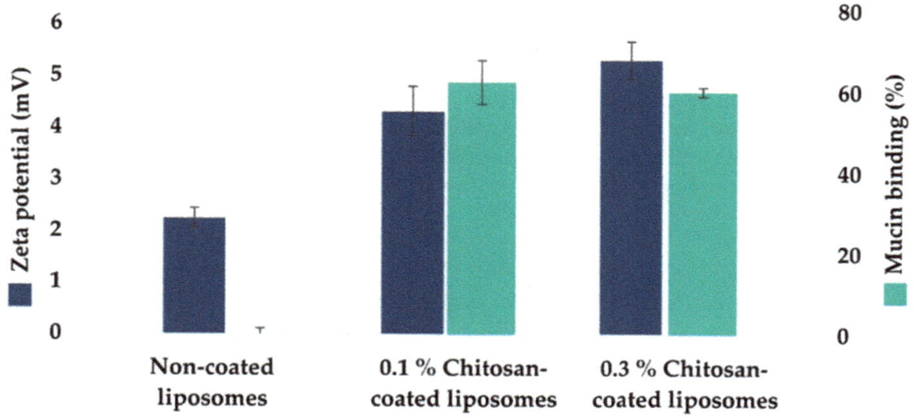

Figure 1. The zeta potential of chitosan-coated liposomes and effect of chitosan coating on mucin binding. In dark blue: The effect of chitosan coating on the zeta potential of liposomes. The values denote the mean of three individual experiments, determined in triplicates, and expressed as the mean ± SD for non-coated liposomes, 0.1 and 0.3% chitosan-coated liposomes, respectively. In light blue: The effect of chitosan coating on the mucin binding efficiency. The values are presented as the mean ± SD (n = 3).

To prolong the residence time of vaginal formulation, it is advantageous to increase the concentration of polymer thereof, enhancing the strength of mucoadhesion [34]. The mucoadhesive properties of chitosan-coated liposomes were determined based on the mucin binding of chitosan-coated liposomes compared to non-coated liposomes (Figure 1) [29]. The mucin binding of chitosan-coated liposomes was significantly higher ($p < 0.001$) than non-coated liposomes, as expected. Results corresponded to earlier findings regarding increased mucin binding due to chitosan coating [28,29,35]. However, the 0.3% (w/v) chitosan concentration did not express significantly increased mucin binding compared to 0.1% (w/v) chitosan-coated liposomes. In our previous work [29], we determined the surface availability of chitosan when two different concentrations of chitosan were used to coat liposomes. The availability of chitosan was higher when the coating was performed with lower chitosan concentrations. The mucin-binding was also superior. It is important to consider that these findings can only provide indirect information about the binding efficiency of chitosan coating on the liposomal surface. The difference between the current and previous work can be contributed to chitosan origin, different molecular weights of chitosan, as well as different size of liposomes that were coated. The longer polymer chains are more likely to interact to a lesser extent with mucin chains, resulting in reduced interpenetration through vaginal mucus, and thus reduced adhesive properties [3].

2.2. *Hydrogel Characteristics*

Chitosan-based hydrogels are considered to be very attractive vehicles for vaginal drug delivery due to their lower pH (4–5), high water content, biodegradability and pronounced mucoadhesiveness [24].

The texture properties of hydrogels, such as the hardness, cohesiveness and adhesiveness, are essential parameters to be evaluated when considering hydrogel as a potential vaginal formulation. In brief, the hardness of the hydrogel indicates the applicability of the hydrogel, considering the ease of application, packaging and storage. The adhesiveness may indicate the contact time between the hydrogel and mucus and therefore the retention within the vaginal cavity. Cohesiveness describes the work required to deform the hydrogel in the downward movement of the probe [36]. The composition of the hydrogels determines their textural properties, which can be further assessed as an indicator to obtain optimal properties suitable for the specific route of administration. Thus, these parameters were investigated for various types of hydrogel formulations to assure that the properties of hydrogels correlate to the desired features. These properties of hydrogels are known to be influenced by the molecular weight of the polymer, and previous findings indicated medium-molecular-weight chitosan to exhibit superior texture properties, considering vaginal administration, compared to the high and low-molecular-weight chitosan [17]. Thus, hydrogels based on medium-molecular-weight chitosan were used in all experiments in this study.

Glycerol was added to hydrogels to maintain the stability of chitosan hydrogels [37]; moreover, glycerol has also shown the ability to improve the texture properties of the hydrogels [17,36]. To avoid possible toxicity and local irritation, we aimed to minimize the acetic acid concentration used in hydrogel preparation. Hydrogels with 0.75 and 1% (w/w) acetic acid were prepared to investigate the effect of acid concentration on texture properties and short time stability. A slight increase in the hardness, cohesiveness and adhesiveness was seen for hydrogels made with 1% (w/w) acetic acid after storage for 5 days at room temperature (Figure 2). The same trend was observed previously [17] for hydrogels stored for 2 months. This was not observed for hydrogels made with a lower concentration (0.75%) of acetic acid (Figure 2). Moreover, the reproducibility of hydrogels comprising 1% (w/w) acetic acid was superior to 0.75% (w/w). This might indicate that 0.75% (w/w) acetic acid is the minimum acid concentration needed to assure chitosan solubility. Additionally, all parameters were increased for the hydrogels comprising an increased concentration of acetic acid, possibly due to enhanced interactions between chitosan and acetic acid [38]. Hence, acetic acid with a concentration of 1% (w/w) was used for the preparation of hydrogels in all further experiments. We did not encounter any toxicity issues for hydrogels prepared with even higher chitosan concentrations (data not shown).

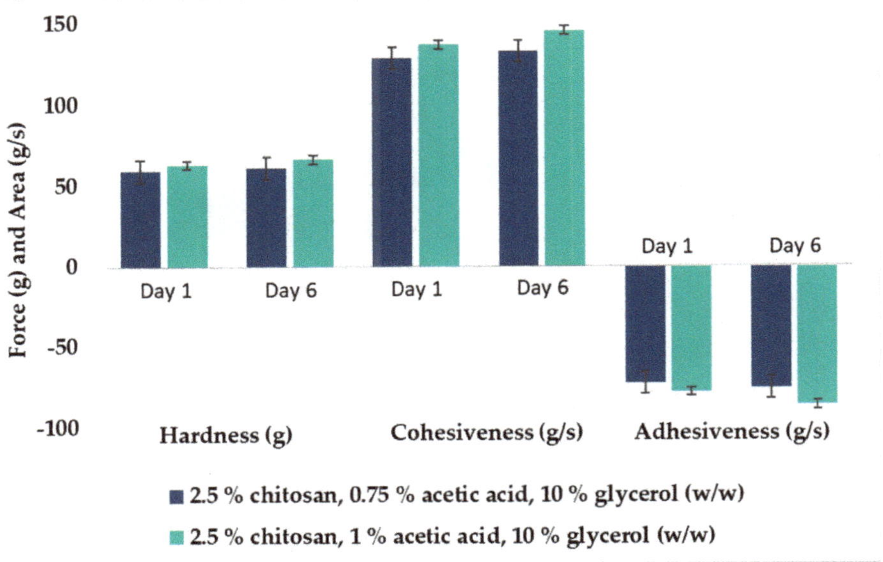

Figure 2. Texture properties of chitosan hydrogels (2.5% w/w) with different compositions determined either as freshly prepared or after storage for 5 days at room temperature (23–25 °C). The values are expressed as the mean ± SD (n = 3).

2.3. Effect of Biological Fluids on The Texture Properties of Chitosan Hydrogels

All formulations administered to the vaginal cavity will be exposed to biological fluids which may affect their properties and consequently their performance [17]. The composition, volume and pH of vaginal fluids varies with women's age and stage in reproductive cycle [39]. The mucoadhesive vaginal drug delivery system can be optimized by utilizing information on texture properties provided by the texture analysis [17,19]. To explore the influence of relevant biological fluids on the texture properties of hydrogels, the hardness, cohesiveness and adhesiveness of hydrogels were determined when the hydrogels were exposed to mucin, vaginal fluid simulant (VFS) and human semen fluid simulant (SFS).

Pig mucin was chosen as a model mucin due to its similarity to human mucin [40]. The cohesiveness and adhesiveness of the chitosan hydrogel was significantly reduced ($p < 0.001$) in the presence of mucin, compared to the non-exposed hydrogels, indicating that mucin is affecting the texture properties (Figure 3). Theoretically, adhesiveness should not be significantly affected due to enhanced adhesion between the polymeric hydrogel and mucin [41]. The hydrogel hardness was not affected by the presence of mucin. However, when hydrogels were exposed to the mixture of biological fluids, all texture parameters were affected and reduced as compared to intact hydrogels. The texture properties of hydrogel in the presence of vaginal fluids may indicate the level of robustness and viscosity of the hydrogel, which can affect the spreadability of the hydrogel and optimal coverage of vaginal mucus. The introduction of vaginal and semen fluid will alter both the viscosity and pH of vaginal mucus, and possibly contribute to improved ability of the hydrogel to spread evenly onto the vaginal mucus, increasing the contact time between mucin and the mucoadhesive hydrogel. However, the strength of the interactions between mucin and hydrogels might be weakened [12]. Similar trends as observed in our testing have been reported for both poloxamer and chitosan-based hydrogels [42,43].

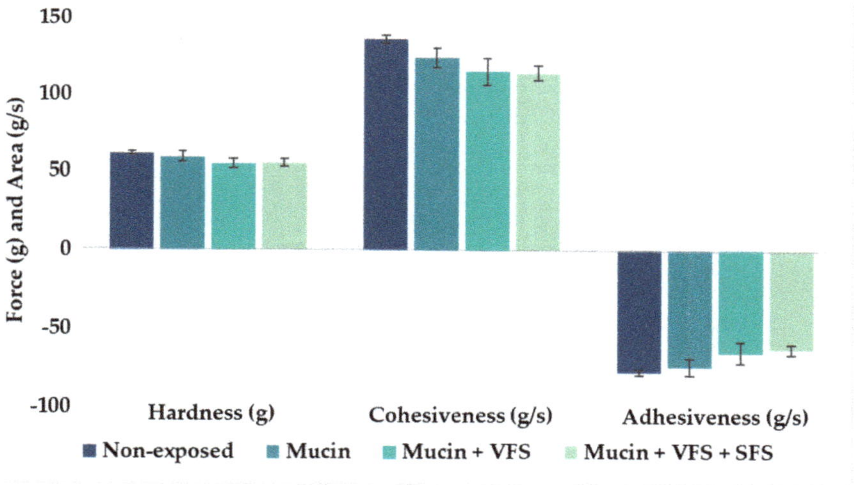

Figure 3. Texture properties of hydrogels (2.5% w/w chitosan) in the presence of mucin, vaginal fluid simulant (VFS) and semen fluid simulant (SFS) as compared to non-exposed hydrogel. The values are shown as the mean ± SD (n = 4).

Many of the active ingredients/drugs destined for localized vaginal therapy are poorly soluble and cannot be dissolved in hydrogels, therefore requiring a carrier able to solubilize them, as well as offer protection against the hydrogel microenvironment [23]. Liposomes are among the most studied carriers for poorly soluble substances/drugs. Due to their liquid nature, liposomes often require secondary vehicles such as a hydrogel to assure prolonged residence time within the vaginal cavity. The incorporation of liposomes in hydrogels has been shown to improve formulation texture properties [17]. Liposomes not only enable the incorporation of poorly soluble drugs, but also act on improved bioavailability and potential controlled drug release. The combination of liposomes and chitosan hydrogel, liposomes-in-hydrogel formulation, provides a prolonged residence time at the vaginal site and improved localized drug therapy. The incorporation of liposomes in hydrogel has also been shown to increase their stability when exposed to vaginal fluids [44]. Hence, we tested how biological fluids influence the texture properties of liposomes-in-hydrogel formulation.

The incorporation of liposomes into hydrogels resulted in hydrogels exhibiting slightly increased adhesiveness and cohesiveness (Figure 4) compared to hydrogels containing buffer in the same concentration as the liposomal suspension (Figure 3). This finding closely corresponded to earlier findings, indicating that liposomes are indeed stabilizing the chitosan network [36]. However, the texture properties of liposomes-in-hydrogel formulation were also affected by the exposure to biological fluids (Figure 4).

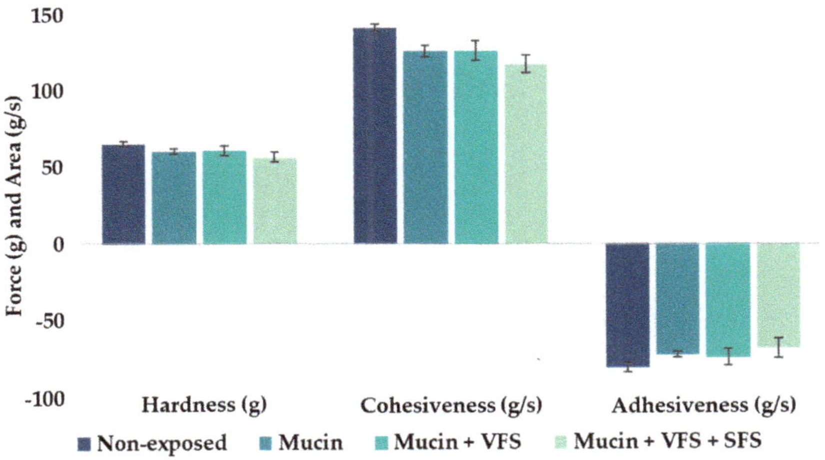

Figure 4. Texture properties of liposomes-in-hydrogels in the presence of mucin, vaginal fluid simulant (VFS) and semen fluid simulant (SFS). The values are shown as the mean ± SD (n = 3).

2.4. Antimicrobial Effects of Chitosan Formulations

After optimizing the two chitosan-based formulations, we evaluated the effect of formulation features on the antimicrobial activity. The antimicrobial properties of chitosan are widely studied [1,7,45]. To characterize the antibacterial activity, we opted to compare two of the most common chitosan-based formulations, namely chitosan-coated liposomes versus chitosan-based hydrogels. The antibacterial effects of chitosan-coated liposomes (0.01%, 0.03%, 0.1% and 0.3%, w/v respectively) and chitosan hydrogel (0.1% and 0.3% w/w, respectively) were tested against methicillin-resistant or sensitive strains of two clinical species of Gram-positive bacteria; namely *S. aureus* and *S. epidermidis*. *Staphylococcus spp*. is naturally found on the human skin and mucosal surfaces. A disturbance in the microbiota can result in *Staphylococcus spp* infections, and poor hygiene, elevated pH, immune deficiency and diabetes can lead to extensive colonization of this bacteria [46]. Few studies have connected *Staphylococcus* to the vaginal environment; however, it is known that *Staphylococci* may contribute to bacterial vaginosis and increase the diversity of bacteria in vaginal microbiota [47]; hence, we chose to use these bacterial species as model organisms to evaluate the effect of the type of chitosan formulation on its antimicrobial properties.

Non-coated (chitosan-free) liposomes were considered as a negative control and, as expected, did not show any antibacterial effect (data not shown). The neutral liposomal membrane is expected to have limited interaction with the bacterial cell membrane, thus, resulting in negligible antibacterial activity, as observed. The antibacterial activities of all liposomal formulations were expressed as a percentage of inhibition compared to a positive control; antibiotic vancomycin. Thus, the antibacterial activity of each formulation was expressed as a percentage of growth inhibition zone relative to the inhibition effect of vancomycin considered to be 100%. No bacterial growth inhibition was observed for liposomes coated with 0.01% chitosan for all bacteria isolates (data not shown) as expected. Interestingly, liposomes coated with chitosan concentration as low as 0.03% did suppress bacteria growth of *S. epidermidis*, whereas the same liposomes did not show the antibacterial effect on *S. aureus* (Figure 5). Those liposomes were very similar in size and zeta potential to non-coated liposomes and were expected to have a very thin layer of coating (Table 1). However, it seems that the available concentration of chitosan on the liposomal surface was sufficient to act as an antimicrobial.

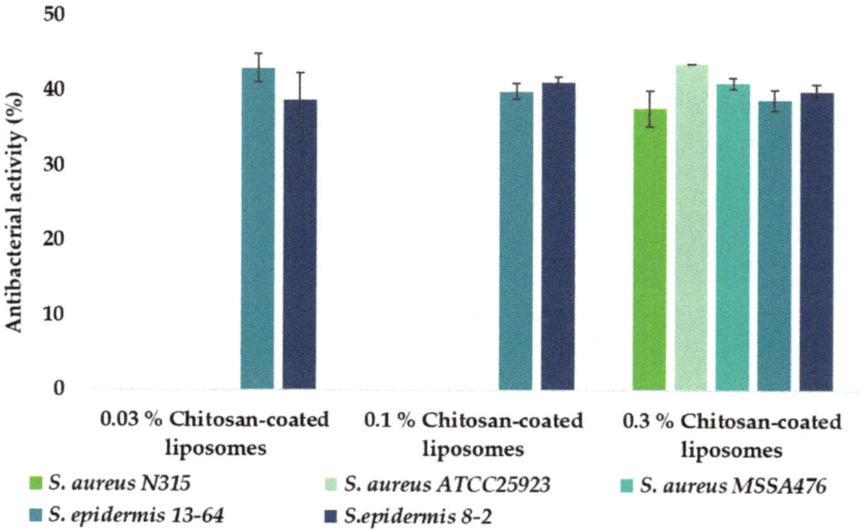

Figure 5. Antibacterial activity of chitosan-coated (%, w/v) liposomes expressed as the percentage of antibacterial activity compared to positive control vancomycin (100%). The values are presented as the mean ± SD (n = 3).

To explain why the same liposomes acted on *S. epidermidis* but not on *S. aureus*, more work should have been included. However, it was shown early on that *S. aureus* is more prone to developing resistance than *S. epidermidis* [48], which could be among the contributing factors for the observed difference. The postulation may be supported by the fact that only the 0.3% chitosan-coated liposomes efficiently inhibited bacterial growth of *S. aureus*, indicating that the growth inhibition potential might be dependent on the chitosan concentration available on the liposomal surface. However, these differences were not statistically significant; and further evaluation of higher concentrations of chitosan-coated liposomes is needed to investigate the hypothesis of increased antibacterial effect at higher concentrations as well as broader antimicrobial spectra when higher chitosan concentrations are used for coating. An additional factor which may be interesting to explore is the size of liposomes. Liposomes coated with the highest chitosan concentration were larger in size than smaller vesicles (Table 1) and more mucoadhesive (Figure 1), which might imply that they were in closer contact with agar.

No significant difference in antibacterial activity was observed between the two concentrations of chitosan hydrogels (0.1% and 0.3%, respectively), indicating that the lower chitosan concentration is sufficient to express an inhibitory effect against both bacterial strains (Figure 6). Hydrogels with 0.1% and 0.3% chitosan were proven to be more effective against *S. aureus* than the chitosan-coated liposomes (Figure 7). Possibly, less chitosan is available on the surface of the chitosan-coated liposomes which are spherical in nature, resulting in reduced electrostatic interactions between chitosan and the negatively charged bacterial cell membrane [26]. Recently, Dumont and colleagues [49] reported that alginate fibers coated with chitosan significantly decreased the bacterial growth of *S. aureus*. Moreover, they were able to confirm that formulation features also play an important role in antimicrobial activity of formulation; longer fibers were found to be better. Although their aim was to develop novel wound dressing, the findings are relevant for our study. It is interesting that the 0.1% chitosan-coated liposomes did not inhibit the growth of *S. aureus* to the same extent as 0.1% chitosan hydrogel, indicating that the type of formulation contributes to the degree of inhibition of this bacterium.

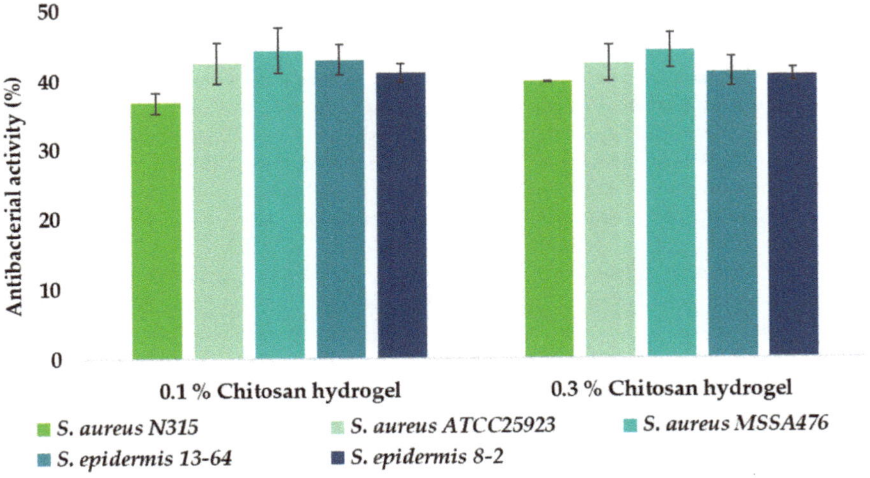

Figure 6. Antibacterial activity of chitosan hydrogels (%, w/w) expressed as the percentage of antibacterial activity compared to positive control vancomycin (100%). The values are presented as the mean ± SD (n = 3).

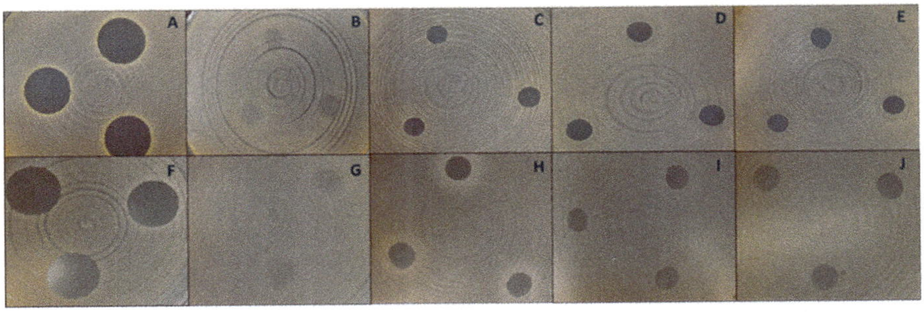

Figure 7. Antibacterial activity of chitosan formulations. Inhibition of *S. aureus MSSA 476* by vancomycin (**A**, positive control), non-coated liposomes (**B**, negative control), 0.3% (w/v) chitosan-coated liposomes (**C**), 0.1% (w/w) chitosan hydrogel (**D**) and 0.3% (w/w) chitosan hydrogel (**E**). Inhibition of *S. aureus ATCC 25923* by vancomycin (**F**, positive control), non-coated liposomes (**G**, negative control), 0.3% (w/v) chitosan-coated liposomes (**H**), 0.1% (w/w) chitosan hydrogel (**I**) and 0.3% (w/w) chitosan hydrogel (**J**).

The zones of inhibition were from 0.00 cm for non-coated liposomes to 1.81 cm for the positive control, vancomycin.

Chitosan can be used as an excipient able to contribute as an antibacterial agent, as suggested by Yang and colleagues [20]. Previous studies have reported that the antimicrobial activity of chitosan depends on parameters such as molecular weight, degree of deacetylation and derivatization [50]. We have shown that the type of chitosan formulation can contribute to the overall antimicrobial performance of the formulation. These promising findings need to be further explored to confirm that the type of formulation affects not only the antibacterial but also antifungal activity of chitosan. Moreover, it would be interesting to evaluate the potential of chitosan derivatives as well as chitosan hybrid nanoparticles. For example, a quaternized chitosan was recently reported to exhibit strong activity against *Escherichia coli* when formulated as a nanofiber membrane [51]. Similarly, hybridization of chitosan with protamine lead to improved activity of chitosan nanoparticles against *E. coli* [52].

3. Materials and Methods

3.1. Materials

Lipoid S 80 (80% phosphatidylcholine from egg) was a gift from Lipoid GmbH, Ludwigshafen, Germany. Chitosan (medium-molecular-weight hydramer HCMF) was a gift from Chitinor AS, Tromsø, Norway. Mucin from porcine stomach (type III, bound sialic acid 0.5%–1.5%, partially purified), acetic acid, ammonium acetate, bovine serum albumin, calcium chloride, calcium hydroxide, fructose, glucose, glycerol, lactic acid, magnesium chloride, potassium chloride, potassium phosphate, sodium chloride, sodium phosphate dibasic, sodium phosphate monobasic monohydrate and vancomycin hydrochloride were all purchased from Sigma Aldrich Chemie GmbH, Steinheim, Germany. Potassium hydroxide and sodium citrate dehydrate were the products of NMD, Oslo, Norway. Urea was the product of Apotekproduksjonen AS, Oslo, Norway. *Staphylococcus aureus* MSSA476 (ATCC® BAA-1721™) was purchased from LGC standard AB, Sweden. *Staphylococcus aureus* N315 was a gift from T. Ito (https://www.ncbi.nlm.nih.gov/pubmed/10348769). *Staphylococcus epidermidis* 8-2 was from Rikshospitalet, The University Hospital, Oslo, Norway, while *Staphylococcus epidermidis* 13-67 and *S. aureus* ATCC25923 were from University Hospital Northern Norway, Tromsø, Norway.

3.2. Preparation of Liposomes

Liposomes were prepared by the conventional thin-film lipid hydration method [29]. Phosphatidylcholine (1 g) was dissolved in excess methanol in a round-bottomed flask. The solvent was evaporated using a rotoevaporator (Büchi rotavapor R-124 with vacuum controller B-721, Büchi Vac® V-500, Büchi Labortechnik, Flawil, Switzerland) for at least 1 h at 60 mBar and 45 °C, forming a thin-film lipid. The lipid film was dislodged from the flask walls by adding 50 mL acetate buffer (pH 4.6, 77.1 g/L CH_3COONH_4, 70 mL glacial acetic acid). The liposomal suspension was kept in a refrigerator (4–6 °C) overnight prior to further experiments.

3.3. Vesicle Size Reduction

The vesicle size of the liposomes was reduced by probe sonication [28]. The liposomal suspension was placed on ice and the needle probe tip inserted approximately 5–7 mm into the liposomal suspension. The sonicator (Ultrasonic processor 500 W, Sigma–Aldrich, St. Louis, MO, USA) was set to 40% amplitude and the samples sonicated 3 times for 1 min, with 1 min resting periods. The samples were stored in the refrigerator (4–6 °C) for at least 6 h prior to further experiments.

3.4. Chitosan Coating of Liposomes

The liposomes were coated with 0.01%, 0.03%, 0.1% and 0.3% (w/v) chitosan solutions, respectively. All solutions were prepared in 0.1% (v/v) glacial acetic acid. The chitosan solution (2 mL) was added drop wise into the liposomal suspension (2 mL) under magnetic stirring at a constant rate, at room temperature for 1 h [29]. Prior to characterization, the chitosan-coated liposomes were stored in a refrigerator (4–6 °C).

3.5. Particle Size Analysis of Liposomes

The particle size distribution of liposomes was determined by photon correlation spectroscopy (NICOMP Submicron particle sizer, model 370, Nicomp Particle Sizing system, Santa Barbara, USA). All analyses were run in the vesicle mode and intensity distribution (NICOMP). Preparation of samples was conducted in laminar air flow bench using particle free equipment to avoid possible exposure to dust particles. Test tubes were rinsed with sterile filtered medium (acetate buffer, using 0.20 µm pore size filter) prior to dilution of the liposomal suspension in the respective medium until the intensity was within 250-350 Hz. Two cycles with a runtime of 15 min were performed.

3.6. Zeta Potential Measurements

Zeta potential measurements were performed on a Malvern Zetasizer Nano ZS (Malvern, Oxford, UK.) The measurement cell was flushed with ethanol and filtrated tap water (0.20 µm pore size filter) before loading of sample. The liposomal suspensions were diluted 1:40 (v/v) with filtered tap water to achieve the optimal measurable concentration. Three cycles for three independent samples of each formulation were performed at 25 °C [53].

3.7. Mucoadhesive Properties of Chitosan-Coated Liposomes

The mucoadhesive properties of chitosan-coated liposomes were determined by measuring the in vitro binding of chitosan to pig mucin (PM) [29]. An aliquot of the liposomal suspension (1 mL) was added to 1 mL PM suspension (400 µg/mL in 0.05 M phosphate buffer) and incubated at room temperature for 2 h, followed by centrifugation (Optima LE-80; Beckman Instruments, Palo Alto, CA, USA) at 10 °C with a speed of 216,000 *g* for 1 h. Volumes of 200 µL (four of each sample) were transferred directly from supernatant in the tubes and over to a microtitre plate (Costar® UV 96-well plate with UV transparent flat bottom, Acrylic, Costar®, Corning, NY, USA) and the amount of PM was measured spectrophotometrically (Microtitre plate reader; Spectra Max 190 Microplate, Spectrophotometer Molecular devices, Sunnyvale, CA, USA) at 251 nm. The PM binding efficiency was calculated according to Naderkhani et al. [35].

3.8. Hydrogel Preparation

Chitosan hydrogels were prepared as previously described [17]. Briefly, medium-molecular-weight chitosan (2.5%, w/w) was dispersed in the blend of glycerol (10% w/w) and acetic acid (0.75% or 1% w/w) and left to swell at room temperature (23–25 °C) for a minimum of 48 h. Hydrogels were diluted in acetate buffer (pH 4.6; comprising 77.1 g/L CH_3COONH_4 and 70 mL glacial acetic acid) to obtain hydrogels with the final chitosan concentrations of 0.1% and 0.3% (w/w), respectively. Hydrogels containing acetate buffer or liposomes (20%, w/w) were prepared with the final chitosan concentration of 2.5% (w/w).

3.9. Preparation of Biological Fluid Simulants

The preparation of the vaginal fluid simulant (VFS) followed the procedure originally published by Owen and Katz [54]. VFS was composed of 3.5 g/L NaCl, 1.40 g/L KOH, 0.222 g/L $Ca(OH)_2$, 0.018g/L bovine serum albumin, 2 g/L lactic acid, 0.16 g/L glycerol, 5.0 g/L glucose, 0.4 g/L urea and 1 g/L acetic acid. The solution was mechanically stirred at room temperature (23–25 °C) to assure a homogenous mixture and the final pH adjusted to 4.5 by addition of 1 M HCl. VFS was stored in the refrigerator (4–6 °C) and was always left for at least 1 h at room temperature prior to experiments.

Semen fluid simulant (SFS) was prepared according to Owen and Katz [55]. In total, four solutions were made separately. Solution 1: 5.24 mL 0.123 M $NaH_2PO_4 \times H_2O$, 49.14 mL 0.123 M Na_2HPO_4,

813 mg sodium citrate dehydrate, 90.8 mg KCl, 88.1 mg KOH, 272 mg fructose, 102 mg glucose anhydrase, 62 mg lactic acid, 45 mg urea and 5.04 mg bovine serum albumin. Solution 2: 101 mg $CaCl_2$ x $2H_2O$, 15.13 mL H_2O. Solution 3: 92 mg $MgCl_2$ x $6H_2O$, 15.13 mL H_2O. Solution 4: 34.4 mg $ZnCl_2$, 15.13 mL H_2O. Solution 2 was added slowly into solution 1 under mechanical stirring, followed by solution 3 and 4, respectively. SFS was filtered (0.20 μm pore size filter) and the pH adjusted to 7.7 with 1 M NaOH. SFS was stored in the refrigerator (4–6 °C) and used after being left at room temperature for 1 h.

3.10. Determination of Texture Properties of Chitosan Hydrogels

The texture properties of chitosan hydrogels were determined according to the method previously described [17] using Texture Analyzer TA.XT plus (Stable micro systems Ltd., Surrey, UK). The freshly made hydrogels were stored at room temperature prior to the analyses and a 40 mm disc was compressed into the hydrogel (40 g) by the backward extrusion. The test was performed in the compression mode with a pretest speed, test speed and posttest speed of 4 mm/sec. Target mode was set to a distance of 10 mm and all measurements were taken at room temperature (23–25 °C). Five measurements were performed for each hydrogel and the hardness, cohesiveness and adhesiveness of the hydrogels were determined. The measurements were repeated after five days.

3.11. Stability Of Hydrogels in the Presence of Biological Fluid Simulants

Hydrogels were exposed to three different types of biological fluid simulants. Mucin solution alone (PM, 700 μL), a mixture of mucin and vaginal fluid simulant (PM, 635 μL + VFS, 65 μL) and a mixture of mucin, a vaginal fluid simulant and a semen fluid simulant (PM, 570 μL + VFS, 65 μL + SFS, 65 μL) were added onto the surface of freshly made hydrogels and left for 30 min prior to analysis. Texture analysis was performed as described above and five measurements were taken for each sample.

3.12. Antibacterial Susceptibility Testing

Chitosan-coated liposomes and hydrogels were assessed for their in vitro antibacterial activity against two clinical species of Gram-positive bacteria, namely *Staphylococcus aureus* and *Staphylococcus epidermidis*, using a modified agar disc-diffusion method [56,57]. Freeze stocks of bacteria isolates were spread on blood agar plates and incubated overnight at 37 °C. A bacterial suspension with a turbidity of 0.5 McFarland was prepared in a saline solution (0.85% w/w). A sterile cotton swab soaked in bacterial suspension was used to draw a cross across the Müller–Hinton agar plates placed on an electrical rotator to achieve uniform plating. Vancomycin (400 μg/mL) was chosen as a positive control due to resistance of chloramphenicol against the bacterial strains. In addition, a negative control was prepared by diluting the non-coated liposomes in same medium as used for coating of liposomes (0.1% w/v acetic acid). Three aliquots (10 μL of samples/controls) were added on the plates, and the plates incubated over night at 37 °C. The inhibition zone was determined by measuring the diameters of the inhibition zones. The antibacterial activity (%) was calculated for each sample based on the inhibition of positive control (100%).

3.13. Statistical Evaluation

The student's t-test was performed to determine the significance of results. The significance level was set to p-value ≤ 0.05.

4. Conclusions

We developed chitosan-based mucoadhesive drug delivery systems for treatment of vaginal infections to assure an increased retention time of the drug at the vaginal site and benefit from the antibacterial effects of chitosan. Two mucoadhesive delivery systems were prepared, namely chitosan-coated liposomes and chitosan-based hydrogels. The mucoadhesive properties of chitosan make it a good potential excipient for a vaginal drug delivery system in improving the residence time at the vaginal site. To evaluate the effect of formulation on antibacterial properties of chitosan-based formulations, we challenged formulations against *Staphylococcus epidermidis* and *Staphylococcus aureus* and confirmed chitosan's antibacterial activity. The antibacterial effect of chitosan appeared to be dependent on the type of bacteria as well as the formulation. Chitosan hydrogels inhibited the growth of both bacteria. The growth of *S. aureus* was only inhibited by 0.3% chitosan-coated liposomes, whereas (0.03%, 0.1% and 0.3%) chitosan-coated liposomes inhibited the growth of *S. epidermidis*. The differences in antibacterial potential need to be further exploited.

Author Contributions: M.W.J. and N.S.-B. contributed to conceptualization, supervision of the master student, data analysis, manuscript preparation and discussions; A.B. conducted the experiments and prepared the draft version of the manuscript; K.J. and M.J. conceptualized the antimicrobial study and contributed to manuscript preparation as well as discussions. All authors have read and agreed to the published version of the manuscript.

Funding: The research received no external funding. The publication charges for this article have been funded by a grant from the publication fund of UiT The Arctic University of Norway.

Acknowledgments: We are indebted to Lipoid GmbH, Germany, for providing the lipids and Chitinor AS, Tromsø, Norway, for chitosan.

Conflicts of Interest: The authors declare no conflict of interest.

References

1. Vanić, Ž.; Škalko-Basnet, N. Hydrogels as intrinsic antimicrobials. In *Hydrogels Based on Natural Polymers*; Elsevier BV: Amsterdam, The Netherlands, 2020; pp. 309–328.
2. Hurler, J.; Sørensen, K.K.; Fallarero, A.; Vuorela, P.; Skalko-Basnet, N. Liposomes-in-Hydrogel Delivery System with Mupirocin: In Vitro Antibiofilm Studies and In Vivo Evaluation in Mice Burn Model. *BioMed. Res. Int.* **2013**, *2013*, 1–8. [CrossRef]
3. Andersen, T.; Bleher, S.; Flaten, G.E.; Tho, I.; Mattsson, S.; Skalko-Basnet, N. Chitosan in Mucoadhesive Drug Delivery: Focus on Local Vaginal Therapy. *Mar. Drugs* **2015**, *13*, 222–236. [CrossRef] [PubMed]
4. Andersen, T.; Mishchenko, E.; Flaten, G.E.; Sollid, J.U.E.; Mattsson, S.; Tho, I.; Škalko-Basnet, N. Chitosan-Based Nanomedicine to Fight Genital Candida Infections: Chitosomes. *Mar. Drugs* **2017**, *15*, 64. [CrossRef] [PubMed]
5. Vanić, Ž.; Škalko-Basnet, N. Hydrogels for vaginal drug delivery. In *Functional Hydrogels in Drug Delivery: Key Features and Future Perspectives*, 1st ed.; Spizzirri, G., Cirillo, G., Eds.; CRC Press: Boca Raton, FL, USA, 2017; pp. 259–300.
6. Rabea, E.I.; Badawy, M.E.-T.; Stevens, C.V.; Smagghe, G.; Steurbaut, W. Chitosan as Antimicrobial Agent: Applications and Mode of Action. *Biomacromolecules* **2003**, *4*, 1457–1465. [CrossRef] [PubMed]
7. Matica, M.A.; Aachmann, F.L.; Tøndervik, A.; Sletta, H.; Ostafe, V. Chitosan as a Wound Dressing Starting Material: Antimicrobial Properties and Mode of Action. *Int. J. Mol. Sci.* **2019**, *20*, 5889. [CrossRef]
8. Tang, H.; Zhang, P.; Kieft, T.L.; Ryan, S.J.; Baker, S.M.; Wiesmann, W.P.; Rogelj, S. Antibacterial action of a novel functionalized chitosan-arginine against Gram-negative bacteria. *Acta. Biomater.* **2010**, *6*, 2562–2571. [CrossRef]
9. Kong, M.; Chen, X.G.; Xing, K.; Park, H.J. Antimicrobial properties of chitosan and mode of action: A state of the art review. *Int. J. Food Microbiol.* **2010**, *144*, 51–63. [CrossRef]
10. Dai, T.; Tanaka, M.; Huang, Y.-Y.; Hamblin, M.R. Chitosan preparations for wounds and burns: Antimicrobial and wound-healing effects. *Expert Rev. Anti-infective Ther.* **2011**, *9*, 857–879. [CrossRef]
11. Kandimalla, K.K.; Borden, E.; Omtri, R.S.; Boyapati, S.P.; Smith, M.; Lebby, K.; Mulpuru, M.; Gadde, M. Ability of Chitosan Gels to Disrupt Bacterial Biofilms and Their Applications in the Treatment of Bacterial Vaginosis. *J. Pharm. Sci.* **2013**, *102*, 2096–2101. [CrossRef]
12. Das Neves, J.; Amiji, M.; Sarmento, B. Mucoadhesive nanosystems for vaginal microbicide development: Friend or foe? *Wiley Interdiscip. Rev. Nanomed. Nanobiotechnol.* **2011**, *3*, 389–399. [CrossRef]
13. Pavelić, Ž.; Skalko-Basnet, N.; Schubert, R.; Jalšenjak, I. Liposomal Gels for Vaginal Drug Delivery. *Methods Enzymol.* **2004**, *387*, 287–299.

14. Vanić, Ž.; Hurler, J.; Ferderber, K.; Golja Gasparovic, P.; Skalko-Basnet, N.; Filipovic-Grcic, J. Novel vaginal drug delivery system: Deformable propylene glycol liposomes-in-hydrogel. *J. Liposome Res.* **2014**, *24*, 27–36.
15. Mesquita, L.; Galante, J.; Nunes, R.; Sarmento, B.; Das Neves, J. Pharmaceutical Vehicles for Vaginal and Rectal Administration of Anti-HIV Microbicide Nanosystems. *Pharmaceutics* **2019**, *11*, 145. [CrossRef] [PubMed]
16. Li, R.; Liu, Q.; Wu, H.; Wang, K.; Li, L.; Zhou, C.; Ao, N. Preparation and characterization of in-situ formable liposome/chitosan composite hydrogels. *Mater. Lett.* **2018**, *220*, 289–292. [CrossRef]
17. Jøraholmen, M.W.; Basnet, P.; Tostrup, M.J.; Moueffaq, S.; Škalko-Basnet, N. Localized Therapy of Vaginal Infections and Inflammation: Liposomes-In-Hydrogel Delivery System for Polyphenols. *Pharmaceutics* **2019**, *11*, 53.
18. Pellá, M.C.; Lima-Tenório, M.K.; Tenório-Neto, E.T.; Guilherme, M.R.; Muniz, E.C.; Rubira, A.F. Chitosan-based hydrogels: From preparation to biomedical applications. *Carbohydr. Polym.* **2018**, *196*, 233–245. [CrossRef]
19. Şenyiğit, Z.A.; Karavana, S.Y.; Erac, B.; Gursel, O.; Limoncu, M.H.; Baloğlu, E. Evaluation of chitosan based vaginal bioadhesive gel formulations for antifungal drugs. *Acta Pharm.* **2014**, *64*, 139–156. [CrossRef]
20. Yang, K.; Han, Q.; Chen, B.; Zheng, Y.; Zhang, K.; Li, Q.; Wang, J. Antimicrobial hydrogels: Promising materials for medical application. *Int. J. Nanomed.* **2018**, *13*, 2217–2263. [CrossRef]
21. Ali, A.; Ahmed, S. A review on chitosan and its nanocomposites in drug delivery. *Int. J. Boil. Macromol.* **2018**, *109*, 273–286. [CrossRef]
22. Yu, T.; Malcolm, K.; Woolfson, D.; Jones, D.S.; Andrews, G.P. Vaginal gel drug delivery systems: Understanding rheological characteristics and performance. *Expert Opin. Drug Deliv.* **2011**, *8*, 1309–1322. [CrossRef]
23. Vanić, Ž; Skalko-Basnet, N. Nanopharmaceuticals for improved topical vaginal therapy: Can they deliver? *Eur. J. Pharm. Sci.* **2013**, *50*, 29–41. [CrossRef] [PubMed]
24. Frank, L.A.; Chaves, P.S.; D'Amore, C.M.; Contri, R.V.; Frank, A.G.; Beck, R.C.; Pohlmann, A.R.; Buffon, A.; Guterres, S.S. The use of chitosan as cationic coating or gel vehicle for polymeric nanocapsules: Increasing penetration and adhesion of imiquimod in vaginal tissue. *Eur. J. Pharm. Biopharm.* **2017**, *114*, 202–212. [CrossRef] [PubMed]
25. Perinelli, D.R.; Fagioli, L.; Campana, R.; Lam, J.K.; Baffone, W.; Palmieri, G.F.; Casettari, L.; Bonacucina, G. Chitosan-based nanosystems and their exploited antimicrobial activity. *Eur. J. Pharm. Sci.* **2018**, *117*, 8–20. [CrossRef] [PubMed]
26. Bozzuto, G.; Molinari, A. Liposomes as nanomedical devices. *Int. J. Nanomed.* **2015**, *10*, 975–999. [CrossRef]
27. Danaei, M.; Dehghankhold, M.; Ataei, S.; Davarani, F.H.; Javanmard, R.; Dokhani, A.; Khorasani, S.; Mozafari, M.R. Impact of Particle Size and Polydispersity Index on the Clinical Applications of Lipidic Nanocarrier Systems. *Pharmaceutics* **2018**, *10*, 57. [CrossRef]
28. Jøraholmen, M.W.; Vanić, Ž.; Tho, I.; Skalko-Basnet, N. Chitosan-coated liposomes for topical vaginal therapy: Assuring localized drug effect. *Int. J. Pharm.* **2014**, *472*, 94–101.
29. Jøraholmen, M.W.; Škalko-Basnet, N.; Acharya, G.; Basnet, P. Resveratrol-loaded liposomes for topical treatment of the vaginal inflammation and infections. *Eur. J. Pharm. Sci.* **2015**, *79*, 112–121. [CrossRef]
30. Karn, P.R.; Vanić, Z.; Pepić, I.; Škalko-Basnet, N. Mucoadhesive liposomal delivery systems: The choice of coating material. *Drug. Dev. Ind. Pharm.* **2011**, *37*, 482–488. [CrossRef]
31. Berginc, K.; Suljaković, S.; Skalko-Basnet, N.; Kristl, A. Mucoadhesive liposomes as new formulation for vaginal delivery of curcumin. *Eur. J. Pharm. Biopharm.* **2014**, *87*, 40–46. [CrossRef]
32. Takeuchi, H.; Matsui, Y.; Sugihara, H.; Yamamoto, H.; Kawashima, Y. Effectiveness of submicron-sized, chitosan-coated liposomes in oral administration of peptide drugs. *Int. J. Pharm.* **2005**, *303*, 160–170. [CrossRef]
33. Smith, M.C.; Crist, R.M.; Clogston, J.D.; McNeil, S.E. Zeta potential: A case study of cationic, anionic, and neutral liposomes. *Anal. Bioanal. Chem.* **2017**, *409*, 5779–5787. [CrossRef] [PubMed]
34. Das Neves, J.; Bahia, M.F.; Amiji, M.M.; Sarmento, B. Mucoadhesive nanomedicines: Characterization and modulation of mucoadhesion at the nanoscale. *Expert Opin. Drug Deliv.* **2011**, *8*, 1085–1104. [CrossRef] [PubMed]
35. Naderkhani, E.; Erber, A.; Škalko-Basnet, N.; Flaten, G.E. Improved Permeability of Acyclovir: Optimization of Mucoadhesive Liposomes Using the Phospholipid Vesicle-Based Permeation Assay. *J. Pharm. Sci.* **2014**, *103*, 661–668. [CrossRef] [PubMed]

36. Hurler, J.; Engesland, A.; Poorahmary Kermany, B.; Škalko-Basnet, N. Improved texture analysis for hydrogel characterization: Gel cohesiveness, adhesiveness, and hardness. *J. Appl. Polym. Sci.* **2012**, *125*, 180–188. [CrossRef]
37. Szymańska, E.; Winnicka, K. Stability of Chitosan—A Challenge for Pharmaceutical and Biomedical Applications. *Mar. Drugs* **2015**, *13*, 1819–1846. [CrossRef]
38. Berger, J.; Reist, M.; Mayer, J.; Felt, O.; Peppas, N.; Gurny, R. Structure and interactions in covalently and ionically crosslinked chitosan hydrogels for biomedical applications. *Eur. J. Pharm. Biopharm.* **2004**, *57*, 19–34. [CrossRef]
39. Das Neves, J.; Bahia, M. Gels as vaginal drug delivery systems. *Int. J. Pharm.* **2006**, *318*, 1–14. [CrossRef]
40. Boegh, M.; Foged, C.; Müllertz, A.; Nielsen, H.M. Mucosal drug delivery: Barriers, in vitro models and formulation strategies. *J. Drug Deliv. Sci. Technol.* **2013**, *23*, 383–391. [CrossRef]
41. Millotti, G.; Hoyer, H.; Engbersen, J.; Bernkop-Schnürch, A. 6-mercaptonicotinamide-functionalized chitosan: A potential excipient for mucoadhesive drug delivery systems. *J. Drug Deliv. Sci. Technol.* **2010**, *20*, 181–186. [CrossRef]
42. Aka-Any-Grah, A.; Bouchemal, K.; Koffi, A.; Agnely, F.; Zhang, M.; Djabourov, M.; Ponchel, G. Formulation of mucoadhesive vaginal hydrogels insensitive to dilution with vaginal fluids. *Eur. J. Pharm. Biopharm.* **2010**, *76*, 296–303. [CrossRef]
43. Rossi, S.; Ferrari, F.; Bonferoni, M.C.; Sandri, G.; Faccendini, A.; Puccio, A.; Caramella, C. Comparison of poloxamer-and chitosan-based thermally sensitive gels for the treatment of vaginal mucositis. *Drug. Dev. Ind. Pharm.* **2014**, *40*, 352–360. [CrossRef] [PubMed]
44. Pavelić, Ž.; Skalko-Basnet, N.; Jalšenjak, I. Characterisation and in vitro evaluation of bioadhesive liposome gels for local therapy of vaginitis. *Int. J. Pharm.* **2005**, *301*, 140–148.
45. Verlee, A.; Mincke, S.; Stevens, C.V. Recent developments in antibacterial and antifungal chitosan and its derivatives. *Carbohydr. Polym.* **2017**, *164*, 268–283. [CrossRef] [PubMed]
46. Cundell, A.M. Microbial ecology of the human skin. *Microb. Ecol.* **2018**, *76*, 113–120. [CrossRef]
47. Fredricks, D.N.; Fiedler, T.L.; Marrazzo, J.M. Molecular Identification of Bacteria Associated with Bacterial Vaginosis. *New Engl. J. Med.* **2005**, *353*, 1899–1911. [CrossRef]
48. Huebner, J.; Goldmann, D.A. Coagulase-negative staphylococci: Role as pathogens. *Annu. Rev. Med.* **1999**, *50*, 223–236. [CrossRef]
49. Dumont, R.; Villet, M.; Guirand, A.; Montembault, A.; Delair, T.; Lack, S.; Barikosky, M.; Crepet, A.; Alcouffe, P.; Laurent, F.; et al. Processing and antimicrobial properties of chitosan-coated alginate fibers. *Carbohydr. Polym.* **2018**, *190*, 31–42. [CrossRef]
50. Tajdini, F.; Amini, M.A.; Nafissi-Varcheh, N.; Faramarzi, M.A. Production, physiochemical and antimicrobial properties of fungal chitosan from Rhizomucor miehei and Mucor racemosus. *Int. J. Boil. Macromol.* **2010**, *47*, 180–183. [CrossRef]
51. Cheah, W.Y.; Show, P.L.; Ng, I.S.; Lin, G.Y.; Chiu, C.Y.; Chang, Y.K. Antimicrobaila activity of quaternized chitosan modified nanofiber membrane. *Int. J. Biol. Macromol.* **2019**, *126*, 569–577. [CrossRef]
52. Tamara, F.R.; Lin, C.; Mi, F.-L.; Ho, Y.-C. Antibacterial Effects of Chitosan/Cationic Peptide Nanoparticles. *Nanomaterials* **2018**, *8*, 88. [CrossRef]
53. Jøraholmen, M.W.; Basnet, P.; Acharya, G.; Škalko-Basnet, N. PEGylated liposomes for topical vaginal therapy improve delivery of interferon alpha. *Eur. J. Pharm. Biopharm.* **2017**, *113*, 132–139. [CrossRef] [PubMed]
54. Owen, D.H.; Katz, D.F. A vaginal fluid simulant. *Contraception* **1999**, *59*, 91–95. [CrossRef]
55. Owen, D.H.; Katz, D.F. A Review of the Physical and Chemical Properties of Human Semen and the Formulation of a Semen Simulant. *J. Androl.* **2005**, *26*, 459–469. [CrossRef] [PubMed]
56. McFarland, J. Nephelometer:an instrument for estimating the number of bacteria in suspensions used for calculating the opsonic index and for vaccines. *JAMA* **1907**, *14*, 1176–1178. [CrossRef]
57. Heatley, N.G. A method for the assay of penicillin. *Biochem. J.* **1944**, *38*, 61–65. [CrossRef]

marine drugs

MDPI

Article

Effects of Chitosan on *Clostridium perfringens* and Application in the Preservation of Pork Sausage

Shun-Hsien Chang [1], Ching-Hung Chen [2] and Guo-Jane Tsai [2,3,*]

1 Institute of Food Safety and Risk Management, National Taiwan Ocean University, Keelung 20224, Taiwan; lewis@mail.ntou.edu.tw

2 Department of Food Science, National Taiwan Ocean University, Keelung 20224, Taiwan; heeves_chen@tty.com.tw

3 Center for Marine Bioenvironment and Biotechnology, National Taiwan Ocean University, Keelung 20224, Taiwan

* Correspondence: b0090@ntou.edu.tw; Tel.: +886-2-2462-2192 (ext. 5150); Fax: +886-2-2462-7954

Received: 30 December 2019; Accepted: 20 January 2020; Published: 22 January 2020

Abstract: The effects of chitosan with 95% deacetylation degree (DD95) on the spore germination, cell proliferation, and heat resistance of *Clostridium perfringens* CCRC 10,648 and CCRC 13,019 were investigated, and its application on pork sausage with sodium nitrite reduction was also evaluated. DD95 chitosan can strongly reduce the heat resistance of both strains. The D_{80} and D_{100} values for strain CCRC 13,019 decreased from 40.98 and 4.64 min to 39.21 and 3.26 min, respectively, as a result of adding 250 ppm DD95; meanwhile, addition of chitosan decreased the D_{80} and D_{100} values for CCRC 10,648 from 41.15 and 6.46 min to 39.52 and 3.78 min, respectively. In pork sausage, addition of 3000 ppm DD95 chitosan considerably slowed down the bacterial proliferation and volatile basic nitrogen production. There were no significant differences in color (L^* and b^* values), shearing force, and hardness in the pork sausages with or without DD95 chitosan during storage at 4 and 25 °C. However, the addition of DD95 chitosan in pork sausage significantly retarded the decrease of the a^* value. Therefore, DD95 chitosan could reduce the concentration of sodium nitrite required in pork sausages for color retention.

Keywords: chitosan; antibacterial activity; *Clostridium perfringens*; pork sausage

---

1. Introduction

The meat processing industry regularly faces many serious challenges regarding the safety and hygiene of various products [1–3]. The pathways for pathogens' transmission into the product could be from throughout handling processes or from the carcass surface [4,5]; however, decontamination or sterilization of the carcass body is very difficult to perform using currently applied antimicrobial agents. Moreover, most commonly used preservatives and antimicrobial agents have a chemical and synthetic nature, giving them many potential side effects and risks on the health of consumers [6–8]. The meat industry continues to seek natural preservatives as antimicrobial agents.

Chitosan, a partially deacetylated chitin (poly-β-(1→4)*N*-acetyl-D-glucosamine) is found in shrimp shells and fungi [9]. This polysaccharide has attracted attention as a biomedical material because of its biocompatibility and various biological activities, including immune-enhancing [10], anti-inflammatory [11], antibacterial [6], and antitumor activities [12]. Because of its excellent antibacterial activity, chitosan has been widely used for food protection [13–16]. Several studies have shown that chitosan's molecular weight (MW) is a crucial factor in its antimicrobial properties, although equivocal results in terms of the correlation between the antibacterial properties and MWs of chitosan have also been observed [17,18]. Our previous report [6] concluded that the correlation between chitosan MW and its antibacterial properties was dependent on the pH value of the reaction mixture.

Clostridium perfringens, an anaerobic spore-forming foodborne pathogen, is widely distributed in various foods, such as meat, seafood, and vegetable products. Due to the heat resistance of *C. perfringens* spores, spores may survive the heating treatment, and then germinate and proliferate in food. After the contaminated food is ingested, this pathogen secretes an enterotoxin in the intestine, which changes the permeability of the cell membrane and causes diarrheal syndrome [19] or even death [20]. Therefore, methods for controlling *C. perfringens*, especially its spores, in various meat products are necessary [21]. Addition of nitrite derivatives, including sodium and potassium nitrite, is the most effective method for controlling the growth of vegetative cells and spores of *Clostridium* species including *C. perfringens* in processed meats. In addition, nitrite also brings a characteristic red color in processed meats [22].

However, the International Agency for Research on Cancer (IARC) reported that consumption of processed meats including sausages may increase the risk for colorectal cancer, and accordingly classified processed meats as carcinogenic to humans. Nitrates and nitrites used as additives in processed meats are sources of *N*-nitroso compounds (NOCs), which have long been known as carcinogenic [23]. Several studies have attempted to develop new methods to inactivate the spores of *Clostridium* as a way to decrease or even avoid the addition of nitrites in processed meats [24].

In this study, we prepared shrimp chitosan with 95% deacetylation (DD95) and demonstrated that DD95 has a strong antibacterial activity against *C. perfringens* and could reduce the heat resistance of *C. perfringens* spores. Moreover, DD95 in pork sausage stored at 4 and 25 °C effectively retarded the increase of both total bacterial and *C. perfringens* counts (CPC), as well as volatile basic nitrogen values. In addition, the synergistic effect of DD95 and sodium nitrite for a favored color development in pork sausage was observed. Thus, the addition of DD95 in pork sausage was able to reduce the amount of sodium nitrite required and extended the shelf life of pork sausage.

2. Result and Discussion

2.1. Antibacterial Activity of Chitosan Against *C. perfringens*

In this study, chitosan with a molecular weight of 220 kDa and 95% degree of deacetylation was prepared from shrimp chitin [6]. The antibacterial effect of DD95 against the vegetative cells of *C. perfringens* CCRC 13,019 and CCRC 10,648 in liver infusion broth (LIB) at 37 °C anaerobically is shown in Figure 1. DD95 at the dosages of 50 and 100 ppm only retarded the growth of *C. perfringens*. However, DD95 at 250 ppm had a bactericidal effect against this pathogen. The strain CCRC 13,019 (Figure 1A) was more susceptible to DD95 compared with the strain CCRC 10,648 (Figure 1B), as evidenced by the exposure time of 5 h for the former and 24 h for the latter, with no survival being observed at 250 ppm DD95.

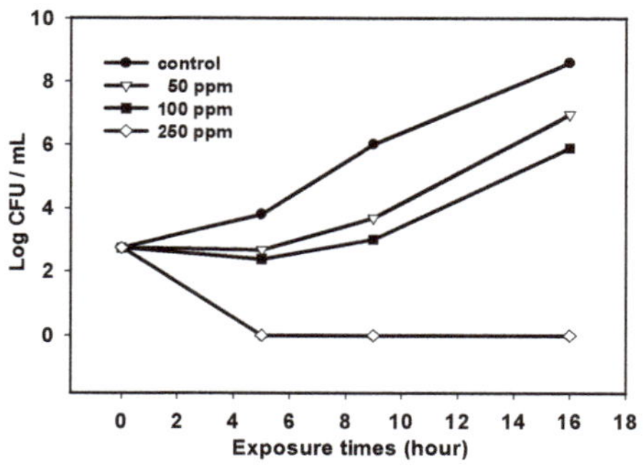

(**A**)

Figure 1. *Cont.*

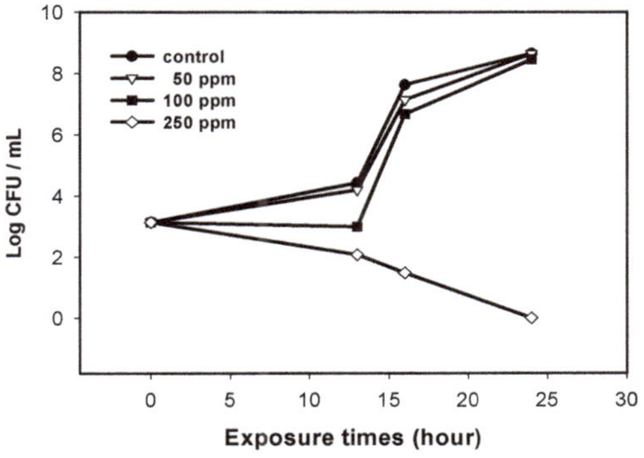

(B)

Figure 1. Survival for *Clostridium perfringens* CCRC 13,019 (**A**) and CCRC 10,648 (**B**) in liver brain broth (LIB) containing various concentrations of chitosan after incubation at 37 °C anaerobically.

2.2. *Effect of Chitosan on Decimal Reduction Time of C. perfringens Spores*

The outbreak of *C. perfringens* poisoning is generally initiated by *C. perfringens* spores that survive the cooking process and are germinated in food, eventually producing enterotoxins in the intestinal tract after ingestion [16]. Therefore, reduction of heat resistance of the spores to decrease spore survival during heating is a preventative approach for *C. perfringens* poisoning [16]. The effect of DD95 at 250 ppm on the decimal reduction time (*D* value) of tested *C. perfringens* strains during heating are shown in Table 1. The *D* values at 80 °C (D_{80}) for spores of *C. perfringens* CCRC 10,648 and CCRC 13,019 were 41.15 and 40.98 min, respectively. In the presence of 250 ppm DD95, D_{80} values decreased to 39.52 and 39.21 min, respectively. Meanwhile, the D_{100} values of these spores decreased from 6.46 and 4.64 min to 3.78 and 3.26 min, respectively, if 250 ppm DD95 was added.

Table 1. Effect of chitosan on the *D* value (min) of *C. perfringens* spores.

Heating Treatment (°C)	DD95 Conc. (ppm)	CCRC 10,648 *	CCRC 13,019
80	0	41.15	40.98
80	250	39.52	39.21
100	0	6.46	4.64
100	250	3.78	3.26

* Data are mean of the duplicate experiments. DD95: 95% deacetylation.

2.3. *Applications of Chitosan in Pork Sausage*

Ground pork containing various amounts of sodium nitrite was spiked with *C. perfringens* CCRC 13,019 spores to have the initial density of approximately 10^4 spore/g for the preparation of pork sausages. For the experimental group, DD95 was added to have the final concentration of 3000 ppm in sausage. The sausages with or without DD95 were stored at 25 and 4 °C. Changes in the total aerobic count (TAC) and *C. perfringens* count (CPC) of pork sausage samples during storage at 25 and 4 °C are shown in Figures 2 and 3. The changes in TAC of sausage samples stored at 25 °C for 48 h were quite similar among the control sample (without sodium nitrite and DD95) and samples containing sodium nitrite only (40–120 ppm); meanwhile, the addition of 3000 ppm DD95 substantially decreased the increase of TAC, regardless of whether or not sodium nitrite was added (Figure 2A). Sodium nitrite alone in the sausage stored at 25 °C was able to retard the increase of CPC, and a dose-dependent effect was observed. The CPC for sausages containing DD95 gradually decreased during storage, regardless of whether or not sodium nitrite was added (Figure 2B).

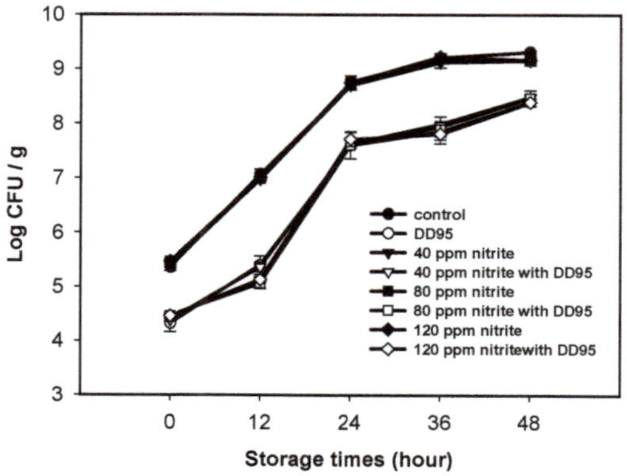

(**A**)

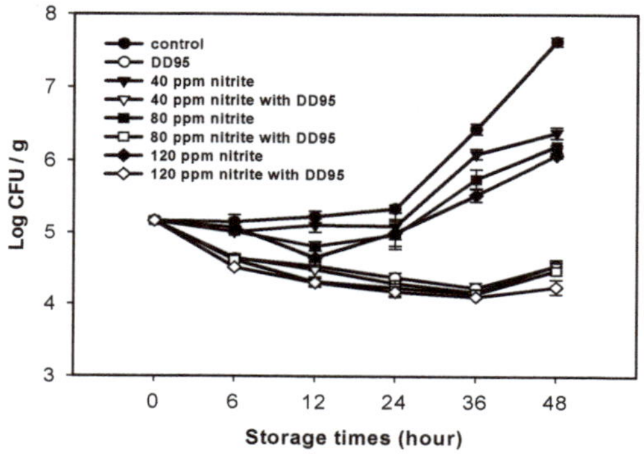

(**B**)

Figure 2. Changes in total aerobic counts (**A**) and *C. perfringens* counts (**B**) of pork sausage containing nitrite and (or) 3000 ppm DD95 chitosan during storage at 25 °C. • and ○, 0 ppm sodium nitrite; ▼ and ▽, 40 ppm sodium nitrite; ■ and □, 80 ppm sodium nitrite; ♦ and ◇, 120 ppm sodium nitrite. Empty symbols, with 3000 ppm DD95; solid symbols, without DD95.

Similar results were observed for sausage samples stored at 4 °C for 10 days (Figure 3). Sodium nitrite alone did not retard the increase of TAC in the sausage samples, whereas DD95 could effectively decrease the increase of TAC (Figure 3A). The dose-dependent effect of sodium nitrite alone on decreasing CPC was also observed, and this CPC decreasing effect was further enhanced by DD95 and sodium nitrite (Figure 3B).

According to Kanner et al. [25], the mechanism of nitrite inhibition in *C. perfringens* is attributable to the destruction of iron–sulfur enzymes such as ferredoxin by nitric oxide (NO), transferred from nitrite by the ferrous ion in meat, and thus inhibition of the synthesis of adenosine triphosphate (ATP). A similar nitrite inhibition effect on other *Clostridium* species, such as *Clostridium botulinum* and *Clostridium sporogenes*, was also reported [26,27]. However, the nitrite effect on *C. perfringens* was almost diminished in the presence of DD95 in sausage (Figures 2B and 3B), probably because of the much stronger activity of DD95 against *C. perfringens* at 3000 ppm, which overwhelmed the inhibition effect of nitrite at 40–120 ppm. Moreover, the iron absorption activity of chitosan may prevent NO production from nitrite [28]. This merits further investigation in the future. The aerobes seemed more resistant to NO produced from nitrite at the dosages tested, probably because of more antioxidant enzymes or compounds present in aerobes to attenuate the NO effect. Therefore, it was observed that nitrite had only a slight effect on TAC in sausages during storage in this study.

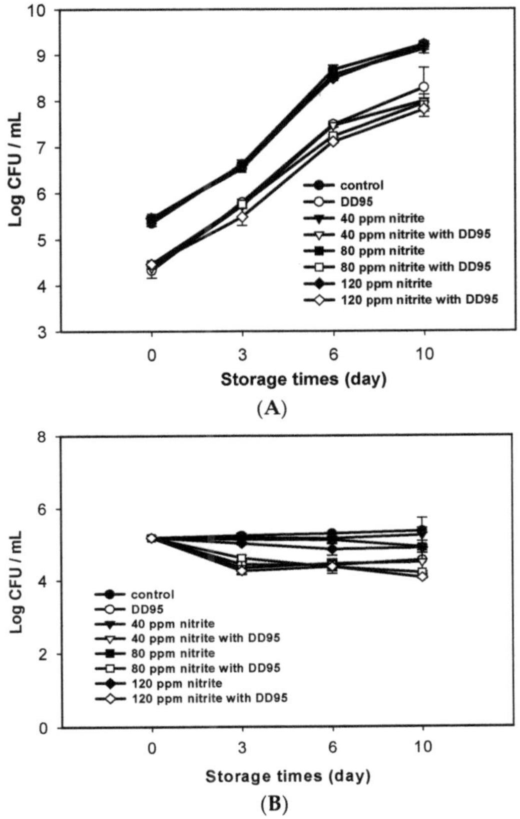

Figure 3. Changes in total aerobic counts (**A**) and *C. perfringens* counts (**B**) of pork sausage containing nitrite and (or) 3000 ppm DD95 chitosan during storage at 4 °C. • and ○, 0 ppm sodium nitrite; ▼ and ▽, 40 ppm sodium nitrite; ■ and □, 80 ppm sodium nitrite; ♦ and ◇, 120 ppm sodium nitrite. Empty symbols, with 3000 ppm DD95; solid symbols, without DD95.

2.4. Color and Color Difference Measurement

Changes in color (L^*, a^*, and b^* values) of pork sausage samples during storage at 25 °C for 48 h and 4 °C for 10 days are shown in Tables 2 and 3, respectively. In general, both L^* and b^* values did not significantly change for all tested samples during storage at 25 °C, and there were no significant differences in L^* values among all tested sausages, regardless of whether or not sodium nitrite and/or DD95 were/was added (Table 2).

Table 2. Changes in *L**, *a**, and *b** values of pork sausage containing chitosan (DD95) and various concentrations of sodium nitrite during storage at 25 °C.

Assay	Group [a]	Nitrite Concentration (ppm)	Values of Pork Sausage after Following Hours of Storage [b,c]				
			0	12	24	36	48
L	Without DD95	0	B42.2 ± 1.8a	A47.5 ± 1.6a	AB44.5 ± 2.3bc	AB46.1 ± 3.3a	AB45.4 ± 3.3a
		40	A45.6 ± 2.1a	A48.9 ± 4.9a	A47.2 ± 2.2abc	A46.4 ± 2.2a	A46.2 ± 1.6a
		80	A45.6 ± 2.1a	A44.9 ± 4.9a	A45.2 ± 5.0bc	A46.4 ± 2.2a	A46.2 ± 3.6a
		120	B44.3 ± 1.7a	AB46.5 ± 1.5a	B43.0 ± 1.5bc	AB46.1 ± 3.5a	A48.6 ± 2.1a
	DD95	0	B46.6 ± 0.7a	AB47.4 ± 1.6a	A50.6 ± 1.5c	AB48.2 ± 3.1a	A50.6 ± 2.2a
		40	A48.6 ± 4.4a	A49.6 ± 2.4a	A45.0 ± 2.1bc	A46.2 ± 0.7a	A46.4 ± 1.6a
		80	A48.8 ± 6.3a	A49.8 ± 3.3a	A48.8 ± 2.8ab	A47.9 ± 1.3a	A49.3 ± 0.9a
		120	A48.0 ± 2.5a	A46.9 ± 1.9a	A46.7 ± 2.1abc	A44.4 ± 1.2a	A48.5 ± 4.8a
a	Without DD95	0	A7.2 ± 0.5a	AB6.60 ± 1.5ab	C3.4 ± 0.8d	BC3.7 ± 3.1d	C2.8 ± 0.5e
		40	AB7.0 ± 0.3a	A7.44 ± 1.2a	A8.1 ± 0.5ab	BC5.8 ± 1.2cd	C5.3 ± 0.5d
		80	A7.0 ± 0.5a	A7.22 ± 1.4a	A7.0 ± 1.4b	A7.2 ± 1.0abc	A6.0 ± 0.7c
		120	AB6.6 ± 1.1a	AB6.84 ± 1.3a	A8.4 ± 0.5ab	B6.5 ± 1.1bc	AB6.5 ± 0.5bc
	DD95	0	A6.5 ± 0.5a	A6.26 ± 0.0ab	AB5.4 ± 1.2c	AB5.2 ± 0.7cd	B4.4 ± 0.5d
		40	B6.1 ± 1.9a	AB6.95 ± 1.6a	A8.7 ± 0.5a	A8.6 ± 0.4ab	AB7.7 ± 1.2bc
		80	B6.4 ± 1.8a	B6.42 ± 0.4ab	A8.0 ± 0.4ab	A8.3 ± 0.5ab	A8.0 ± 1.2ab
		120	B6.7 ± 0.6a	B6.61 ± 0.3b	A8.3 ± 0.8ab	A9.3 ± 0.4a	A9.4 ± 0.8a
b	Without DD95	0	A8.3 ± 0.5b	A9.48 ± 0.7a	A8.1 ± 0.3a	A8.4 ± 1.3b	A8.5 ± 0.7b
		40	A9.4 ± 0.5ab	A9.42 ± 0.9a	A10.2 ± 0.5a	A9.4 ± 0.7ab	A9.3 ± 0.4a
		80	A9.6 ± 0.8a	A9.18 ± 0.4a	A9.4 ± 0.8a	A9.2 ± 0.4ab	A9.3 ± 0.9ab
		120	A9.3 ± 0.5ab	A9.64 ± 0.4a	A9.7 ± 0.6a	A9.7 ± 0.3ab	A10.0 ± 0.8a
	DD95	0	A9.1 ± 0.5ab	A9.21 ± 0.4a	A9.8 ± 0.3a	A9.2 ± 0.8ab	A9.5 ± 0.9ab
		40	A9.8 ± 1.0a	A9.80 ± 0.2a	A9.8 ± 0.3a	A9.8 ± 0.4a	A8.9 ± 0.6ab
		80	A9.2 ± 0.7ab	A10.2 ± 1.2a	A10.0 ± 1.1a	A9.7 ± 0.46ab	A9.9 ± 0.2a
		120	A9.3 ± 0.6ab	A8.96 ± 0.4a	A9.7 ± 0.6a	A9.1 ± 0.7ab	A9.8 ± 0.9ab

[a] DD95, 3000 ppm chitosan with 95% deacetylation degree added. [b] Data are mean ± standard deviation ($n = 3$). [c] a–c, different letters in the column for the same test item are significantly different ($p < 0.05$); A,B, different letters in the same row with are significantly different ($p < 0.05$).

Table 3. Changes in *L**, *a**, and *b** values of pork sausage containing chitosan (DD95) and various concentrations of sodium nitrite during storage at 4 °C.

Assay	Group [a]	Nitrite Concentration (ppm)	Values of Pork Sausage after Following Days of Storage [b,c]			
			0	3	6	10
L	Without DD95	0	B42.2 ± 1.8a	AB45.3 ± 2.3abc	A47.0 ± 1.5a	A48.0 ± 1.0a
		40	A45.6 ± 2.1a	A42.8 ± 1.1c	A45.9 ± 2.9a	A47.5 ± 4.3a
		80	A45.6 ± 2.1a	A44.5 ± 3.0bc	A48.3 ± 2.1a	A45.2 ± 1.4a
		120	B44.3 ± 1.7a	A46.3 ± 2.1abc	A47.5 ± 2.7a	A44.3 ± 1.7a
	DD95	0	A46.6 ± 0.7a	A48.6 ± 1.8ab	A45.7 ± 3.5a	A47.1 ± 2.1a
		40	A48.6 ± 4.4a	A47.2 ± 4.2ab	A49.2 ± 1.6a	A45.3 ± 3.7a
		80	A48.8 ± 6.3a	A49.6 ± 2.4a	A49.8 ± 3.2a	A48.8 ± 1.7a
		120	A47.9 ± 2.5a	A46.0 ± 2.6abc	A48.0 ± 1.8a	A45.5 ± 2.4a
a	Without DD95	0	A7.18 ± 0.5a	A6.9 ± 0.4abc	AB6.2 ± 1.9a	B4.3 ± 1.6d
		40	AB6.95 ± 0.3a	A7.3 ± 0.9a	AB6.8 ± 0.7a	B5.3 ± 2.2cd
		80	A6.95 ± 0.5a	A7.5 ± 0.4ab	A7.7 ± 0.1a	A8.0 ± 0.8ab
		120	A6.62 ± 1.1a	A6.4 ± 0.7abc	A6.0 ± 1.6a	A7.8 ± 1.4abc
	DD95	0	A6.46 ± 0.5a	A6.4 ± 0.2abc	A6.2 ± 0.4a	A5.7 ± 1.2bcd
		40	A7.10 ± 1.9a	A7.5 ± 2.3bc	A7.6 ± 1.3b	A8.7 ± 1.7a
		80	A7.37 ± 1.8a	A7.2 ± 1.5bc	A7.3 ± 0.6b	A7.9 ± 0.8bcd
		120	A7.66 ± 0.6a	A8.0 ± 1.6c	A7.0 ± 0.3b	A7.9 ± 0.1d
b	Without DD95	0	A8.25 ± 0.5a	A8.9 ± 0.6b	A9.3 ± 1.3a	A9.0 ± 0.5c
		40	B9.38 ± 0.5a	B9.1 ± 0.3ab	B9.1 ± 0.7a	A10.5 ± 0.4a
		80	A9.58 ± 0.8a	A9.5 ± 0.3ab	A10.4 ± 0.5a	A10.2 ± 0.6a
		120	A9.27 ± 0.5a	A10.0 ± 0.5a	A10.0 ± 0.9a	A9.8 ± 0.3abc
	DD95	0	A9.10 ± 0.5a	A9.6 ± 0.6ab	A8.9 ± 1.3a	A9.1 ± 0.4c
		40	A9.76 ± 1.1a	A9.4 ± 0.9ab	A9.7 ± 0.5a	A10.1 ± 0.2ab
		80	A9.17 ± 0.7a	A9.5 ± 0.7ab	A9.8 ± 1.0a	A9.3 ± 0.4bc
		120	A9.26 ± 0.6a	A8.9 ± 0.5b	A9.5 ± 0.9a	A9.3 ± 0.6bc

[a] DD95, 3000 ppm chitosan with 95% deacetylation degree added. [b] Data are mean ± standard deviation ($n = 3$). [c] a–d, different letters in the column for the same test item are significantly different ($p < 0.05$); A,B, different letters in the same row are significantly different ($p < 0.05$).

The a^* value (representing the red color) for the control sausage (without nitrite and DD95) was substantially decreased with the increase in incubation time at 25 °C, from 7.18 ± 0.45 at the beginning to 2.76 ± 0.53 at the end of storage. At the beginning, the addition of sodium nitrite at 40–120 ppm did not significantly change the a^* value in sausage without DD95. The retention of a^* value was significantly enhanced with the increasing amount of nitrite added during storage. After 48 h of incubation, the a^* values for sausages containing 80 and 120 ppm nitrite were significantly higher than those for sausages containing 0 and 40 ppm nitrite. The a^* value was further enhanced by DD95 addition in nitrite-containing sausage. The sausage containing DD95 and 120 ppm nitrite had the highest a^* value after incubation for 48 h. In addition, at this moment there was no significant difference in a^* value between the sausage containing 120 ppm nitrite only and the sausage containing DD95 and 40 ppm nitrite (Table 2).

Similarly, all L^* values were not significantly different for all sausage samples during storage at 4 °C (Table 3). Although there was some variation in the b^* value of sausage samples during storage, these b^* values were still quite similar (in the range of 8.97–10.45) after incubation for 10 days. For the control sausage (without DD95 and nitrite), the a^* value significantly decreased with the increase in incubation time. Nitrite addition, especially at 80 and 120 ppm, substantially increased the a^* value after incubation for 10 days. There was no significant difference in a^* value between the sausage containing 120 ppm nitrite only and the sausage containing DD95 and 40 ppm nitrite (Table 3).

After storage at 25 °C for 48 h, the appearances of pork sausages containing 0–120 ppm sodium nitrite and with/without 3000 ppm DD95 are shown in Figure 4. The control sausage (without nitrite and DD95) became greenish. The attenuation of green color and increase of red color for sausages with increasing concentration of sodium nitrite were observed (Figure 4A). Moreover, less green color for sausage with DD95 only (sample no. 5 in Figure 4) was observed in comparison with the control sausage (sample no. 1). The light red color for sausages with DD95 and nitrite (40–120 ppm) was observed (Figure 4B). In addition, a similar or even better appearance for the sausages containing DD95 and 40 ppm nitrite (sample no. 6) was observed in comparison with that for the sausage containing 120 ppm nitrite only (sample no. 4). The color appearance of sausages shown here correlated well with the a^* values shown in Table 2.

In this study, except for sodium nitrite and/or DD95, we did not add any other curing agents such as salt and sugar to eliminate the probable combination effects of these curing agents with nitrite and DD95 on color development in pork sausage. It is well known that the oxidation of deoxymyoglobin (red color) to metmyoglobin (brown color) in meat causes the decrease of a^* value. The nitrosomyoglobin formation after nitrite reaction with myoglobin results in red color formation [29]—that is, it increased the a^* value. The antioxidant activity of chitosan may retard the oxidation of myoglobin [30]. Accordingly, the higher a^* value was obtained in sausages containing DD95 after storage at 25 and 4 °C in this study.

In addition, sulfmyoglobin formation by H_2S induced by some putrefactive bacteria including *Pseudomonas* spp. [31] causes the greenish color of meat. This study clearly demonstrates that the addition of DD95 in sausage during storage not only retards the increase of TAC, because of its strong antibacterial activity [18], but also effectively prevents green color formation in sausages.

Owing to the carcinogenic potential of nitrite in sausages, the consumers' interest in "synthetic nitrite-free" meat products is continuously increasing nowadays [31]. As a result, several studies have tried to use natural ingredients, such as potato paste and cured brine, to replace nitrite. However, lower L^* and a^* values were obtained for these products, compared to sausage added with sodium nitrite [32,33].

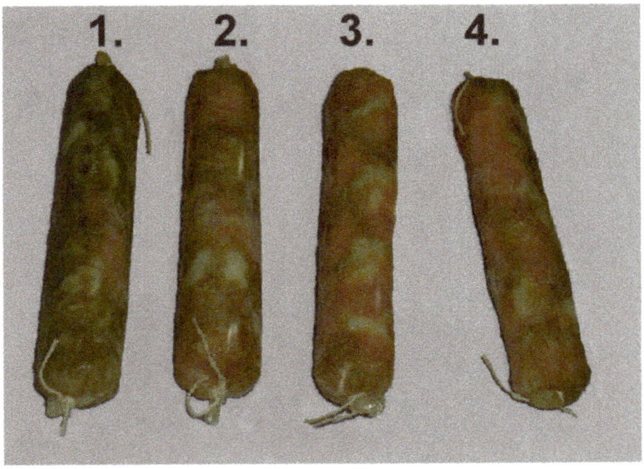

(A)

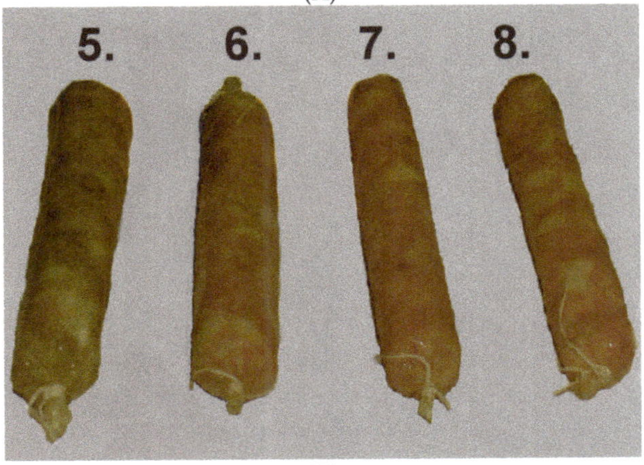

(B)

Figure 4. Appearance of pork sausage containing various concentrations of sodium nitrite only (**A**) and sodium nitrite plus 3000 ppm chitosan (**B**) after storage at 25 °C for 2 days. No. 1, no. 2, no. 3, and no. 4, containing 0, 40, 80, and 120 ppm nitrite only, respectively; no. 5, no. 6, no. 7, and no. 8, containing chitosan plus 0, 40, 80, and 120 ppm nitrite, respectively.

2.5. Volatile Basic Nitrogen (VBN)

In the meat industry, the VBN value is used to indicate the level of putrefaction. As shown in Figure 5, the VBN values in sausages usually increased during storage at 25 °C (Figure 5A) and 4 °C (Figure 5B). Nitrite addition at 40–120 ppm significantly retarded the increase of VBN values, and a dose-dependent response was observed. The VBN values were further decreased by adding both DD95 and nitrite in sausage. We also observed that VBN values between the sausage with DD95 and 40 ppm nitrite and the sausages with 120 ppm nitrite only were quite similar after storage at 25 °C for 48 h (Figure 5A) and 4 °C for 6 days (Figure 5B). In addition, the shearing force and hardness of pork sausages with or without DD95 and nitrite during storage at 25 and 4 °C were not significantly different (data not shown).

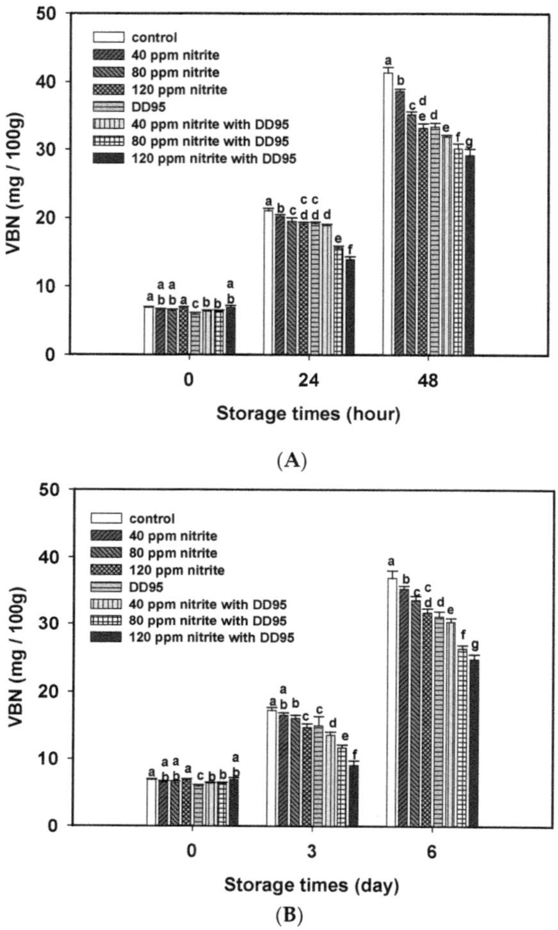

Figure 5. Changes in the volatile basic nitrogen (VBN) of pork sausage containing various concentrations of sodium nitrite and/or 3000 ppm chitosan (DD95) during storage at 25 °C (**A**) and 4 °C (**B**).

3. Material and Methods

3.1. Bacterial Strains and Chemicals

C. perfringens CCRC 10,648 and CCRC 13,019 were purchased from the Biosources Collection and Research Center (Hsinchu, Taiwan, China). Acetic acid, acetonitrile, dimethyl sulfoxide (DMSO), glycerol, methanol, and sodium hydroxide (NaOH) were purchased from Fluka (Garage Gmbh, Buchs, Switzerland). Meanwhile, sodium azide (NaN_3), phenol red, and sodium bicarbonate ($NaHCO_3$) were purchased from Sigma Chemical Co. (Gillingham, UK). Cellulase (3000 U/g) from *Trichoderma viride* was purchased from Challenge Bioproducts Co., Ltd. (Taichung, Taiwan, China), whereas chitin powder was obtained from Applied Chemical Co., Ltd. (Kaohsiung, Taiwan, China). LIB, plate count agar (PCA), tryptose–sulfite–cycloserine (TSC) agar base, bacto agar, proteose peptone no. 3, yeast extract, and 50% egg yolk saline were supplied by Becton Dickinson (Sparks, MD, USA).

3.2. DD95 Chitosan Preparation

On the basis of the method described by Chang, Lin, Wu and Tsai [6], chitosan with 95.0% deacetylation degree, as measured using the colloid titration method [34], was obtained after deacetylation of a shrimp chitin powder suspension in 50% NaOH (1.0 g chitin per 13 mL NaOH) at 140 °C for 1 h. DD95 chitosan MW was 300 kDa, as determined by size-exclusion high-performance liquid chromatography using a column packed with TSKgel G4000 PWXL and G5000 PWXL [35].

3.3. Culture Conditions

C. perfringens CCRC 10,648 and CCRC 13,019 were stored in LIB containing 50% sterile glycerol at −80 °C. To prepare the bacteria cultures, the strains stored at −80 °C were inoculated into 50 mL LIB and anaerobically incubated at 37 °C for 18–24 h. All strains were subcultured twice in LIB at 37 °C for 18–24 h, and the cultures were diluted to 1.0×10^8 CFU/mL with sterile 0.1% peptone water before use.

3.4. Spore Preparation

Briefly, 1 mL of the 18–24 h *C. perfringens* culture in LIB was added in 9.0 mL of the modified Ducan–Strong (DS) medium [36], and incubated for 18–24 h under anaerobic conditions. Next, 1 mL of the cultivated DS medium broth was added into 9 mL fresh modified DS medium and heated at 70 °C for 20 min, then incubated anaerobically for 20–24 h; the process was repeated twice. Cultivated broths were subsequently placed under centrifugation at 1500× *g* for 30 min; precipitates were washed under suspension in 10 mL phosphate-buffered saline (PBS) and heated at 70 °C for 20 min to inactivate the cells, and then spores were collected and stored at 4 °C until use.

3.5. Antibacterial Test

A 1% chitosan stock solution was prepared by adding 0.2 g of DD95 chitosan to 10 mL distilled water, sterilizing at 121 °C for 15 min, and then adding 10 mL sterile 0.2 N HCl. In 50 mL flasks containing 10 mL of LIB, DD95 chitosan in 0.1 N HCl was added to obtain concentrations of 50, 100, and 250 ppm. Next, 1 mL of *C. perfringens* spore suspension was added into a flask to an initial spore density of ca. 10^3 CFU/mL, and incubated at 37 °C for 24 h under anaerobic conditions. Then, 0.1 mL aliquots of decimal dilutions of LIB culture were spread onto LIB agar plates, which were incubated under anaerobic conditions at 37 °C for 24 h before colonies were counted. For evaluation of chitosan against spores, spores of two strains were collected into PBS added with 250 ppm DD95 chitosan, and further incubation was performed as described in the above test. The experiments were run in triplicate.

3.6. Measurement of Heat Resistance of C. perfringens Spores

On the basis of the method of Tsai, Tsai, Lee and Zhong [16], 1 mL of *C. perfringens* spore suspension (1×10^7 spore/mL) in sterile saline alone or in sterile saline containing 250 ppm chitosan was injected into glass microhematocrit tubes (inside diameter, 5 mm; length, 20 cm; wall thickness, 0.5 mm) and submerged in an oil bath at 90 or 100 °C. Three tubes for each strain were removed at intervals and cooled immediately in ice water. The initial spore concentration and the number of spores that survived heating were determined by spreading 0.1 mL of decimal dilutions of spore suspension on LIB agar. Colonies were counted after incubation at 37 °C for 2 days. The log transformed number of surviving spores was plotted against the corresponding heating time. Data points were fitted using the least squares method, and the reciprocal of the slope was taken as the D value.

3.7. Application of DD95 Chitosan to Pork Sausage

Raw pork sausage was added to an equal amount (w/w) of chitosan at the final concentration of 3000 and 6000 ppm. The two sausages with or without DD95 chitosan were added with *C. perfringens* strain spore cells to a density of ca. 10^4 spore/g, then vacuum-packed and stored at 4 and 25 °C during storage until use. Then, 25 g of vacuum-packed pork sausage was poured into a sterile stomacher bag with 225 mL of 0.1% peptone water and homogenized with a stomacher (Stomacher 400 Lab Blender; Seward Medical, London, UK), and the resulting solution was diluted serially with 0.1% peptone water. The total aerobic bacterial count and the CPC for each sample were determined by spread plating 0.1 mL of sample decimal dilutions onto PCA at 37 °C for 48 h and TSC agar (250 mL TSC agar base +20 mL 50% egg yolk saline +20 mL cycloserine (0.5%)) under anaerobic conditions at 37 °C for 24 h.

3.8. Application of DD95 Chitosan and Nitrite for Pork Sausage

Pork sausage was added to an equal amount (w/w) of chitosan and finally to 3000 ppm of DD95 chitosan and 0, 40, 80, and 120 ppm of nitrite substitution for pork sausage. The two sausages with or without DD95 chitosan were added with *C. perfringens* strain spore cells to a density of ca. 10^4 spore/g, then vacuum-packed and stored at 4 and 25 °C during storage until use. The survival counts were measured as described in Section 3.7.

3.9. Color and Color Difference Measurement

On the basis of the method described by [37,38], samples were cut into 2 cm-thick pieces and measured on the plate of the Color Difference Meter (Spectrophotometer CM-3500d; Minolta Co., Ltd., Osaka, Japan). The instrument was calibrated to standard black and white tiles before analysis. Eight pieces per treatment were evaluated, and mean values were used for replication. A medium-size aperture was used, and the measurement was duplicated. The Hunter color L^*, a^*, and b^* values were reported through the computerized system using Spectra Magic software (version 2.11; Minolta Cyberchrom Inc. Osaka, Japan).

3.10. Volatile Basic Nitrogen

According to the method described by Saito et al. [39], 5 g of the sample was homogenized with 45 mL 7% trichloroacetic acid (TCA) to obtain a final concentration of 50 mL. A volume of 0.02 N boric acid as a VBN absorber was placed in the inner section of a Conway microdiffusion cell [40]. Then, 1 mL of the homogenized solution was pipetted to the Conway dish containing 1 mL saturated K_2CO_3 solution and allowed for reaction at 37 °C for 90 min. The boric acid solution containing indicator (methyl red and bromocresol green) was used to absorb volatile nitrogen. The solution was titrated with 0.01 N HCl. The VBN value, expressed as mg %, was calculated as follows: VBN value (mg %) = $0.02 \times 14 \times (a - b) \times F \times V/W \times 100$, where a is the titration volume of sample solution, b is the titration volume of water blank, V is the final volume with TCA of sample after extraction, W is the mass of the sample (g), and F is the unit of 0.02 HCl.

3.11. Statistical Analysis

Data were analyzed using the general linear model (GLM) of Statistical Analysis System's Procedures (SAS Institute Inc., Cary, NC, USA) with a 5% level of significance. Means were separated using Duncan's new multiple range test.

4. Conclusions

Sodium nitrite at 40–120 ppm significantly retarded the proliferation of *C. perfringens* and VBN values, and increased red color retention in pork sausage during storage. However, sodium nitrite at the tested concentration had little inhibition effect on the growth of the aerobes. DD95 chitosan clearly inhibited the growth of *C. perfringens* and reduced the heat resistance of the spore of this pathogen. The addition of DD95 chitosan effectively slowed down the increase of TAC and VBN values, preserved the red color, and inhibited the growth of *C. perfringens*. In effect, DD95 chitosan could serve as a substitute for part of the total amount of sodium nitrite used in pork sausages as a way to reduce the sodium nitrite content in pork sausages. DD95 chitosan shows strong potential as an alternative natural preservative and can help maintain the stability of color in pork sausages.

Author Contributions: S.-H.C. performed the experiments and wrote the initial version of the manuscript; C.-H.C. designed the experiments and analyzed the data; G.-J.T. conceived the experiments, formally analyzed the data, and wrote, reviewed, and edited the paper. All authors have read and agreed to the published version of the manuscript.

Funding: This research was funded by the Ministry of Science and Technology of Republic of China, grant number [MOST 107-2321-B-019-003].

Conflicts of Interest: The authors declare no conflict of interest.

References

1. D'Ostuni, V.; Tristezza, M.; De Giorgi, M.G.; Rampino, P.; Grieco, F.; Perrotta, C. Occurrence of Listeria monocytogenes and Salmonella spp. in meat processed products from industrial plants in Southern Italy. *Food Control* **2016**, *62*, 104–109. [CrossRef]
2. Lee, S.; Lee, H.; Kim, S.; Lee, J.; Ha, J.; Choi, Y.; Oh, H.; Choi, K.-H.; Yoon, Y. Microbiological safety of processed meat products formulated with low nitrite concentration—A review. *Asian Australas. J. Anim. Sci.* **2018**, *31*, 1073–1077. [CrossRef] [PubMed]
3. Ruiz-Capillas, C.; Herrero, A.M. Impact of biogenic amines on food quality and safety. *Foods* **2019**, *8*, 62. [CrossRef] [PubMed]
4. Craven, S.; Stern, N.; Bailey, J.; Cox, N. Incidence of Clostridium perfringens in broiler chickens and their environment during production and processing. *Avian Dis* **2001**, *45*, 887–896. [CrossRef]
5. Palmer, J.; Flint, S.; Brooks, J. Bacterial cell attachment, the beginning of a biofilm. *J. Ind. Microbiol. Biotechnol.* **2007**, *34*, 577–588. [CrossRef]
6. Chang, S.-H.; Lin, H.-T.V.; Wu, G.-J.; Tsai, G.J. pH Effects on solubility, zeta potential, and correlation between antibacterial activity and molecular weight of chitosan. *Carbohydr. Polym.* **2015**, *134*, 74–81. [CrossRef]
7. Hosseinnejad, M.; Jafari, S.M. Evaluation of different factors affecting antimicrobial properties of chitosan. *Int. J. Biol. Macromol.* **2016**, *85*, 467–475. [CrossRef]
8. Li, Q.; Tan, W.; Zhang, C.; Gu, G.; Guo, Z. Synthesis of water soluble chitosan derivatives with halogeno-1,2,3-triazole and their antifungal activity. *Int. J. Biol. Macromol.* **2016**, *91*, 623–629. [CrossRef]
9. Marpu, S.B.; Benton, E.N. Shining light on chitosan: A review on the usage of chitosan for photonics and nanomaterials research. *Int. J. Mol. Sci.* **2018**, *19*, 1795. [CrossRef] [PubMed]
10. Smith, A.; Perelman, M.; Hinchcliffe, M. Chitosan: A promising safe and immune-enhancing adjuvant for intranasal vaccines. *Hum. Vaccines Immunother.* **2014**, *10*, 797–807. [CrossRef] [PubMed]
11. Chang, S.-H.; Lin, Y.-Y.; Wu, G.-J.; Huang, C.-H.; Tsai, G.J. Effect of chitosan molecular weight on anti-inflammatory activity in the RAW 264.7 macrophage model. *Int. J. Biol. Macromol.* **2019**, *131*, 167–175. [CrossRef] [PubMed]
12. Liang, J.; Li, F.; Fang, Y.; Yang, W.; An, X.; Zhao, L.; Xin, Z.; Cao, L.; Hu, Q. Cytotoxicity and apoptotic effects of tea polyphenol-loaded chitosan nanoparticles on human hepatoma HepG2 cells. *Mater. Sci. Eng. C* **2014**, *36*, 7–13. [CrossRef]
13. El Ghaouth, A.; Arul, J.; Grenier, J.; Asselin, A. Antifungal activity of chitosan on two postharvest pathogens of strawberry fruits. *Phytopathology* **1992**, *82*, 398–402. [CrossRef]
14. Knorr, D. Use of chitinous polymers in food: A challenge for food research and development. *Food Technol. (USA)* **1984**, *38*, 85–97.
15. Muzzarelli, R. Enzymatic synthesis of chitin and chitosan. Occurrence of chitin. *Chitin* **1977**, 5–17.
16. Tsai, G.-J.; Tsai, M.-T.; Lee, J.-M.; Zhong, M.-Z. Effects of chitosan and a low-molecular-weight chitosan on Bacillus cereus and application in the preservation of cooked rice. *J. Food Prot.* **2006**, *69*, 2168–2175. [CrossRef] [PubMed]
17. Cheng, Y.; Kang, J.; Shih, Y.; Lo, Y.; Wang, C. Cholesterol-3-beta, 5-alpha, 6-beta-triol induced genotoxicity through reactive oxygen species formation. *Food Chem. Toxicol.* **2005**, *43*, 617–622. [CrossRef]
18. Tsai, G.-J.; Zhang, S.-L.; Shieh, P.-L. Antimicrobial activity of a low-molecular-weight chitosan obtained from cellulase digestion of chitosan. *J. Food Prot.* **2004**, *67*, 396–398. [CrossRef]

19. Limbo, S.; Torri, L.; Sinelli, N.; Franzetti, L.; Casiraghi, E. Evaluation and predictive modeling of shelf life of minced beef stored in high-oxygen modified atmosphere packaging at different temperatures. *Meat Sci.* **2010**, *84*, 129–136. [CrossRef]
20. Grass, J.E.; Gould, L.H.; Mahon, B.E. Epidemiology of Foodborne Disease Outbreaks Caused by Clostridium perfringens, United States, 1998–2010. *Foodborne Pathog. Dis.* **2013**, *10*, 131–136. [CrossRef]
21. Juneja, V.K.; Gonzales-Barron, U.; Butler, F.; Yadav, A.S.; Friedman, M. Predictive thermal inactivation model for the combined effect of temperature, cinnamaldehyde and carvacrol on starvation-stressed multiple Salmonella serotypes in ground chicken. *Int. J. Food Microbiol.* **2013**, *165*, 184–199. [CrossRef] [PubMed]
22. Choi, Y.S.; Kim, T.K.; Jeon, K.H.; Park, J.D.; Kim, H.W.; Hwang, K.E.; Kim, Y.B. Effects of Pre-Converted Nitrite from Red Beet and Ascorbic Acid on Quality Characteristics in Meat Emulsions. *Korean J. Food Sci. Anim. Resour.* **2017**, *37*, 288–296. [CrossRef] [PubMed]
23. Wang, J.; Yang, H.J.; Shi, H.Z.; Zhou, J.; Bai, R.S.; Zhang, M.Y.; Jin, T. Nitrate and Nitrite Promote Formation of Tobacco-Specific Nitrosamines via Nitrogen Oxides Intermediates during Postcured Storage under Warm Temperature. *J. Chem.* **2017**, *2017*, 1–11. [CrossRef]
24. Dutra, M.P.; Aleixo, G.D.; Ramos, A.D.S.; Silva, M.H.L.; Pereira, M.T.; Piccoli, R.H.; Ramos, E.M. Use of gamma radiation on control of Clostridium botulinum in mortadella formulated with different nitrite levels. *Radiat. Phys. Chem.* **2016**, *119*, 125–129. [CrossRef]
25. Kanner, J.; Shpaizer, A.; Nelgas, L.; Tirosh, O. S-Nitroso-N-acetylcysteine (NAC-SNO) as an Antioxidant in Cured Meat and Stomach Medium. *J. Agric. Food Chem.* **2019**, *67*, 10930–10936. [CrossRef] [PubMed]
26. Woods, L.F.; Wood, J. A note on the effect of nitrite inhibition on the metabolism of Clostridium botulinum. *J. Appl. Bacteriol.* **1982**, *52*, 109–110. [CrossRef]
27. Woods, L.F.; Wood, J.M.; Gibbs, P.A. The involvement of nitric oxide in the inhibition of the phosphoroclastic system in Clostridium sporogenes by sodium nitrite. *Microbiology* **1981**, *125*, 399–406. [CrossRef]
28. Burke, A.; Yilmaz, E.; Hasirci, N.; Yilmaz, O. Iron (III) ion removal from solution through adsorption on chitosan. *J. Appl. Polym. Sci.* **2002**, *84*, 1185–1192. [CrossRef]
29. Yong, H.I.; Han, M.; Kim, H.-J.; Suh, J.-Y.; Jo, C. Mechanism underlying green discolouration of myoglobin induced by atmospheric pressure plasma. *Sci. Rep.* **2018**, *8*, 9790. [CrossRef]
30. Chang, S.-H.; Wu, C.-H.; Tsai, G.-J. Effects of chitosan molecular weight on its antioxidant and antimutagenic properties. *Carbohydr. Polym.* **2018**, *181*, 1026–1032. [CrossRef]
31. Yong, H.I.; Park, J.; Kim, H.J.; Jung, S.; Park, S.; Lee, H.J.; Choe, W.; Jo, C. An innovative curing process with plasma-treated water for production of loin ham and for its quality and safety. *Plasma Process Polym.* **2018**, *15*. [CrossRef]
32. Deda, M.S.; Bloukas, J.G.; Fista, G.A. Effect of tomato paste and nitrite level on processing and quality characteristics of frankfurters. *Meat Sci.* **2007**, *76*, 501–508. [CrossRef]
33. Krause, B.L.; Sebranek, J.G.; Rust, R.E.; Mendonca, A. Incubation of curing brines for the production of ready-to-eat, uncured, no-nitrite-or-nitrate-added, ground, cooked and sliced ham. *Meat Sci.* **2011**, *89*, 507–513. [CrossRef] [PubMed]
34. Tôei, K.; Kohara, T. A conductometric method for colloid titrations. *Anal. Chim. Acta* **1976**, *83*, 59–65. [CrossRef]
35. Tsai, M.L.; Bai, S.W.; Chen, R.H. Cavitation effects versus stretch effects resulted in different size and polydispersity of ionotropic gelation chitosan–sodium tripolyphosphate nanoparticle. *Carbohydr. Polym.* **2008**, *71*, 448–457. [CrossRef]
36. Miwa, N.; Masuda, T.; Kwamura, A.; Terai, K.; Akiyama, M. Survival and growth of enterotoxin-positive and enterotoxin-negative Clostridium perfringens in laboratory media. *Int. J. Food Microbiol.* **2002**, *72*, 233–238. [CrossRef]
37. Jang, S.I.; Lillehoj, H.S.; Lee, S.H.; Lee, K.W.; Lillehoj, E.P.; Hong, Y.H.; An, D.J.; Jeoung, H.Y.; Chun, J.E. Relative Disease Susceptibility and Clostridial Toxin Antibody Responses in Three Commercial Broiler Lines Coinfected with Clostridium perfringens and Eimeria maxima Using an Experimental Model of Necrotic Enteritis. *Avian Dis.* **2013**, *57*, 684–687. [CrossRef]
38. Lee, S.H.; Choe, J.; Shin, D.J.; Yong, H.I.; Choi, Y.; Yoon, Y.; Jo, C. Combined effect of high pressure and vinegar addition on the control of Clostridium perfringens and quality in nitrite-free emulsion-type sausage. *Innov. Food Sci. Emerg.* **2019**, *52*, 429–437. [CrossRef]

39. Saito, K.; Ahhmed, A.M.; Kawahara, S.; Sugimoto, Y.; Aoki, T.; Muguruma, M. Evaluation of the performance of osmotic dehydration sheets on freshness parameters in cold-stored beef biceps femoris muscle. *Meat Sci.* **2009**, *82*, 260–265. [CrossRef]
40. Conway, E.J. *Microdiffusion Analysis and Volumetric Error*, 4th ed.; Crosby Lockwood: London, UK, 1947.

marine drugs

MDPI

Article

Vaginal Polyelectrolyte Layer-by-Layer Films Based on Chitosan Derivatives and Eudragit® S100 for pH Responsive Release of Tenofovir

Raúl Cazorla-Luna [1], Araceli Martín-Illana [1], Fernando Notario-Pérez [1], Luis Miguel Bedoya [2], Aitana Tamayo [3], Roberto Ruiz-Caro [1], Juan Rubio [3] and María-Dolores Veiga [1,*]

1 Department of Pharmaceutics and Food Technology, Faculty of Pharmacy, Complutense University of Madrid, 28040 Madrid, Spain; racazorl@ucm.es (R.C.-L.); aracelimartin@ucm.es (A.M.-I.); fnotar01@ucm.es (F.N.-P.); rruizcar@ucm.es (R.R.-C.)

2 Department of Pharmacology, Pharmacognosy and Botany, Faculty of Pharmacy, Complutense University of Madrid, 28040 Madrid, Spain; lmbedoya@ucm.es

3 Institute of Ceramics and Glass, Spanish National Research Council, 28049 Madrid, Spain; aitanath@icv.csic.es (A.T.); jrubio@icv.csic.es (J.R.)

* Correspondence: mdveiga@ucm.es

Received: 11 December 2019; Accepted: 6 January 2020; Published: 9 January 2020

Abstract: Women are still at high risk of contracting the human immunodeficiency virus (HIV) virus due to the lack of protection methods under their control, especially in sub-Saharan countries. Polyelectrolyte multilayer smart vaginal films based on chitosan derivatives (chitosan lactate, chitosan tartate, and chitosan citrate) and Eudragit® S100 were developed for the pH-sensitive release of Tenofovir. Films were characterized through texture analysis and scanning electron microscopy (SEM). Swelling and drug release studies were carried out in simulated vaginal fluid and a mixture of simulated vaginal and seminal fluids. Ex vivo mucoadhesion was evaluated in bovine vaginal mucosa. SEM micrographs revealed the formation of multilayer films. According to texture analysis, chitosan citrate was the most flexible compared to chitosan tartrate and lactate. The swelling studies showed a moderate water uptake (<300% in all cases), leading to the sustained release of Tenofovir in simulated vaginal fluid (up to 120 h), which was accelerated in the simulated fluid mixture (4–6 h). The films had high mucoadhesion in bovine vaginal mucosa. The multilayer films formed by a mixture of chitosan citrate and Eudragit® S100 proved to be the most promising, with zero toxicity, excellent mechanical properties, moderate swelling (<100%), high mucoadhesion capacity, and Tenofovir release of 120 h and 4 h in vaginal fluid and the simulated fluid mixture respectively.

Keywords: chitosan lactate; chitosan tartrate; chitosan citrate; Eudragit® S100; layer-by-layer film; mucoadhesive film; Tenofovir controlled release; pH responsive release; vaginal preexposure prophylaxis; HIV sexual transmission

1. Introduction

Acquired immunodeficiency syndrome (AIDS) is still the leading cause of death among young women. According to United Nations Joint Programme on HIV/AIDS (UNAIDS), 460 adolescent women contract human immunodeficiency virus (HIV) each day and 350 women of the same age group die weekly of AIDS-related complications. In fact, almost 80% of people infected with HIV in the 10–19 age group in sub-Saharan Africa in 2017 were women [1]. Unfortunately, women in these countries do not benefit from options to prevent the sexual transmission of HIV such as condoms, due to gender differences which prevent them from negotiating with their sexual partners. This highlights the need to develop prevention systems that women can initiate without their partner's consent [2]. In this scenario, topical preexposure prophylaxis (PrEP) with antiretroviral drugs is one option to prevent the sexual transmission of HIV, since they can be applied in the vagina and serve as a method of protection that can be controlled by women themselves, thus empowering them in the fight against HIV-1 infection without the consent of their sexual partner [3].

Tenofovir (TFV) is an ideal candidate for use as a topical microbicide for preventing the sexual transmission of HIV due to its efficacy, long half-life, and safety profile [4]. Clinical trials have been carried out with this drug in different dosage forms such as rings [5] and gels [6].

However, adherence is central to PrEP effectiveness, and it is essential to develop products that are easy to use and support high adherence [7]. Vaginal films are emerging as a promising option among the pharmaceutical dosage forms in developmental stages, as they are preferred over other dosage forms due to their advantages of portability, storage and handling, and also ensure comfort and ease of insertion [8,9]. Fast dissolving films based on TFV have been produced and show lower leakage and similar vaginal drug concentrations to those obtained with vaginal gels for pericoital administration. Nevertheless, sustained release formulations must be developed to provide lasting protection to women [7].

One approach to obtaining films for the sustained release of drugs is the use of the layer-by-layer (LbL) technique, which produces films composed of two or more layers of different polymers. This offers great versatility, since it combines the properties of the constituent polymers of each layer [10]. For instance, the combination of a highly mucoadhesive polymer to increase vaginal retention [11] with another polymer capable of modulating the release of the drug [12] can achieve effective and long-lasting drug release in the vaginal mucosa. The combination of polyanionic polymeric layers with polycationic polymeric layers by means of this technique also produces polyelectrolyte multilayers (PEM) [13,14], with the advantage that these polymers have a pH-dependent behaviour [15,16]. This is of great interest when developing formulations for the prevention of sexual transmission of HIV, since accelerating vaginal drug release at the time of ejaculation can increase the effectiveness of the protection [17].

Among the polycationic polymers that are being explored, chitosan is a copolymer composed of β(1→4)-linked 2-acetamido-2-deoxy-β-D-glucopyranose (N-acetylglucosamine) and α(1→4)-linked 2-amino-2-deoxy-β-D-glucospyranose (glucosamine). Chitosan has been widely explored in the development of several pharmaceutical dosage forms such as tablets [11,18], hydrogels [19] and bigels [17], and attempts have recently been made to develop chitosan-based films as drug delivery systems [20,21]. Chitosan has mucoadhesive properties and antimicrobial activity; is from a renewable source and is completely devoid of toxicity, and has many applications in the pharmaceutical industry such as wound dressing and drug delivery systems [22,23]. This polymer has a pH-dependent solubility due to the presence of the amine groups in its structure [24], and the protonation of these groups in dilute acids allows the gelation of the polymer. Acetic acid is widely used among the various acids applied for the gelation of chitosan [25], although its strong and unpleasant smell induces rejection when applying the formulations [26]. For this reason, other acids are beginning to be used that allow the gelation of chitosan with better organoleptic properties, such as lactic acid [26], tartaric acid [27], and citric acid [28]. It has even been proven that the dilute acid used to dissolve the chitosan can condition the polymer's properties [29].

In order to improve its properties, it possible to add suitable fillers [30,31] or combine it with different polymers such as hypromellose [32], sodium alginate [33], pectin [18], poly(vinyl alcohol) [34] and different types of Eudragit® [35,36], among which it is particularly worth highlighting Eudragit® S100 (ES100), a polyanionic copolymer derived from metacrylic acid and methyl metacrylate. It is non-soluble in acids and water but soluble in dissolutions with a pH of over 7 [37]. This behaviour makes it an interesting candidate for the development of pH-sensitive drug delivery systems for oral, ocular, vaginal and topical administration [38]. Mixtures of chitosan and ES100 have been explored with promising results, due to their ability to form polyelectrolyte complexes [39].

Although nowadays films are a promising tool for vaginal administration, the development of controlled release films is a field yet to be explored. Furthermore, the use of pH-sensitive polymers may allow obtaining novel drug delivery systems for the prevention of sexually transmitted diseases [40]. Against this backdrop, the aim of this study is to develop PEM vaginal films based on optimized chitosan derivatives and ES100 using the LbL technique and evaluate them through scanning electron microscopy, texture analysis, swelling, ex vivo mucoadhesion and drug release tests and materials citotoxicity. These films would allow a high mucoadhesion capacity due to the presence of the chitosan-based layer, and a sustained release in the vaginal environment thanks to the ES100 layer. After ejaculation during intercourse, the release of the drug would accelerate, thus maximizing the effectiveness of the formulations in the prevention of the sexual transmission of HIV.

2. Results and Discussion

2.1. Characterization of Chitosan Gels

The results of the characterization of the gels are shown in Figure 1.

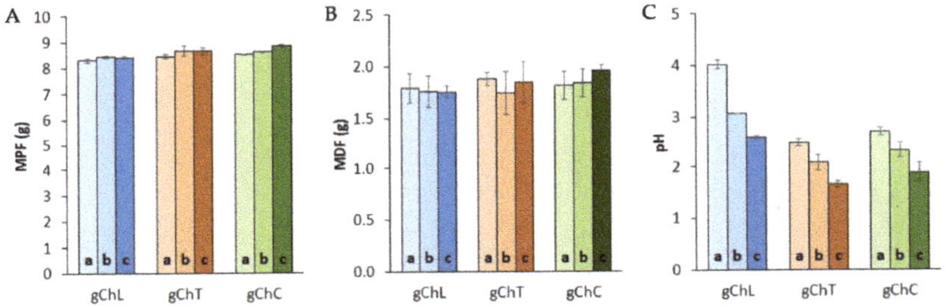

Figure 1. Results of the characterization of the chitosan gels prepared with lactic acid (gChL), tartaric acid (gChT) and citric acid (gChC) at different concentrations (0.25 M (a), 0.5 M (b) and 1 M (c)). (**A**) and (**B**) show the texture analysis results (maximum penetration force (MPF) and maximum detachment force (MDF) respectively). (**C**) shows the pH values obtained for the gels.

According to these data, all the gels had identical results for maximum penetration force (MPF, Figure 1A) and maximum detachment force (MDF, Figure 1B), indicating that the consistency of chitosan gels, represented by the MPF, is not modified by the acid used for its gelation. The adhesiveness of the gel, represented by the MDF, is also equal in all the gels. These properties are therefore characteristic of the polymer and are not modified by the acid. Previously published results show that pure water has similar values of MPF and MDF (7.90 ± 00 g and 1.49 ± 0.07 g) [41], so at these concentrations, chitosan gels have a similar consistency and adhesiveness to pure water. However, a comparison of the pH of the different gels in Figure 1C reveals some differences. In all cases an increase in the acid concentration leads to a decrease in the pH of the gel. The gels prepared with lactic acid show the highest values of pH (≈2.5–4), while citric acid and tartaric acid generate more acid gels, with pH values in the range of ≈2–3. According to the literature, the use of acidic substances in the vaginal environment may be beneficial for the prevention of sexually transmitted infections [42,43]. These formulations would therefore allow the acidification of the medium after administration, making them interesting candidates for the development of formulations for the prevention of sexual transmission of HIV.

2.2. Chitosan Derivative-Based Films

2.2.1. Attenuated Total Reflection Fourier Transform Infrared (FTIR-ATR) Spectroscopy

Figure 2 shows the spectra obtained for the raw materials. In the spectrum corresponding to raw chitosan, bands are observed at 1655 cm^{-1} and 1325 cm^{-1}, corresponding to the C=O bond of amide I and the N-H bond of amide III respectively. A band appears at 1585 cm^{-1}, corresponding to the free amine [44]. In the lactic acid spectrum, a peak can be observed at 1720 cm^{-1} corresponding to the C=O bond of the acid group, and a band at 1210 cm^{-1} that can be attributed to the C-O carboxylic acid bond [45]. In tartaric acid, the peak observed at 1720 cm^{-1} corresponds to the C=O bond of the carboxylic acid. Another peak at 1445 cm^{-1} corresponds to the O-H bond of the carboxylic groups. The peaks at 1185 cm^{-1}, 3328 cm^{-1} and 3400 cm^{-1} are also attributable to O-H links [46]. In the citric acid spectrum, the peaks that appear around 1720 cm^{-1} are due to the C=O bonds of carboxylic acids. A band corresponding to the O-H bond of carboxylic acids is observed at 1390 cm^{-1}. The 3492 cm^{-1} peak is also attributable to free hydroxyls [47].

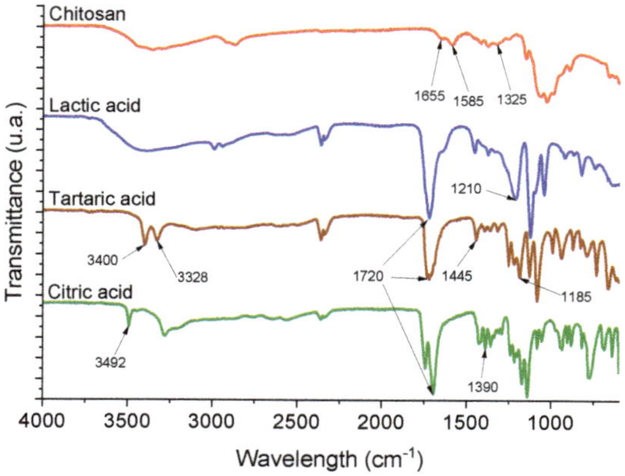

Figure 2. Spectra obtained through FTIR-ATR for the raw materials used to manufacture the chitosan derivative films.

The spectra corresponding to chitosan films prepared with different amounts of lactic acid (ChL-a, ChL-b and ChL-c) are shown in Figure 3. All have a broad band between 1660–1475 cm^{-1}, caused by the overlapping of the chitosan amide (1655 cm^{-1}) and the C=O bond corresponding to the amide formed with lactic acid [48]. Since the carbonyl in the acid (1720 cm^{-1}) changes to amide, a reduction in the intensity of this peak can be seen in samples ChL-a and ChL-b. The peak is also observed to decrease to 1210 cm^{-1}, due to the replacement of hydroxyl in the formation of this amide (Scheme 1a). When the amount of lactic acid in the film is increased (especially in ChL-c), esters form between the lactic acid molecules, creating oligomers of polylactic acid (Scheme 1b) [48] and causing the intensity of the band to increase at 1720 cm^{-1} due to the C=O bonds corresponding to the esters. The formation of these esters is favoured by the high concentration of lactic acid, so this peak is more intense than the peak attributable to the C=O of the amide. The band at 1210 cm^{-1} also increases, indicating the presence of the C-O bond, which is absent in the amide but present in the ester [48].

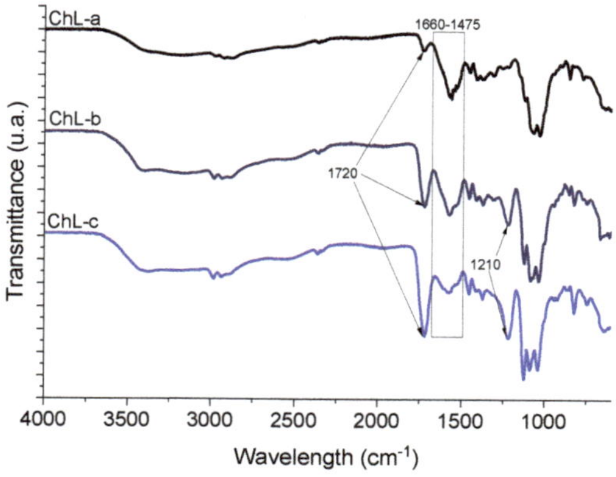

Figure 3. Spectra obtained through FTIR for the films manufactured by solvent casting chitosan gels prepared with different concentrations of lactic acid: 0.25 M (ChL-a), 0.5 M (ChL-b), and 1 M (ChL-c).

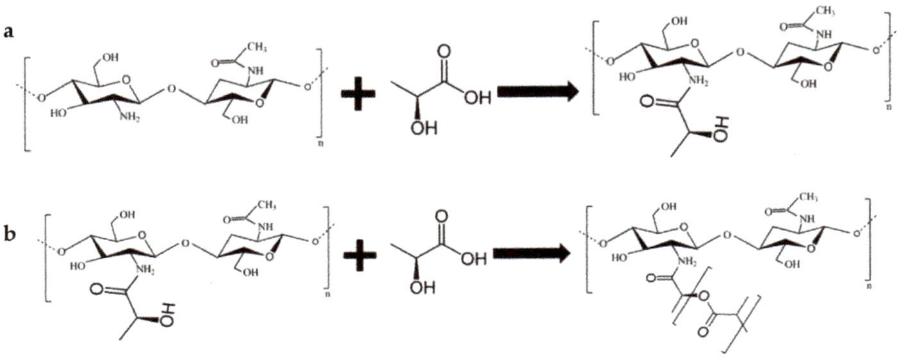

Scheme 1. Chemical reaction between chitosan and lactic acid. First, the carboxylic group of lactic acid reacts with the amine group of chitosan, forming the corresponding amide (henceforth chitosan lactate) (**a**). If there is an excess of lactic acid, the carboxylic groups of free molecules react with the free hydroxyl of the lactic group in chitosan lactate, forming polylactate groups (**b**).

The spectra corresponding to chitosan films prepared with tartaric acid are shown in Figure 4. A broad band appears between 1660 cm^{-1} and 1475 cm^{-1}, with two peaks attributable to the amide group [49]. In ChT-a and ChT-b, the peak disappears at 1445 cm^{-1}, corresponding to the O-H bond of the carboxylic acid of the tartaric acid. Other peaks that disappear with the lowest proportions of tartaric acid are 1185 cm^{-1}, 3400 cm^{-1} and 3328 cm^{-1}, which also indicates the replacement of hydroxyls in tartaric acid and confirms the formation of the amide between chitosan and tartaric acid (Scheme 2) [27]. The absence of these peaks corresponding to the O-H bonds of the carboxylic acids indicates that all acid groups react with the chitosan amines, suggesting that tartaric acid acts as a crosslinker of the chitosan chains. The peaks corresponding to O-H bonds (1445 cm^{-1}, 1185 cm^{-1}, 3328 cm^{-1}, and 3400 cm^{-1}) [46] reappear with the highest amount of tartaric acid (ChT-c), indicating that not all the tartaric acid is used in the reaction at this proportion.

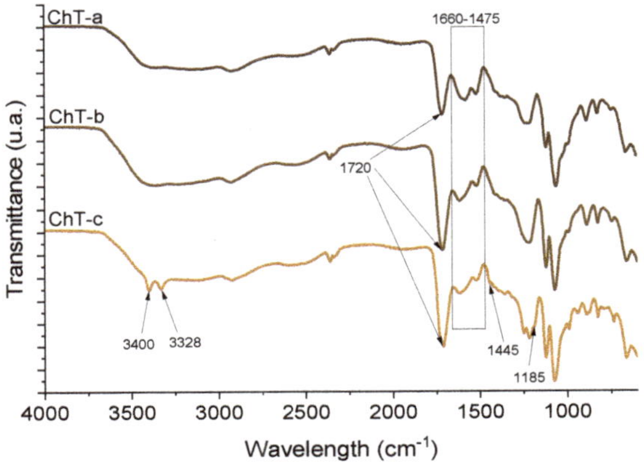

Figure 4. Spectra obtained through FTIR for the films manufactured by solvent casting chitosan gels prepared with different concentrations of tartaric acid: 0.25 M (ChT-a), 0.5 M (ChT-b) and 1 M (ChT-c).

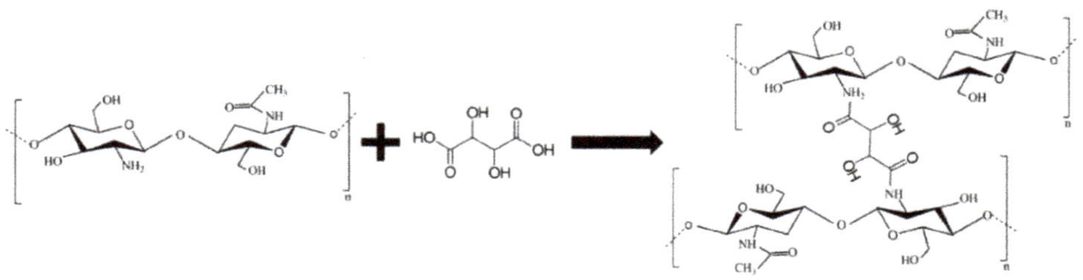

Scheme 2. Chemical reaction between chitosan and tartaric acid. The carboxylic groups of tartaric acid react with the amine group of chitosan, forming the corresponding amide (henceforth chitosan tartrate). The complete reaction with the two carboxylic groups in the molecule of tartaric acid leads to the crosslinking of chitosan.

According to the spectra obtained for the chitosan films prepared with citric acid shown in Figure 5, a wide band appears between 1660 cm^{-1} and 1475 cm^{-1}, attributable to the formation of the amide group [50]. The bands at 1390 cm^{-1} and 3492 cm^{-1} disappear in samples ChC-a and ChC-b due to the replacement of all free carboxylic hydroxyls by the chitosan amines. This indicates that amide is formed between chitosan and citric acid, and that citric acid acts as a crosslinker for chitosan chains through an amide formed between both compounds (Scheme 3) [51]. The peaks at 1390 cm^{-1} and 3492 cm^{-1} reappear in the sample with the highest proportion of citric acid (ChC-c), suggesting that the reaction with citric acid in these proportions is incomplete.

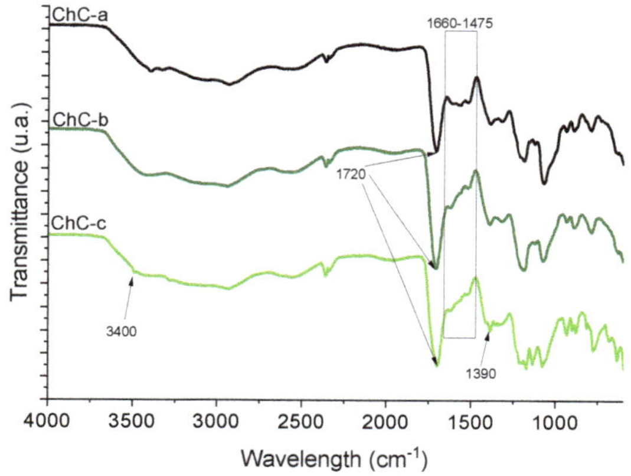

Figure 5. Spectra obtained through FTIR for the films manufactured by solvent casting chitosan gels prepared with different concentrations of citric acid: 0.25 M (ChC-a), 0.5 M (ChC-b), and 1 M (ChC-c).

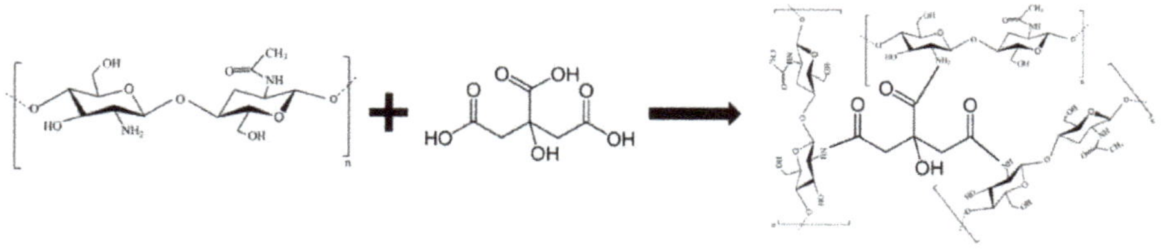

Scheme 3. Chemical reaction between chitosan and citric acid. The carboxylic groups of citric acid react with the amine group of chitosan, forming the corresponding amide (henceforth chitosan citrate). The complete reaction with the three carboxylic groups in the citric acid molecule leads to the crosslinking of chitosan.

2.2.2. Appearance and Mechanical Properties

The films made with chitosan derivatives were visually evaluated. The pliability and organoleptic characteristics of each batch are shown in Table 1.

Table 1. Characteristics observed by visual evaluation of films based on chitosan derivatives.

Batch	Pliability	Organoleptic Characteristics	Comments
ChL-a	✓	Homogeneous. Translucent, yellowish and shiny. Odourless. Soft touch.	Although somewhat flexible, it breaks if folded in half.
ChL-b	✓✓	Homogeneous. Translucent, yellowish and shiny. Odourless. Soft touch.	
ChL-c	✗	Homogeneous. Translucent, yellowish and shiny. Odourless. Sticky touch.	The film can barely be handled due to its stickiness.
ChT-a	✓✓	Homogeneous. Translucent, yellowish and shiny. Odourless. Soft touch.	
ChT-b	✓✓✓	Homogeneous. Translucent, yellowish and shiny. Odourless. Soft touch.	
ChT-c	✗	Heterogeneous. Opaque, yellowish and matt. Odourless. Rough touch.	Completely rigid, it breaks when even slight force is applied.
ChC-a	✓✓	Homogeneous. Translucent, yellowish and shiny. Odourless. Soft touch.	
ChC-b	✓✓✓	Homogeneous. Translucent, yellowish and shiny. Odourless. Soft touch.	
ChC-c	✗	Heterogeneous. Opaque, yellowish and matt. Odourless. Rough touch.	Completely rigid, it breaks when even slight force is applied.

✗: Unacceptable; ✓: Acceptable; ✓✓: Good; ✓✓✓: Excellent.

The mechanical properties of the system must be taken into account when developing films for vaginal administration, as they can determine comfort and acceptability for the patient and may even be related to the performance of the film once administered. In the case of ChL-c, the formation of polylactic acid is so pronounced that the film is sticky and becomes impossible to handle. ChT-c and ChC-c films were also observed to be rigid and irregular, which can be attributed to the excess of acid during the reaction, as corroborated by FTIR studies (Section 2.2.1). The excess of tartaric acid or citric acid stiffens the film, as they are solid substances. These films were therefore discarded from further studies.

The comparison of the other films in terms of the acid used for their preparation revealed that the films with chitosan lactate had the lowest deformation capacity, while those containing chitosan tartrate or chitosan citrate had a higher capacity. This may be related to the ability of tartaric acid and citric acid to act as crosslinkers, possibly facilitating the mobility of the chitosan chains [52]. In all cases the films prepared with the diluted acids at 0.5 M (CaL-b, ChT-b, and ChC-b) were more flexible than those obtained with the diluted acids at 0.25 M (ChL-a, ChT-a, and ChC-a).

2.2.3. Drug Release Assessment

Chitosan derivative films prepared with the previously determined optimal concentration of diluted acids (ChL-b, ChT-b, ChC-b) were loaded with 30 mg of TFV (batches ChL-TFV, ChT-TFV and ChC-TFV). The drug release profiles from these chitosan derivative-based films are shown in Figure 6.

In all cases, the entire Tenofovir dose is released in 6 h, revealing the inability of these films to control the release of the drug. The crosslinking of chitosan chains generates complex three-dimensional structures, so ChC-TFV and ChT-TFV could be expected to show a greater capacity for controlled drug release than ChL-TFV, which should release the drug at the fastest rate. While this behaviour is indeed observed, there are insufficient differences between the formulations. This can be explained by the fact that they form gels with a very low consistency, as was observed in the gel characterization studies (Section 2.1). For this reason, and to modulate the gelation rate of chitosan derivatives, and consequently the release of TFV, it was decided to prepare LbL films using ES100.

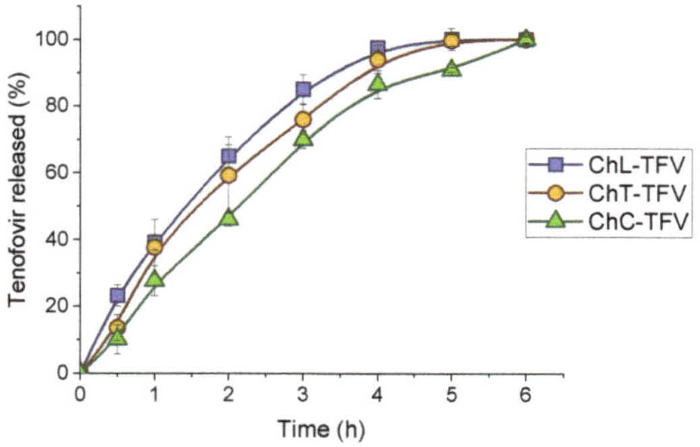

Figure 6. Tenofovir release from the films containing chitosan lactate (ChL-TFV), chitosan tartrate (ChT-TFV) and chitosan citrate (ChC-TFV).

2.3. *Layer-by-Layer Films*

In order to improve the properties of the chitosan derivatives, LbL films were prepared using the previously selected chitosan derivative-based films (ChL-TFV, ChT-TFV and ChC-TFV). Six different batches were obtained by adding a layer of ES100 (plasticized with Triethylcitrate (TEC)) of 75 mg (ChL/E-a, ChT/E-a and ChC/E-a) or 150 mg (ChL/E-b, ChT/E-b and ChC/E-b). As seen in the SEM micrographs (Figure 7), the layers were tightly joined and LbL films were obtained.

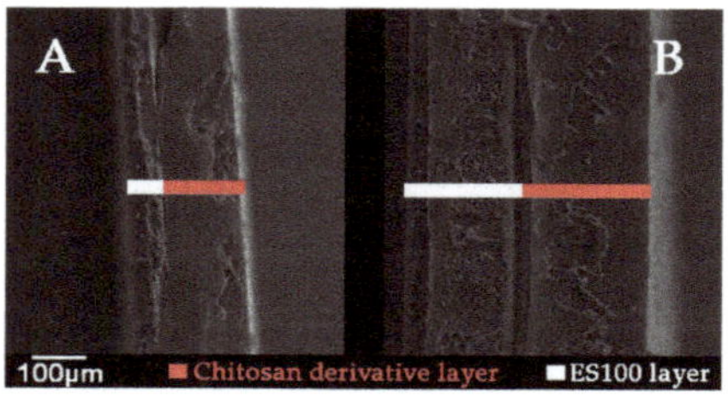

Figure 7. Micrographs of the cross-section of LbL films at 100 times magnification, with 75 mg of ES100 (**A**) and 150 mg of ES100 (**B**).

2.3.1. Texture Analysis

Figure 8 shows the deformability of the films, determined through texture analysis.

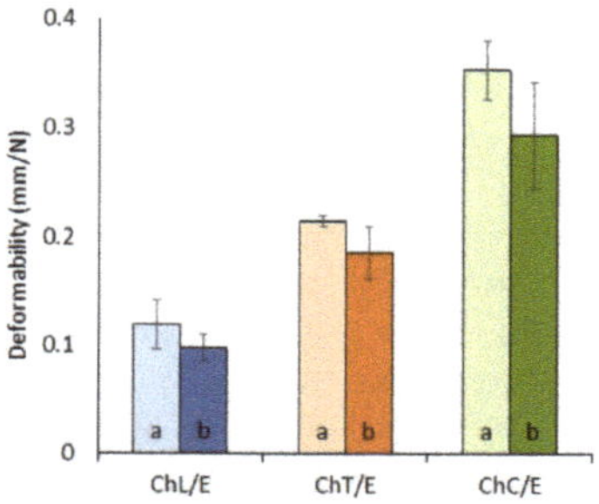

Figure 8. Results of the deformability of the LbL films containing chitosan derivatives and ES100, determined through texture analysis.

The films containing chitosan lactate (ChL/E 1 and ChL/E 2) have the lowest deformability values. Films based on chitosan tartrate (ChT/E 1 and ChT/E 2) exhibit a higher deformation capacity compared to ChL/E films. Chitosan citrate-based films (ChC/E 1 and ChC/E 2) have the highest deformability. According to the ANOVA processing, the differences are statistically significant (p-value = 1.85×10^{-11}). The proportion of ES100 also conditions the deformability of the systems with statistically significant differences (p-value = 7.73×10^{-3}), which can be attributed to the thickness of the ES100 layer. It is therefore necessary to apply a slightly greater force to obtain the same deformation when this layer is double the thickness.

These results can be explained by the fact that lactic acid is unable to crosslink chitosan chains. Conversely, tartaric acid and citric acid act as crosslinkers for chitosan, which is why these films (ChT/E and ChC/E) present better mechanical properties, as the mobility of the polymer chains may be enhanced by the presence of crosslinkers [52]. Among the films evaluated, those based on chitosan citrate (ChC/E-a and ChC/E-b) can therefore be considered to have the best mechanical properties, followed by films based on chitosan tartrate (ChT/E-a and ChT/E-b); films prepared with chitosan lactate (ChL/E-a and ChL/E-b) are the least appealing. However, all the films show good properties for handling and application, since they are highly resistant and flexible.

2.3.2. Swelling Behaviour

The results of the swelling behaviour assessment in simulated vaginal fluid (SVF) are shown in Figure 9. In the case of films based on chitosan lactate and ES100, it can be observed that the maximum amount of water imbibed is significantly greater when the ES100 layer is thicker. ChL/E-a shows a maximum swelling ratio (SR_{max}) of ≈ 200% while ChL/E-b has a SR_{max} of ≈ 320%. The complete dissolution of the derivative (which leads to the constant weight of the formulation) occurs in both cases at 168 h. These results show a certain incompatibility between the layers, since an increase in the thickness of the ES100 layer leads to an increase in the water uptake rate and in the SR_{max}.

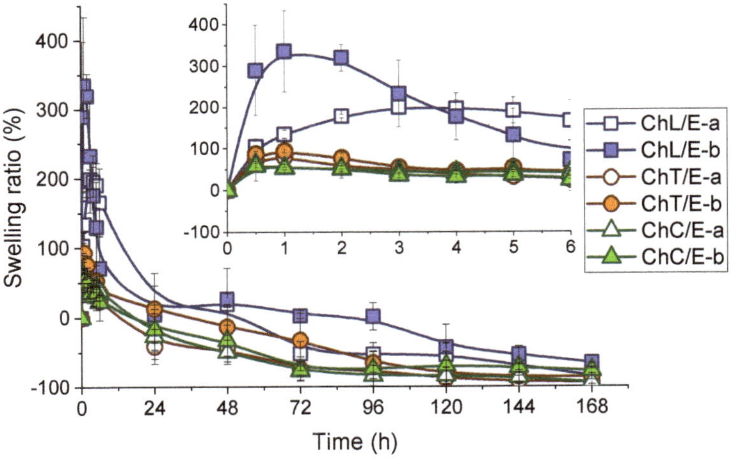

Figure 9. Swelling profiles of the LbL films in SVF.

The profiles of the batches based on chitosan tartrate (ChT/E-a, ChT/E-b) are practically overlapping, which implies that the presence of the ES100 layer does not condition the swelling process in this medium. Their low SR_{max} (less than 100%) indicate that these films swell very little. The swelling profiles of the films based on chitosan citrate and ES100 (ChC/E-a and ChC/E-b) also overlap, suggesting that the thickness of the ES100 layer does not condition the water uptake capacity, as observed in ChT/E films. These films also have the lowest SRmax values in SVF (less than 75%).

These results can be explained by the fact that that the three-dimensional structure generated by crosslinkers in chitosan hinders water penetration [53], so although CL/E films show a higher swelling capacity, all the films could be useful for developing mucoadhesive vaginal formulations, since they swell so little that they would be extremely comfortable for the patient.

2.3.3. Ex Vivo Mucoadhesion

Ex vivo mucoadhesion was determined through texture analysis on excised bovine vaginal mucosa in SVF, and the data are shown in Figure 10. According to the results, ChL/E films have the lowest values for mucosal stickiness (represented by the work required to detach them) and adhesiveness (detachment force). This is because these films show the highest SR_{max}. According to previously published results [54], the amount of water imbibed is inversely related to the mucoadhesion capacity of a formulation, as water hinders the interaction between the polymer and the mucosa. ChT/E and ChC/E therefore show higher values for mucosal stickiness, adhesiveness or both. The results reveal that the amount of ES100 also conditions the mucoadhesion capacity of the ChT/E and ChC/E films, probably because ES100 acts as a support capable of holding the chitosan derivative. Thus the greater the amount of ES100, the greater the ability of the chitosan to bind to the mucosa. In the case of ChC/E films, the difference between the formulations points to a synergy between the layers, and shows that increasing the thickness of the ES100 layer substantially improves the mucoadhesion capacity of the chitosan derivative-based layer. Finally, it should be noted that ChC/E-b shows a slightly higher mucoadhesion capacity than ChT/E-b. The ChC/E-b film thus has a high mucoadhesion capacity, superior to the formulations previously developed, which remained mucoadhered for 120 h [18].

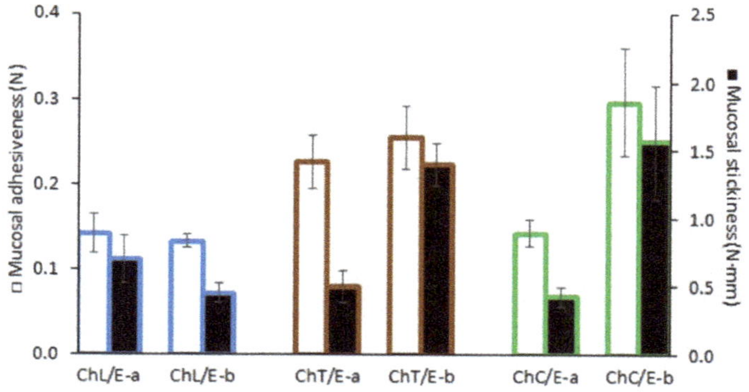

Figure 10. Ex vivo mucosal adhesiveness and stickiness obtained for the LbL films, determined in excised vaginal bovine mucosa and SVF. Mucosal adhesiveness is represented by the white bars (values on the left axis), and mucosal stickiness is by the black bars (values on the right axis).

2.3.4. Drug Release

Drug release data from the systems in SVF and SVF/SSF are shown in Figure 11. All the systems exhibited an ability to release the drug in a controlled manner in SVF (in all cases the release lasts more than 48 h), while a burst release is observed in SVF/SSF for all the systems (the complete amount of drug is released in less than 6 h).

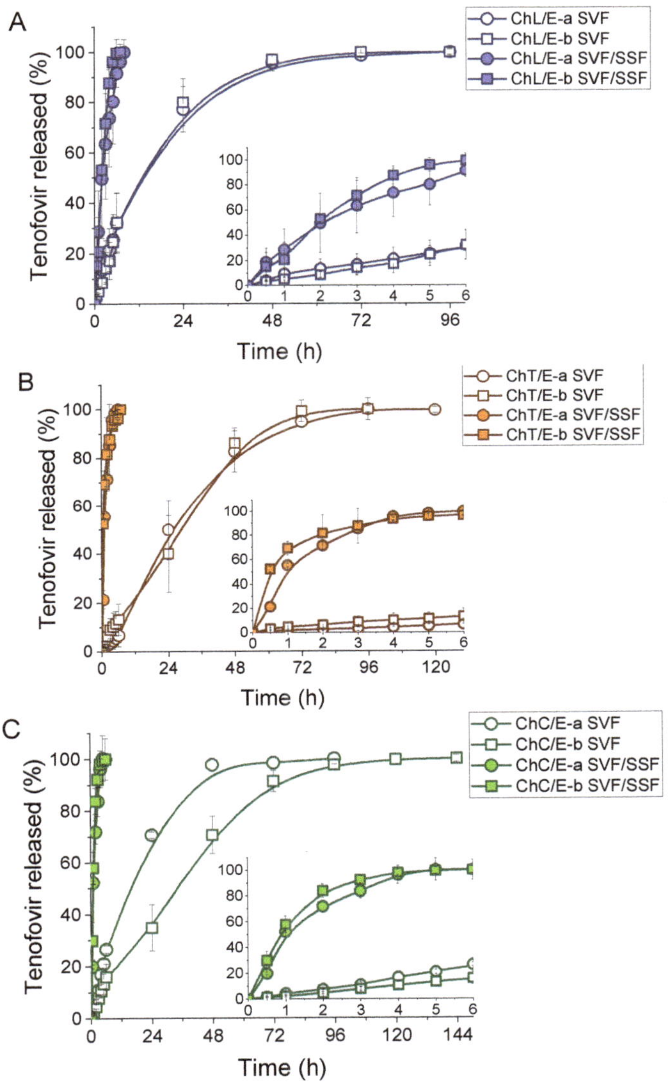

Figure 11. TFV release profiles in SVF and SVF/SSF from the LbL films based on chitosan lactate (**A**), chitosan tartrate (**B**) and chitosan citrate (**C**). The first 6 h of testing are amplified in the lower right corner of each graph.

According to Figure 11A, films based on chitosan lactate (ChL/E-a and ChL/E-b) show a sustained release of TFV of up to 48 h in SVF and 6h in SVF/SSF. In films based on chitosan tartrate (ChT/E-a and ChT/E-b), whose release profiles are shown in Figure 11B, TFV release in SVF extends up to 96 h, and 4 h in SVF/SSF. In films containing chitosan citrate (ChC/E-a and ChC/E-b), the release of TFV in SVF is maintained for 120 h, while in SVF/SSF the totality of the drug is released in 4 h, as seen in Figure 11C. These findings are closely related to the swelling behaviour of LbL films, where the swelling of ChL/E-a and ChL/E-b is greater in SVF; as they have the highest penetration of water in the system, the TFV molecules are more easily accessed by the water in the medium, accelerating the drug dissolution.

The SRmax is slightly higher in ChT/E films than in ChC/E films, which explains why ChC/E films show the most extended release and also confirms that crosslinking chitosan improves the capacity to control drug release, as chitosan tartrate and chitosan citrate-based films show better controlled release than chitosan lactate-based films. A comparison of tartaric acid and citric acid suggests that citric acid is the best crosslinker and has the most persistent TFV release. However, this confirms the need for an upper layer based on ES100 to enhance the properties of the crosslinked chitosan.

According to the f_2 statistic (Table 2), no significant differences are observed in the release profiles for ChL/E and ChT/E in SVF when comparing the release from films in SVF based on the amount of ES100 in the upper layer. As seen in the swelling test results, this implies that the entry of water into the formulation is modulated by the presence of ES100 regardless of the thickness of the layer, which is key to the capacity to modulate drug release. However, ChC/E films show differences in release depending on the thickness of the ES100 layer, once again indicating a synergy between the chitosan citrate and ES100, as was observed in the mucoadhesion studies (Section 2.3.3). In SVF/SSF the entry of water is so accelerated that the difference in release based on the thickness of this layer is negligible, and they all release the drug in similar times. It is verified by statistical f_2 that the release profiles of LbL films are strongly conditioned by pH, due to the fact that ES100 is a pH-sensitive polymer that becomes soluble in aqueous media at a pH of over 7 [55]. In consequence, the dissolution of the ES100 in the medium leaves the chitosan solely responsible for the release of Tenofovir, and this polymer will release the drug in less than 8 h, as already verified in the release profiles of chitosan derivative-based films (Section 2.2.3).

Table 2. Results of f2 processing for drug release from LbL films.

	ChL/E-a SVF	**ChL/E-b SVF/SSF**
ChL/E-a SVF/SSF	19.68	59.96
ChL/E-b SVF	73.63	21.21
	ChT/E-a SVF	**ChT/E-b SVF/SSF**
ChT/E-a SVF/SSF	14.34	34.43
ChT/E-b SVF	64.99	9.72
	ChC/E-a SVF	**ChC/E-b SVF/SSF**
ChC/E-a SVF/SSF	13.00	50.80
ChC/E-b SVF	43.01	11.71

The interest of this finding lies in the ability of the ChC/E-b film to offer women effective protection for a maximum of 120 h, generating a much higher concentration of TFV in the vaginal environment after ejaculation during sexual intercourse. This points to a high efficiency in the prevention of sexual transmission of HIV, and therefore justifies future evaluations.

2.4. Material Cytotoxicity

To study cell toxicity, the materials were incubated in culture media at 37 °C and 5% CO_2 for 48 h before the assay to ensure that any potential toxic component would be present in the dilutions to be tested. The cell culture was then treated with a suspension of base 5 serial dilutions of the most concentrated suspension (1000 μg/mL). Experiments were performed in lymphoblastic (MT-2) and macrophage-monocyte (THP-1) derived cell lines to evaluate toxicity on the immune cells present in vaginal or uterine mucosae, and in a uterine epithelial cell line (HEC-1A) to evaluate the potential damage to mucosal integrity (Figure 12).

As shown in Figure 12 and Table 3, lactic acid and ES100 were biocompatible in the three cell types, displaying CC_{50} values of over 1000 μg/mL, the maximum concentration tested. Citric acid CC_{50} value in THP-1 was around 1000 μg/mL, which is high enough to rule out a toxic effect in vivo, since it must pass through the epithelium layers at that concentration to reach the monocytes/macrophages that are only present on the inside of the epithelium. The same can be said of TEC since its CC_{50} of around 1000 μg/mL is only seen in MT-2 cells, which is a lymphocyte type cell line. The only compound showing cell toxicity below 1000 μg/mL was tartaric acid, with a CC_{50} of around 200 μg/mL in HEC-1A cells, with no effect on THP-1 and MT-2 cells. In this case tartaric acid is toxic to the epithelium cells, which could lead to the disruption of the layer and to a potential inflammatory response, facilitating viral entry through the vaginal mucosa, as other substances as nonoxynol-9 have been found to do [56]. Therefore, although the concentration needed to obtain the toxic effect is quite high (200 μg/mL), tartaric acid should be avoided in any formulation to be applied to the vaginal and/or uterine epithelium.

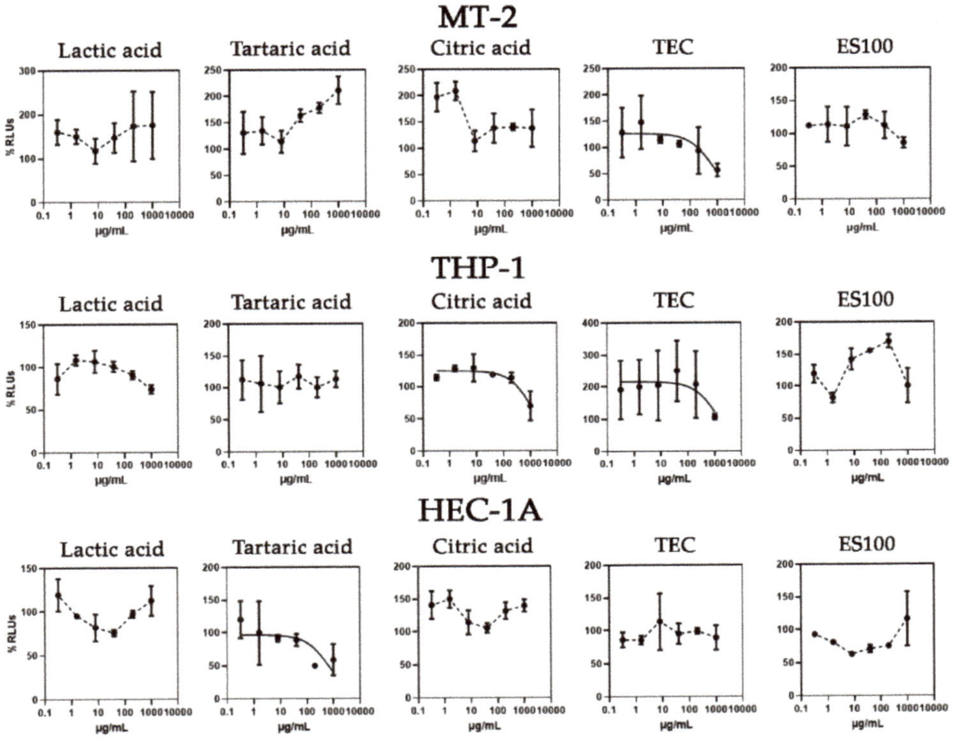

Figure 12. Graphic representation of the cytotoxic evaluation of lactic acid, tartaric acid, citric acid, TEC and ES100 in MT-2, THP-1 and HEC-1A cells. Cell viability is expressed as a percentage of living cells (%RLUs) as compared to a non-treated control (100%). RLUs: relative luminescence units.

Table 3. Results of the cytotoxicity analysis of lactic acid, tartaric acid, citric acid, TEC and ES100 in MT-2, THP-1 and HEC-1A cells. Cytotoxic concentrations 50 (CC_{50}) were calculated using GraphPad Prism software.

	CC_{50} μg/mL (CI95%; R^2)		
	HEC-1A	*THP1*	*MT-2*
Lactic acid	>1000	>1000	>1000
Tartaric acid	≈200	>1000	>1000
Citric acid	>1000	≈1000	>1000
TEC	>1000	>1000	≈1000
ES100	>1000	>1000	>1000

3. Materials and Methods

3.1. Materials

Tenofovir (TFV, lot: FT104801401, MW: 287.21 g/mol, purity ≥ 98%) was provided by Carbosynth Limited (Berkshire, UK). Low molecular weight chitosan [18] (CH, lot: 0055790, MW ≈ 32KDa, purity ≥ 90%) was supplied by Guinama (Valencia, Spain). L(+)-Lactic acid (lot: 0001552193, MW: 90.08 g/mol, purity = 90.8%) was purchased from PanReac AppliChem (Barcelona, Spain). L(+)-Tartaric acid (lot: BCBW8050, MW: 150.09 g/mol, purity = 99.97%), citric acid (lot: BCBV9045, MW: 192.12 g/mol, purity ≥ 99.5%) and triethylcitrate (TEC, Lot: BCBN8745V, MW: 276.28 g/mol, purity = 99.9%) were supplied by Sigma Aldrich (Saint Louis, MO, USA). Eudragit® S100 (ES100, lot: B071005090, MW = 135KDa [57]) was a kind gift from Evonik (Darmstadt, Germany). All other reagents used in this study were of analytical grade and used without further purification. Demineralized water was used in all cases.

3.2. Methods

3.2.1. Manufacture and Characterization of Chitosan Gels

Diluted acids must be used to obtain chitosan gels in aqueous media [54]. 50 mL of chitosan gels were therefore prepared with three different organic acids (lactic acid, tartaric acid and citric acid) at three concentrations, as shown in Table 4. The gels obtained were stored for 24 h at room temperature to ensure the correct hydration of the polymer, then immediately evaluated.

Table 4. Composition of the chitosan gels.

Batch	Chitosan (%)	Lactic Acid (M)	Tartaric Acid (M)	Citric Acid (M)
gChL-a	3	0.25		
gChL-b	3	0.5		
gChL-c	3	1		
gChT-a	3		0.25	
gChT-b	3		0.5	
gChT-c	3		1	
gChC-a	3			0.25
gChC-b	3			0.5
gChC-c	3			1

The influence of the acid used and its concentration on the chitosan gels was studied by evaluating their textural properties with a TA.XTplus Texture Analyser (Stable Micro Systems, Surrey, UK) using a 5 kg load cell, and following a previously described method [54]. A 20 mm-diameter stainless-steel probe with an activation force of 2 g was introduced in each gel at a rate of 0.5 mm/s to a depth of 15 mm, and returned to the initial height at the same rate. 500 points per second were monitored during data collection, and the maximum penetration force (MPF)—an accurate prediction of gel consistency—was calculated. The maximum detachment force (MDF), said to be a predictor of adhesive performance, was also recorded. The test was performed in triplicate for all the gels evaluated.

The pH of the gels was also determined using a pH-meter (GLP 21, Crison Instruments® S.A., Barcelona, Spain).

3.2.2. Chitosan Derivative-Based Films

Film Manufacture

Films were obtained from 5 mL of the previously prepared and evaluated gels using the solvent casting method [9] (Table 5) in silicon moulds. Once the solvent was completely dried at room temperature, 45-mm diameter circular films were stored until further analysis.

Table 5. Composition of the chitosan derivative films manufactured with the solvent casting method.

Batch	Chitosan (mg)	Lactic Acid (mg)	Tartaric Acid (mg)	Citric Acid (mg)	TFV (mg)
ChL-a	150	112.5 (0.25 M)			
ChL-b	150	225 (0.5 M)			
ChL-c	150	450 (1 M)			
ChT-a	150		187.5 (0.25 M)		
ChT-b	150		375 (0.5 M)		
ChT-c	150		750 (1 M)		
ChC-a	150			240 (0.25 M)	
ChC-b	150			480 (0.5 M)	
ChC-c	150			960 (1 M)	
ChL-TFV	150	225 (0.5 M)			30
ChT-TFV	150		375 (0.5 M)		30
ChC-TFV	150			480 (0.5 M)	30

The films were visually assessed to determine the optimum concentration of the different acids to obtain films based on chitosan derivatives. Their organoleptic properties were observed and their pliability was determined by folding the films, considering their capacity to deform and recover their form. The optimal proportions were then prepared using the same method with the addition of 30 mg of TFV to the gel. The amount of TFV for the development of the films was carefully selected according to literature and previous evaluations. Among the different dosage forms for the vaginal administration of this drug in clinical trials, lower and higher doses have been tested, showing adequate efficacy and security [7]. It has also been proved that extremely low cervicovaginal fluid concentration of TFV (1000 ng/mL) confer protection against HIV in women, ensuring the efficacy of these films during the release period [58]. As for the security of the films, it was confirmed in cytotoxicity studies that the dose included is not toxic for the vaginal tissue [59].

Attenuated Total Reflection Fourier Transform Infrared (FTIR-ATR) Spectroscopy

Attenuated total reflection Fourier transform infrared (FTIR-ATR) spectroscopy was used to characterize raw materials and chitosan derivative-based films with a Perkin-Elmer spectrophotometer, equipped with a MIRacle™ accessory designed for measurements (Perkin-Elmer). 16 scans were recorded for all the spectra at a resolution of 4 cm^{-1}.

Drug Release

Drug release was evaluated following the method described by Sánchez-Sánchez et al. [60]. Each sample was inserted in a borosilicate glass bottle with a 45 mm diameter base containing 80 mL of SVF and then placed in a shaking water bath (37 °C, 15 opm). Samples were taken every hour until the release of TFV was completed. 5 mL aliquots were removed and filtered, and the medium was replaced with the same volume of SVF at the same temperature. TFV concentrations were quantified by UV spectroscopy at a wavelength of 260 nm (Abs_{SVF} = 482.05·C(mg/mL)−0.0019; r^2 = 0.9996) in an Evolution 60S spectrophotometer (Thermo Scientific, Kyoto, Japan). The test was performed in triplicate.

3.2.3. Layer-by-Layer Films

Manufacture

Although the chitosan derivative-based films had an acceptable texture, they appear unable to sufficiently modulate the release of the drug. The optimal proportions of each chitosan derivative-based film were selected to prepare LbL films, adding different proportions of ES100 to prepare the second layer (Table 6). Since ES100 is an acidic polymer, the interaction between the surface of the chitosan film and the film based on ES100 occurs through electrostatic interactions, and both layers become tightly joined. These systems were obtained using the solvent casting method. First, chitosan derivative-based films containing TFV were prepared according to the method described above, then after the complete evaporation of water, a solution of ES100 in 10 mL acetone was added with TEC as a plasticizer. When this solvent was completely dry at room temperature, the resulting films were stored until further assessment.

Table 6. Composition of the LbL films manufactured with the solvent casting method.

		ChL/E-a	ChL/E-b	ChT/E-a	ChT/E-b	ChC/E-a	ChC/E-b
CHITOSAN DERIVATIVE-BASED LAYER	Chitosan (mg)	150	150	150	150	150	150
	Lactic acid (mg)	225	225				
	Tartaric acid (mg)			375	375		
	Citric acid (mg)					480	480
	Tenofovir (mg)	30	30	30	30	30	30
EUDRAGIT® S100-BASED LAYER	Eudragit® S100 (mg)	75	150	75	150	75	150
	Triethylcitrate (mg)	37.5	75	37.5	75	37.5	75

SEM Microscopy

To verify the structure of the film and the arrangement of the layers, the cross-sections of the films were analysed by electron microscopy using a field emission scanning electron microscope (JEOL JSM-6335F, Tokyo, Japan) at an accelerating voltage of 20 V and a work distance of 15 mm.

Texture Analysis

Although the pliability of the chitosan derivative-based films has already been assessed, the incorporation of the ES100-based layer may lead to a significant modification in the mechanical properties of the system. The texture of the LbL films was therefore evaluated according to a previously set up methodology [61] using a TA.XTplus Texture Analyser (Stable Micro Systems, Surrey, UK) with a 30 kg load cell. Before starting the experiments, each film was fixed to a support rig. A 5mm-diameter spherical stainless probe with an activation force of 5 g applied increasing force to each film to maintain a moving rate of 0.5 mm/s. 500 points per second were monitored during data collection, and the force applied (N) and the distance travelled by the probe (mm) were registered at each point. The measurement ended when the film burst at the maximum registered force. The distance travelled by the probe at the burst of the films was also recorded. The deformability of the systems was then determined as the average distance travelled by the probe when applying a force of 1 N.

All assays were performed in quadruplicate, and the data were statistically processed using two-way ANOVA (p-value 0.05) with the nature of the chitosan derivative and the proportion of ES100 as factors.

Swelling Behaviour

Swelling studies were performed on the LbL films to characterize the swelling of the formulations in SVF as a function of time.

The swelling processes of the different batches in SVF were analysed following the method described by Mamani et al. [62]. Fragments of each formulation with a diameter of 3 cm were fixed with cyanoacrylate adhesive to stainless steel discs of the same size, with the chitosan derivative-based layer facing the disc and the ES100 layer facing outwards, thus reproducing the expected conditions after administration. They were then placed in beakers containing 100 mL of SVF and introduced in a shaking water bath (37 °C, 15 opm). At given times (every hour during the first six hours and once a day up to constant weight), the discs were extracted from the medium and weighed after removing excess liquid. Swelling ratio (SR) was calculated according to Equation (1):

$$SR\ (\%) = [(F_s - F_d)/(F_d \cdot SF)] \cdot 100, \quad (1)$$

where F_s and F_d correspond to the swollen and dry film weights respectively, and SF represents the swellable fraction of the film. All the assays were performed in triplicate.

Ex Vivo Mucoadhesion

The mucoadhesion force and work were assessed ex vivo using the TA.XTplus Texture Analyser (Stable Micro Systems) to check whether the formulations show sufficient mucoadhesion capacity to adhere to the vaginal mucosa at the time of administration, using a modification of a previously described method [17]. A 2 × 2 cm fragment of excised bovine vaginal mucosa (obtained from a local slaughterhouse) was fixed to the bottom of a Petri dish and hydrated with 5 mL of SVF. The LbL film was fixed to a 1 cm-diameter cylindrical probe, with the chitosan derivative layer facing the vaginal mucosa, as expected at the time of administration. The preparation was moved at a speed of 1 mm/s until it came into contact with the vaginal mucosa, applying a contact force of 500 g for 30 s. The probe was then separated from the sample at a speed of 1 mm/s up to the starting height of the test. The maximum force required to separate the film from the vaginal mucosa (detachment force) was recorded as the mucosal adhesiveness. The area under the curve between the force-distance profiles (detachment work) was determined, which is considered to be the mucosal stickiness. Each batch was evaluated in triplicate.

Drug Release

To verify that the release of TFV from the films is pH dependent, the drug release from the LbL films was evaluated in SVF (pH = 4.2) and in a SVF and simulated seminal fluid mixture (SVF/SSF, ratio 1:4, pH = 7.5 [63]) to reproduce the conditions after ejaculation during intercourse. Each sample was inserted in a borosilicate glass bottle with a 45-mm diameter base containing 80 mL of medium, with the hydrophilic layer of the film in contact with the glass and the hydrophobic layer in contact with the medium, as it would be positioned in the vagina. The preparation was then placed in a shaking water bath (37 °C, 15 opm). Samples were taken every hour during the first six hours and every day after that at given times. 5mL aliquots were removed and filtered, and the medium was replaced with the same volume of either SVF or SVF/SSF at the same temperature. TFV concentrations were quantified by UV spectroscopy at a wavelength of 260nm ($Abs_{SVF/SSF} = 482.23 \cdot C(mg/mL) - 0.0145$; $r^2 = 0.9990$) in an Evolution 60S spectrophotometer (Thermo Scientific, Kyoto, Japan). The test was performed in triplicate.

The release profiles of the LbL films were compared using a f_2 statistic [64] in order to determine whether there are significant differences between the two media, and whether the thickness of the ES100 layer determines the release of the drug.

3.2.4. Material Cytotoxicity

Three human cell lines were used: a lymphoblastic cell line, MT-2 [65], a macrophage-monocyte derived cell line, THP-1 (ATCC® TIB-202) and a uterine/endometrial epithelial cell line, HEC-1A (ATCC® HTB-112™) (kindly provided by Maria Angeles Muñoz). All the cell lines were cultured in RPMI 1640 medium supplemented with 10 % (*v/v*) fetal bovine serum, 2 mM L-glutamine and 50 mg/mL streptomycin (all Whittaker M.A. Bio-Products, Walkerville, MD, USA) at 37 °C in a humidified atmosphere of 5 % CO_2. To detach the HEC-1-A cells, the medium was removed and the flask was rinsed during 10 min with 1 to 2 mL of trypsin 0.25%—EDTA 0.03% solution. The medium was replaced every three days after cell centrifugation at 1500 rpm for 5 min.

Cell toxicity was measured using the CellTiter Glo kit (Promega, Madison, WI, USA). Cells were incubated in 96-well plates at a density of 10×10^5 cells per well (MT-2 and THP-1) and 2×10^4 (HEC-1A) in complete medium. To assess the cytotoxic effect, cells were exposed to fresh medium containing different concentrations of lactic acid, tartaric acid, citric acid, TEC and ES100 suspensions, or the same concentration of PBS 1× as control. Experiments were performed in triplicate and the culture was maintained at 37 °C and 5% CO_2 humidified atmosphere for 48 h. A standard method was followed to suspend the materials in PBS 1× [66]. After incubation for 48 h, the medium was removed from cell cultures and 50 μL of CellTiter Glo reactive was added to each well on the plate. Relative luminescence units (RLUs) were measured in a luminometer (Sirius, Berthold Detection Systems). Cytotoxic concentration 50 (CC_{50}) values were calculated using GraphPad Prism Software (non-linear regression, log inhibitor versus response). The results of the cytotoxic assay are shown as the average of at least three individual experiments.

4. Conclusions

The gelation of chitosan in different diluted acids allows the production of chitosan derivative-based films with different mechanical properties without the need to include plasticizers. It has been confirmed that the crosslinking of the chitosan chains with tartaric acid or citric acid generates films with improved mechanical properties. The combination of these films with a polymer with pH-sensitive solubility (Eudragit® S100) produces formulations that exhibit a pH-dependant Tenofovir release, high mucoadhesion, and a moderate swelling profile, which would make them comfortable for the patient.

Among the films obtained through the layer-by-layer technique, those based on the combination of chitosan citrate and Eudragit® S100 in a 1:1 ratio (ChC/E-b) allow a sustained release of Tenofovir for up to five days in simulated vaginal fluid and release all the drug in less than 4 h after sexual intercourse, with very moderate swelling and a high mucoadhesion capacity. The materials used were also non-toxic in the vaginal environment. These formulations are thus a future option for the prevention of the sexual transmission of HIV in women.

Author Contributions: Conceptualization, R.C.-L., R.R.-C., and M.-D.V.; Funding acquisition, M.-D.V.; Investigation, R.C.-L., A.M.-I., F.N.-P., L.M.B. and A.T.; Methodology, R.C.-L., R.R.-C., J.R. and M.-D.V.; Project administration, R.R.-C., and M.-D.V.; Supervision, J.R., R.R.-C., and M.-D.V.; Writing—original draft, R.C.-L.; Writing—review & editing, M.-D.V., and R.R.-C. All authors have read and agreed to the published version of the manuscript.

Funding: This work was supported by project MAT2016-76416-R financed by the Spanish Research Agency and the European Regional Development Fund (AEI/FEDER, UE).

Acknowledgments: Raúl Cazorla-Luna and Araceli Martín-Illana are beneficiaries of university professor training fellowships granted by the Spanish Ministry of Education, Culture and Sport. Fernando Notario-Pérez is the beneficiary of a research training fellowship granted by the Spanish Ministry of Science, Innovation and Universities. We are grateful to the Carnes Barbero slaughterhouse (El Barraco, Ávila, Spain) for supplying the bovine vaginal mucosa samples. We would also like to thank María Hernando, veterinarian of the Junta de Castilla y León, for verifying the suitability of these biological samples. Scanning electron microscopy was done at the National Electron Microscopy Centre, part of the Research Support Centres and Unique Science and Technology Facility at the Complutense University of Madrid.

Conflicts of Interest: The authors declare no conflict of interest.

References

1. United Nations Joint Programme on HIV/AIDS (UNAIDS). *On International Women's Day, UNAIDS Calls for Greater Action to Protect Young Women and Adolescent Girls*; United Nations Joint Programme on HIV/AIDS (UNAIDS): Geneva, Switzerland, 2019.
2. Stankevitz, K.; Schwartz, K.; Hoke, T.; Li, Y.; Lanham, M.; Mahaka, I.; Mullick, S. Reaching at-risk women for PrEP delivery: What can we learn from clinical trials in sub-Saharan Africa? *PLoS ONE* **2019**, *14*, e0218556. [CrossRef] [PubMed]
3. Yang, H.; Li, J.; Patel, S.K.; Palmer, K.E.; Devlin, B.; Rohan, L.C. Design of Poly(lactic-co-glycolic Acid) (PLGA) Nanoparticles for Vaginal Co-Delivery of Griffithsin and Dapivirine and Their Synergistic Effect for HIV Prophylaxis. *Pharmaceutics* **2019**, *11*, 184. [CrossRef]
4. McConville, C.; Boyd, P.; Major, I. Efficacy of Tenofovir 1% Vaginal Gel in Reducing the Risk of HIV-1 and HSV-2 Infection. *Clin. Med. Insights Women's Heal.* **2014**, *7*, 1–8. [CrossRef]

5. Thurman, A.R.; Schwartz, J.L.; Brache, V.; Clark, M.R.; McCormick, T.; Chandra, N.; Marzinke, M.A.; Stanczyk, F.Z.; Dezzutti, C.S.; Hillier, S.L.; et al. Randomized, placebo controlled phase I trial of safety, pharmacokinetics, pharmacodynamics and acceptability of tenofovir and tenofovir plus levonorgestrel vaginal rings in women. *PLoS ONE* **2018**, *13*, e0199778. [CrossRef]
6. Delany-Moretlwe, S.; Lombard, C.; Baron, D.; Bekker, L.-G.; Nkala, B.; Ahmed, K.; Sebe, M.; Brumskine, W.; Nchabeleng, M.; Palanee-Philips, T.; et al. Tenofovir 1% vaginal gel for prevention of HIV-1 infection in women in South Africa (FACTS-001): A phase 3, randomised, double-blind, placebo-controlled trial. *Lancet Infect. Dis.* **2018**, *18*, 1241–1250. [CrossRef]
7. Marzinke, M.A.; Moncla, B.J.; Hendrix, C.W.; Richardson-Harman, N.; Dezzutti, C.S.; Schwartz, J.L.; Spiegel, H.M.L.; Hillier, S.L.; Bunge, K.E.; Meyn, L.A.; et al. FAME-04: A Phase 1 trial to assess the safety, acceptability, pharmacokinetics and pharmacodynamics of film and gel formulations of tenofovir. *J. Int. AIDS Soc.* **2018**, *21*, e25156.
8. Jalil, A.; Asim, M.H.; Le, N.-M.N.; Laffleur, F.; Matuszczak, B.; Tribus, M.; Bernkop-Schnürch, A. S-protected gellan gum: Decisive approach towards mucoadhesive antimicrobial vaginal films. *Int. J. Biol. Macromol.* **2019**, *130*, 148–157. [CrossRef]
9. Machado, R.M.; Palmeira-De-Oliveira, A.; Martinez-De-Oliveira, J.; Palmeira-De-Oliveira, R. Vaginal films for drug delivery. *J. Pharm. Sci.* **2013**, *102*, 2069–2081. [CrossRef]
10. Guzmán, E.; Mateos-Maroto, A.; Ruano, M.; Ortega, F.; Rubio, R.G. Layer-by-Layer polyelectrolyte assemblies for encapsulation and release of active compounds. *Adv. Colloid Interface Sci.* **2017**, *249*, 290–307. [CrossRef]
11. Notario-Pérez, F.; Martín-Illana, A.; Cazorla-Luna, R.; Ruiz-Caro, R.; Peña, J.; Veiga, M.D. Improvement of Tenofovir vaginal release from hydrophilic matrices through drug granulation with hydrophobic polymers. *Eur. J. Pharm. Sci.* **2018**, *117*, 204–215. [CrossRef]
12. Melegari, C.; Bertoni, S.; Genovesi, A.; Hughes, K.; Rajabi-Siahboomi, A.R.; Passerini, N.; Albertini, B. Ethylcellulose film coating of guaifenesin-loaded pellets: A comprehensive evaluation of the manufacturing process to prevent drug migration. *Eur. J. Pharm. Biopharm.* **2016**, *100*, 15–26. [CrossRef]
13. Volodkin, D.; von Klitzing, R. Competing mechanisms in polyelectrolyte multilayer formation and swelling: Polycation–polyanion pairing vs. polyelectrolyte–ion pairing. *Curr. Opin. Colloid Interface Sci.* **2014**, *19*, 25–31. [CrossRef]
14. Jeganathan, B.; Prakya, V.; Deshmukh, A. Preparation and Evaluation of Diclofenac Sodium Tablet Coated with Polyelectrolyte Multilayer Film Using Hypromellose Acetate Succinate and Polymethacrylates for pH-Dependent, Modified Release Drug Delivery. *AAPS PharmSciTech* **2016**, *17*, 578–587. [CrossRef]
15. Lokova, A.Y.; Zaborova, O.V. Modification of fliposomes with a polycation can enhance the control of pH-induced release. *Int. J. Nanomed.* **2019**, *14*, 1039–1049. [CrossRef]
16. Wang, X.-Q.; Zhang, Q. pH-sensitive polymeric nanoparticles to improve oral bioavailability of peptide/protein drugs and poorly water-soluble drugs. *Eur. J. Pharm. Biopharm.* **2012**, *82*, 219–229. [CrossRef]
17. Martín-Illana, A.; Notario-Pérez, F.; Cazorla-Luna, R.; Ruiz-Caro, R.; Veiga, M.D. Smart Freeze-Dried Bigels for the Prevention of the Sexual Transmission of HIV by Accelerating the Vaginal Release of Tenofovir during Intercourse. *Pharmaceutics* **2019**, *11*, 232. [CrossRef]
18. Cazorla-Luna, R.; Notario-Pérez, F.; Martín-Illana, A.; Tamayo, A.; Rubio, J.; Ruiz-Caro, R.; Veiga, M.D. Chitosan-Based Mucoadhesive Vaginal Tablets for Controlled Release of the Anti-HIV Drug Tenofovir. *Pharmaceutics* **2019**, *11*, 20. [CrossRef]
19. Frank, L.A.; Sandri, G.; D'Autilia, F.; Contri, R.V.; Bonferoni, M.C.; Caramella, C.; Frank, A.G.; Pohlmann, A.R.; Guterres, S.S. Chitosan gel containing polymeric nanocapsules: A new formulation for vaginal drug delivery. *Int. J. Nanomedicine* **2014**, *9*, 3151. [PubMed]
20. Kilicarslan, M.; Ilhan, M.; Inal, O.; Orhan, K. Preparation and evaluation of clindamycin phosphate loaded chitosan/alginate polyelectrolyte complex film as mucoadhesive drug delivery system for periodontal therapy. *Eur. J. Pharm. Sci.* **2018**, *123*, 441–451. [CrossRef] [PubMed]
21. Layek, B.; Rahman Nirzhor, S.S.; Rathi, S.; Kandimalla, K.K.; Wiedmann, T.S.; Prabha, S. Design, Development, and Characterization of Imiquimod-Loaded Chitosan Films for Topical Delivery. *AAPS PharmSciTech* **2019**, *20*, 58. [CrossRef]
22. Ali, A.; Ahmed, S. A review on chitosan and its nanocomposites in drug delivery. *Int. J. Biol. Macromol.* **2018**, *109*, 273–286. [CrossRef] [PubMed]

23. Valenta, C. The use of mucoadhesive polymers in vaginal delivery. *Adv. Drug Deliv. Rev.* **2005**, *57*, 1692–1712. [CrossRef] [PubMed]
24. Cheung, R.C.F.; Ng, T.B.; Wong, J.H.; Chan, W.Y. Chitosan: An Update on Potential Biomedical and Pharmaceutical Applications. *Mar. Drugs* **2015**, *13*, 5156–5186. [CrossRef] [PubMed]
25. Furuike, T.; Komoto, D.; Hashimoto, H.; Tamura, H. Preparation of chitosan hydrogel and its solubility in organic acids. *Int. J. Biol. Macromol.* **2017**, *104*, 1620–1625. [CrossRef]
26. Soares, L.S.; Perim, R.B.; de Alvarenga, E.S.; Guimarães, L.M.; Teixeira, A.V.N.C.; Coimbra, J.S.D.R.; de Oliveira, E.B. Insights on physicochemical aspects of chitosan dispersion in aqueous solutions of acetic, glycolic, propionic or lactic acid. *Int. J. Biol. Macromol.* **2019**, *128*, 140–148. [CrossRef]
27. Tronci, G.; Ajiro, H.; Russell, S.J.; Wood, D.J.; Akashi, M. Tunable drug-loading capability of chitosan hydrogels with varied network architectures. *Acta Biomater.* **2014**, *10*, 821–830. [CrossRef]
28. Libio, I.C.; Demori, R.; Ferrão, M.F.; Lionzo, M.I.Z.; da Silveira, N.P. Films based on neutralized chitosan citrate as innovative composition for cosmetic application. *Mater. Sci. Eng. C* **2016**, *67*, 115–124. [CrossRef]
29. Stie, M.B.; Jones, M.; Sørensen, H.O.; Jacobsen, J.; Chronakis, I.S.; Nielsen, H.M. Acids 'generally recognized as safe' affect morphology and biocompatibility of electrospun chitosan/polyethylene oxide nanofibers. *Carbohydr. Polym.* **2019**, *215*, 253–262. [CrossRef]
30. Benucci, I.; Liburdi, K.; Cacciotti, I.; Lombardelli, C.; Zappino, M.; Nanni, F.; Esti, M. Chitosan/clay nanocomposite films as supports for enzyme immobilization: An innovative green approach for winemaking applications. *Food Hydrocoll.* **2018**, *74*, 124–131. [CrossRef]
31. Cacciotti, I.; Lombardelli, C.; Benucci, I.; Esti, M. Clay/chitosan biocomposite systems as novel green carriers for covalent immobilization of food enzymes. *J. Mater. Res. Technol.* **2019**, *8*, 3644–3652. [CrossRef]
32. Notario-Pérez, F.; Cazorla-Luna, R.; Martín-Illana, A.; Ruiz-Caro, R.; Tamayo, A.; Rubio, J.; Veiga, M.D. Optimization of tenofovir release from mucoadhesive vaginal tablets by polymer combination to prevent sexual transmission of HIV. *Carbohydr. Polym.* **2018**, *179*, 305–316. [CrossRef] [PubMed]
33. Kyzioł, A.; Mazgała, A.; Michna, J.; Regiel-Futyra, A.; Sebastian, V. Preparation and characterization of alginate/chitosan formulations for ciprofloxacin-controlled delivery. *J. Biomater. Appl.* **2017**, *32*, 162–174. [CrossRef]
34. Ali, A.; Shahid, M.A.; Hossain, M.D.; Islam, M.N. Antibacterial bi-layered polyvinyl alcohol (PVA)-chitosan blend nanofibrous mat loaded with Azadirachta indica (neem) extract. *Int. J. Biol. Macromol.* **2019**, *138*, 13–20. [CrossRef]
35. Ubaid, M.; Shah, S.N.H.; Khan, S.A.; Murtaza, G. Synthesis and Characterization of pH-Sensitive Genipin Cross-Linked Chitosan/Eudragit® L100 Hydrogel for Metformin Release Study Using Response Surface Methodology. *Curr. Drug Deliv.* **2018**, *15*, 1343–1358. [CrossRef] [PubMed]
36. Chen, S.; Guo, F.; Deng, T.; Zhu, S.; Liu, W.; Zhong, H.; Yu, H.; Luo, R.; Deng, Z. Eudragit S100-Coated Chitosan Nanoparticles Co-loading Tat for Enhanced Oral Colon Absorption of Insulin. *AAPS PharmSciTech* **2017**, *18*, 1277–1287. [CrossRef] [PubMed]
37. Ansari, F.; Pourjafar, H.; Jodat, V.; Sahebi, J.; Ataei, A. Effect of Eudragit S100 nanoparticles and alginate chitosan encapsulation on the viability of Lactobacillus acidophilus and Lactobacillus rhamnosus. *AMB Express* **2017**, *7*, 144. [CrossRef]
38. Qindeel, M.; Ahmed, N.; Sabir, F.; Khan, S.; Ur-Rehman, A. Development of novel pH-sensitive nanoparticles loaded hydrogel for transdermal drug delivery. *Drug Dev. Ind. Pharm.* **2019**, *45*, 629–641. [CrossRef]
39. Prasad, S.; Dangi, J.S. Development and characterization of pH responsive polymeric nanoparticles of SN-38 for colon cancer. *Artif. Cells Nanomed.Biotechnol.* **2016**, *44*, 1824–1834. [CrossRef]
40. Solanki, A.; Thakore, S. Cellulose crosslinked pH-responsive polyurethanes for drug delivery: α-hydroxy acids as drug release modifiers. *Int. J. Biol. Macromol.* **2015**, *80*, 683–691. [CrossRef]
41. Martín-illana, A.; Cazorla-luna, R.; Notario-pérez, F.; Bedoya, L.M.; Ruiz-caro, R.; Dolores, M. Freeze-dried bioadhesive vaginal bigels for controlled release of Tenofovir. *Eur. J. Pharm. Sci.* **2019**, *127*, 38–51. [CrossRef]
42. Nelson, A.L. An overview of properties of Amphora (Acidform) contraceptive vaginal gel. *Expert Opin. Drug Saf.* **2018**, *17*, 935–943. [CrossRef] [PubMed]
43. Notario-Pérez, F.; Ruiz-Caro, R.; Veiga-Ochoa, M.D. Historical development of vaginal microbicides to prevent sexual transmission of HIV in women: From past failures to future hopes. *Drug Des. Devel. Ther.* **2017**, *11*, 1767–1787. [CrossRef] [PubMed]

44. Benucci, I.; Lombardelli, C.; Cacciotti, I.; Liburdi, K.; Nanni, F.; Esti, M. Chitosan beads from microbial and animal sources as enzyme supports for wine application. *Food Hydrocoll.* **2016**, *61*, 191–200. [CrossRef]
45. Kowalczyk, D.; Kordowska-Wiater, M.; Nowak, J.; Baraniak, B. Characterization of films based on chitosan lactate and its blends with oxidized starch and gelatin. *Int. J. Biol. Macromol.* **2015**, *77*, 350–359. [CrossRef]
46. Izutsu, H.; Mizukami, F.; Kiyozumi, Y.; Maeda, K. Preparation and characterization ofL-tartaric acid–silica composites recognizing molecular asymmetry. *J. Mater. Chem.* **1997**, *7*, 1519–1525. [CrossRef]
47. Lin, H.; Su, J.; Kankala, R.K.; Zeng, M.; Zhou, S.-F.; Lin, X. Using pH-Activable Carbon Nanoparticles as Cell Imaging Probes. *Micromachines* **2019**, *10*, 568. [CrossRef]
48. Bhattarai, N.; Ramay, H.R.; Chou, S.H.; Zhang, M. Chitosan and lactic acid-grafted chitosan nanoparticles as carriers for prolonged drug delivery. *Int. J. Nanomed.* **2006**, *1*, 181–187. [CrossRef]
49. Basumallick, S.; Gabriela Nogueira Campos, M.; Richardson, D.; Gesquiere, A.; Santra, S. Hydrothermally treated chitosan spontaneously forms water-soluble spherical particles stable at a wide pH range. *Int. J. Polym. Mater. Polym. Biomater.* **2016**, *65*, 751–758. [CrossRef]
50. Gylienė, O.; Nivinskienė, O.; Vengris, T. Sorption of tartrate, citrate, and EDTA onto chitosan and its regeneration applying electrolysis. *Carbohydr. Res.* **2008**, *343*, 1324–1332. [CrossRef]
51. Bagheri, M.; Younesi, H.; Hajati, S.; Borghei, S.M. Application of chitosan-citric acid nanoparticles for removal of chromium (VI). *Int. J. Biol. Macromol.* **2015**, *80*, 431–444. [CrossRef]
52. Miles, K.B.; Ball, R.L.; Matthew, H.W.T. Chitosan films with improved tensile strength and toughness from N-acetyl-cysteine mediated disulfide bonds. *Carbohydr. Polym.* **2016**, *139*, 1–9. [CrossRef] [PubMed]
53. Xu, S.; Li, H.; Ding, H.; Fan, Z.; Pi, P.; Cheng, J.; Wen, X. Allylated chitosan-poly(N-isopropylacrylamide) hydrogel based on a functionalized double network for controlled drug release. *Carbohydr. Polym.* **2019**, *214*, 8–14. [CrossRef] [PubMed]
54. Cazorla-Luna, R.; Martín-Illana, A.; Notario-Pérez, F.; Bedoya, L.-M.; Bermejo, P.; Ruiz-Caro, R.; Veiga, M.-D. Dapivirine Bioadhesive Vaginal Tablets Based on Natural Polymers for the Prevention of Sexual Transmission of HIV. *Polymers (Basel)* **2019**, *11*, 483. [CrossRef] [PubMed]
55. Mehta, R.; Chawla, A.; Sharma, P.; Pawar, P. Formulation and in vitro evaluation of Eudragit S-100 coated naproxen matrix tablets for colon-targeted drug delivery system. *J. Adv. Pharm. Technol. Res.* **2019**, *4*, 31–41.
56. Wilkinson, D.; Ramjee, G.; Tholandi, M.; Rutherford, G.W. Nonoxynol-9 for preventing vaginal acquisition of HIV infection by women from men. *Cochrane Database Syst. Rev.* **2002**, *4*, CD003939. [CrossRef]
57. Ai, Z.; Jiang, Z.; Li, L.; Deng, W.; Kusakabe, I.; Li, H. Immobilization of Streptomyces olivaceoviridis E-86 xylanase on Eudragit S-100 for xylo-oligosaccharide production. *Process Biochem.* **2005**, *40*, 2707–2714. [CrossRef]
58. Moss, J.A.; Malone, A.M.; Smith, T.J.; Butkyavichene, I.; Cortez, C.; Gilman, J.; Kennedy, S.; Kopin, E.; Nguyen, C.; Sinha, P.; et al. Safety and pharmacokinetics of intravaginal rings delivering tenofovir in pig-tailed macaques. *Antimicrob. Agents Chemother.* **2012**, *56*, 5952–5960. [CrossRef]
59. Notario-Pérez, F.; Martín-Illana, A.; Cazorla-Luna, R.; Ruiz-Caro, R.; Bedoya, L.M.; Tamayo, A.; Rubio, J.; Veiga, M.D. Influence of chitosan swelling behaviour on controlled release of tenofovir from mucoadhesive vaginal systems for prevention of sexual transmission of HIV. *Mar. Drugs* **2017**, *15*, 50. [CrossRef]
60. Bermejo, P.; Rubio, J.; Martín-Illana, A.; Sánchez-Sánchez, M.-P.; Bedoya, L.-M.; Otero-Espinar, F.; Fernández-Ferreiro, A.; Carro, R.; Veiga, M.-D.; Ruiz-Caro, R.; et al. Chitosan and Kappa-Carrageenan Vaginal Acyclovir Formulations for Prevention of Genital Herpes. In Vitro and Ex Vivo Evaluation. *Mar. Drugs* **2015**, *13*, 5976–5992.
61. Notario-Pérez, F.; Martín-Illana, A.; Cazorla-Luna, R.; Ruiz-Caro, R.; Bedoya, L.-M.; Peña, J.; Veiga, M.-D. Development of mucoadhesive vaginal films based on HPMC and zein as novel formulations to prevent sexual transmission of HIV. *Int. J. Pharm.* **2019**, *570*, 118643. [CrossRef]
62. Mamani, P.L.; Ruiz-Caro, R.; Veiga, M.D. Matrix Tablets: The Effect of Hydroxypropyl Methylcellulose/Anhydrous Dibasic Calcium Phosphate Ratio on the Release Rate of a Water-Soluble Drug Through the Gastrointestinal Tract I. In Vitro Tests. *AAPS PharmSciTech* **2012**, *13*, 1073–1083. [CrossRef]
63. Owen, D.H.; Katz, D.F. A review of the physical and chemical properties of human semen and the formulation of a semen simulant. *J. Androl.* **2005**, *26*, 459–469. [CrossRef]
64. Shah, V.P.; Tsong, Y.; Sathe, P.; Liu, J.P. In vitro dissolution profile comparison- Statistics and analysis of the similarity factor, f2. *Pharm. Res.* **1998**, *15*, 889–896. [CrossRef]

65. Harada, S.; Koyanagi, Y.; Yamamoto, N. Infection of HTLV-III/LAV in HTLV-I-carrying cells MT-2 and MT-4 and application in a plaque assay. *Science* **1985**, *229*, 563–566. [CrossRef]

66. Krug, H.F. *Handbook Standard Procedures for Nanoparticle Testing*; Comprehensive Assessment of Hazardous Effects of Engineering Nanomaterials on the Immune System Quality; EMPA: Dübendorf, Switzerland, 2011; p. 225.

marine drugs

MDPI

Article

Different Molecular Interaction between Collagen and α- or β-Chitin in Mechanically Improved Electrospun Composite

Hyunwoo Moon [1,†], Seunghwan Choy [2,†], Yeonju Park [3], Young Mee Jung [3], Jun Mo Koo [4,*] and Dong Soo Hwang [1,2,*]

1 Division of Environmental Science and Engineering, Pohang University of Science and Technology (POSTECH), 77 Chengam-ro, Nam-gu, Pohang 37673, Korea; lbemmoon@postech.ac.kr
2 Division of Integrative Biosciences and Biotechnology, Pohang University of Science and Technology (POSTECH), 77 Chengam-ro, Nam-gu, Pohang 37673, Korea; lbemchoi@postech.ac.kr
3 Department of Chemistry, Institute for Molecular Science and Fusion Technology, Kangwon National University, Chuncheon 24341, Korea; yeonju4453@kangwon.ac.kr (Y.P.); ymjung@kangwon.ac.kr (Y.M.J.)
4 Department of Fibre and Polymer Technology, KTH Royal Institute of Technology, Teknikringen 58, SE-100 44 Stockholm, Sweden
* Correspondence: jmkoo071128@gmail.com (J.M.K.); dshwang@postech.ac.kr (D.S.H.)
† These authors are equally contributed.

Received: 10 May 2019; Accepted: 28 May 2019; Published: 30 May 2019

Abstract: Although collagens from vertebrates are mainly used in regenerative medicine, the most elusive issue in the collagen-based biomedical scaffolds is its insufficient mechanical strength. To solve this problem, electrospun collagen composites with chitins were prepared and molecular interactions which are the cause of the mechanical improvement in the composites were investigated by two-dimensional correlation spectroscopy (2DCOS). The electrospun collagen is composed of two kinds of polymorphs, α- and β-chitin, showing different mechanical enhancement and molecular interactions due to different inherent configurations in the crystal structure, resulting in solvent and polymer susceptibility. The collagen/α-chitin has two distinctive phases in the composite, but β-chitin composite has a relatively homogeneous phase. The β-chitin composite showed better tensile strength with ~41% and ~14% higher strength compared to collagen and α-chitin composites, respectively, due to a favorable secondary interaction, i.e., inter- rather than intra-molecular hydrogen bonds. The revealed molecular interaction indicates that β-chitin prefers to form inter-molecular hydrogen bonds with collagen by rearranging their uncrumpled crystalline regions, unlike α-chitin.

Keywords: chitin; collagen; electrospinning; mechanical property; 2D correlation spectroscopy; polymorph

1. Introduction

Collagen is one of the most popular materials used as a tissue scaffold, drug carrier, cosmetic ingredient, bio-ink, dentistry and guide membrane in regenerative medicine and has been significantly utilized in medical fields [1–5]. Collagen mainly consists of repeating units of triplet sequence [Gly–Xaa–Yaa] with a hierarchically assembled triple helix and forms matrices of most of the vertebrate organs [6,7]. Collagen xenografts that are generally extracted from bovine or pig are non-cytotoxic, biocompatible, and easily resorbable in the human body; which is why clinicians prefer using collagen for human tissue regeneration [8,9]. However, the collagen xenografts have inherently lower mechanical strength than the native collagen tissues in humans with the hierarchical structure reinforced by Ca-based biomineralization [10,11].

To overcome the mechanical weakness of the collagen xenograft, without the cost of the fibrous feature, researchers have been trying to make collagen composites with varied synthetic and natural polymers including polycaprolactone, polylactic acid, polyvinyl alcohol, silk fibroin, chitosan, cellulose, and chitin [12–16]. Among them, chitin is the second most abundant natural polymer on Earth and can be acquired from marine creatures such as crab, shrimp, and squid. In addition, chitin has several attractive bioactivities, including environmental friendliness, biocompatibility, antibacterial activity, cost-effectiveness, and stiffness [17,18]. However, practical applications of chitin as a reinforcing material for mechanically weak polymers, such as collagen, have been impeded due to its insolubility in common solvent systems [19]. A highly crystalline structure which results from tight chain arrangement with multiple hydrogen bonds in chitin [20], limits its solubility in common organic solvent systems, thus only relatively low molecular weight and low concentrations of chitin could be dissolved in hexafluoro-2-propanol (HFIP). HFIP is a well-established halogenated solvent for electrospinning by dissolving the internal structure of polymers. However, in the case of chitin, HFIP is not a good solvent because strong hydrogen bonds in chitin prevent HFIP from infiltrating into its structure. However, it was suggested that chitin is electrospinable in acidic solvents, such as formic acid, methanesulfonic acid, basic lithium chloride (LiCl)/dimethylacetamide (DMAc), or ionic liquids [21,22]. However, only a small amount of chitin (<1%) is soluble in the above solvent systems.

In addition, the type of chitin resource that can be utilized for making the composite has been overlooked. Chitin has two naturally occurring polymorphs that are in the α and β phase. Two different phases occur by different inter- and intra-hydrogen bonds from a myriad of hydroxyl and amide groups, resulting in α- and β-chitin having different solvent susceptibilities. Therefore, it is a prerequisite to explore which solvent system can be used for dissolving both the chitins and collagen to make a mechanically reinforced composite material. Furthermore, we investigated which chitin phase will form inter-chain interactions with collagen which are preferential for the resultant mechanical prowess. Until now, molecular interactions that determine the mechanical properties have scarcely been investigated for a chitin adjuvant.

The aim of this work is exploring the solvent system that dissolves both the chitins as well as collagen and unraveling different molecular interactions for mechanical improvement. We electrospun the composite of chitins and collagen and investigated which chitin phase is more effective to improve the mechanical stability of the collagen and further estimated the molecular interactions behind the improvement.

2. Results and Discussion

Relatively high molecular weights of α- and β-chitin were adopted as an adjuvant for generating collagen composites to investigate the different molecular interactions. Depending on the intrinsic crystal structure and inter- and intra-chain hydrogen bonds, chitins showed different solvent susceptibilities as well as blending properties. Before blending with collagen, an appropriate solvent ratio for chitins was found by an α-chitin dissolution test at various ratios between HFIP and trifluoroacetic acid (TFA) (Figure S1). We found that the combination of a halogenated solvent with a small amount of acidic solvent is effective to dissolve chitin. In the HFIP/TFA (85:15, *v*/*v*) chitin was dissolved at a maximum concentration of 5% (*w*/*v*). In Figure 1, α- and β-chitin that had been dissolved in HFIP/TFA (85:15, *v*/*v*) showed distinct film morphologies which were cast on Teflon-covered dishes in the same conditions. Interestingly, the cast film of α-chitin was opaque and had broccoli-like grain structures (~5 μm), as observed in the scanning electron microscopy (SEM) image (Figure 1a). On the contrary, β-chitin formed a relatively unstructured smooth surface, resulting in a transparent film (Figure 1b). This means that different chain arrangements and crystal structures derived from different hydrogen bond configurations affect the solvation properties and reconstructing factors. Generally, α-chitin has an orthorhombic crystal structure with unit cell dimensions of a = 4.74 Å, b = 18.86 Å, and c = 10.32 Å from the anti-parallel chain configuration and tight hydrogen bonds [18] (Figure 1c). However, a relatively loose configuration by the parallel assembly of β-chitin with a particularly short inter-plane distance, b, equal to 9.26 Å, compared to that of α-chitin makes a monoclinic crystal structure. Consequently, we hypothesized that the collagen/chitin composite probably exhibits different fiber formations and macroscopic mechanical properties depending on the type of chitin added to the composite.

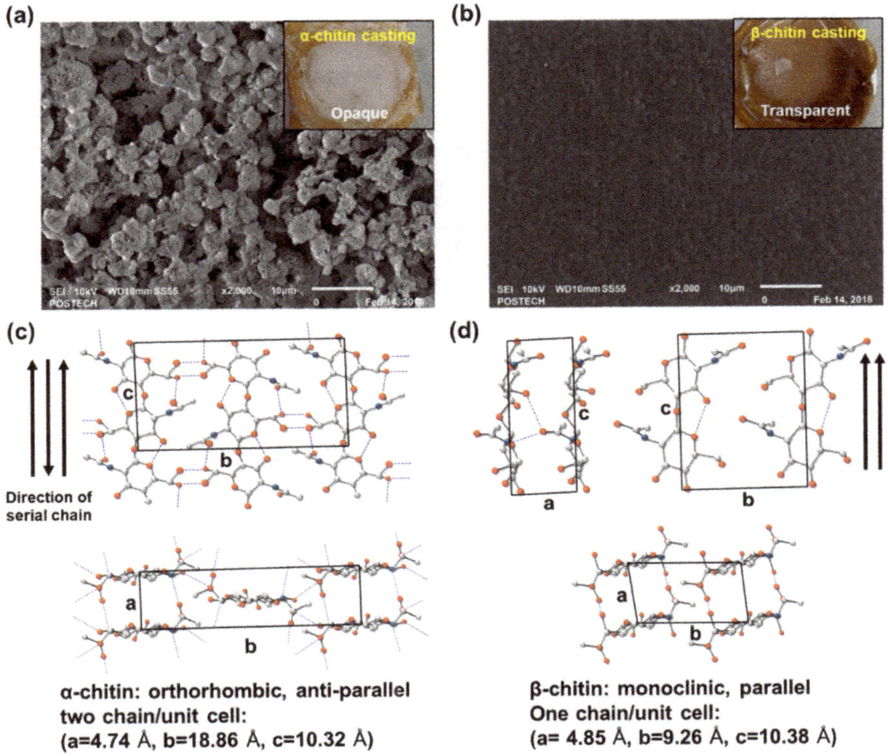

Figure 1. Scanning electron microscopy (SEM) micrographs of cast (**a**) α-chitin (opaque) and (**b**) β-chitin (transparent) film for different solvent susceptibilities to hexafluoro-2-propanol (HFIP)/ trifluoroacetic acid (TFA) solvent systems (magnification: 2000×). Different chain arrangements and crystal structures of (**c**) α-chitin and (**d**) β-chitin [18].

To confirm the macroscopic mechanical effect achieved by adding the chitins into collagen, electrospinning was utilized to obtain well-blended composites [23]. For the mat formation, relevant electrospinning conditions were evaluated in terms of the voltage, pumping speed, and needle tip-to-collector distance. A custom-made iron block was placed on the collector to harvest homogeneously made mats, as illustrated in Figure 2a. The tip-to-plate distance was set at 8 cm, otherwise, the fiber would snap (>8 cm) or it would be too difficult to form fiber, due to lack of the solvent vaporization (<8 cm). Furthermore, optimized electrospinning conditions of applied voltage and flow rate were 25–30 kV and 0.25 mL/h, respectively. The concentration of chitin and collagen was set to 1% (*w*/*v*) and 13% (*w*/*v*), respectively, for electrospinability. As a result, we successfully made three kinds of mats—collagen (Col), collagen/α-chitin (Col/α-Chi), and collagen/β-chitin (Col/β-Chi). The Col composed of collagen nanofibers which had a fiber diameter of ~0.210 μm (Figure 2b). However, changes in the diameter of the nanofiber by adding different chitins showed a different appearance, which can be determined by the pattern of molecular interaction, including molecular distance, the nanocrystalline structure, and distribution of the crystalline phase [24]. The Col/α-Chi showed a diameter that was ~29% greater than that of Col (~0.271 μm) (Figure 2c). This increase was due to the added crystalline phase α-chitin, which probably indicates that inhomogeneous blending of collagen and α-chitin occurred. On the other hand, nanofibers in Col/β-Chi showed a similar diameter to that of Col, achieving a slight increase to ~0.223 μm.

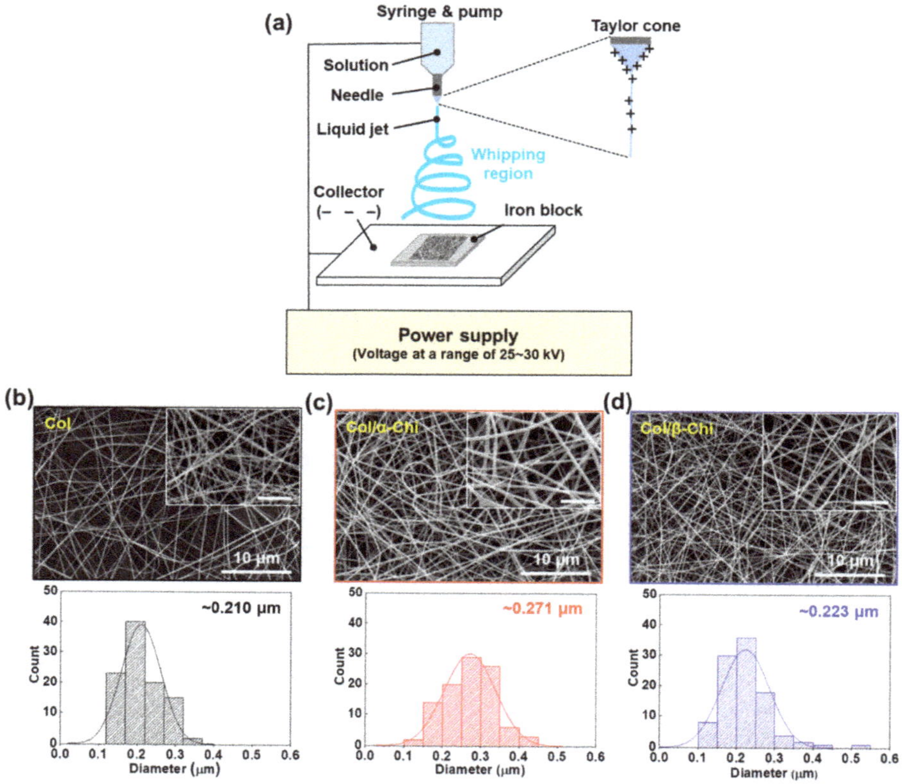

Figure 2. (**a**) Schematic illustration for electrospinning on iron block in HFIP/TFA (85:15, *v*/*v*). SEM observation of electrospun (**b**) Col, (**c**) Col/α-Chi, and (**d**) Col/β-Chi mats and corresponding width distributions constituting the nanofibers (n = 100, inset: magnified images and all scale bars are 3 μm).

To reveal how the blending characteristics at the molecular level and interactions between collagen and chitin affect the macroscopic mechanical properties, electrospun mats were subjected to a uniaxial tensile test (Figure 3a). The tensile strength was increased from 3.4 ± 0.7 to 3.9 ± 0.3 and 4.8 ± 0.3 MPa for Col/α- and Col/β-Chi, respectively (Figure 3b). As expected, Col/β-Chi showed better tensile strength, with a value that was ~41% and ~14% greater than Col and Col/α-Chi, respectively, due to a favorable secondary interaction, i.e., intermolecular hydrogen bonds. This could be explained by homogeneous crystal dissolution and the formation of new hydrogen bonds. Furthermore, increased uncrumpled regions of β-chitin enable more collagen–chitin interactions than intra-molecular interactions within the chitin. It manifests as an effective energy dissipation by collaborating between collagen and chitin despite the loss of the crystalline phase of β-chitin. However, Young's modulus of Col/β-Chi (177.3 ± 16.6 MPa) was comparable to that of Col/α-Chi (180.6 ± 14.07 MPa), even though both the mats were stiffer than Col (116.2 ± 0.7 MPa) (Figure 1c). We anticipate that these interesting features are probably due to solvent susceptibility, which could originate from the inherently developed chain arrangement and the resultant crystal structure.

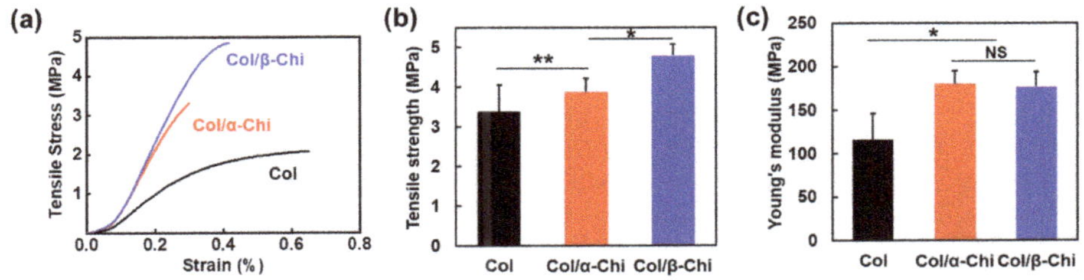

Figure 3. Mechanical improvement of Col by adding α- and β-chitin. (**a**) Representative stress–strain curves of electrospun mats during uniaxial tensile test. Statistical evaluation of (**b**) tensile strength and (**c**) Young's modulus (the mean value ± SD; n = 6, * $p < 0.05$; ** $p < 0.01$; NS, not significant).

To understand the mechanical behavior derived from α- and β-chitin, it is important to re-evaluate the structural properties of chitins and collagen. As mentioned, chitin has two major naturally occurring crystalline polymorphs, α- and β-chitin. The proposed unit cell for α-chitin is orthorhombic with an antiparallel arrangement [25]. This structure allows α-chitin to have a three-dimensional cooperative hydrogen bond network that includes inter-sheet hydrogen bonds, making it thermodynamically more stable than β-chitin [26]. The unit cell of β-chitin is monoclinic with a parallel chain arrangement. It consists of well-defined sheets but lacks hydrogen bonding. Such an anisotropic nature and weak association of the sheets leads to an unstable state, which results in the superior susceptibility to other materials compared to the susceptibility of α-chitin [27,28]. In detail, there are three major hydrogen bonds, two intermolecular and one intramolecular, that are not cooperative. Unlike α-chitin, unoccupied hydrogen-bonding acceptors in β-chitin are isolated, which act as hydrogen bonding terminators [29].

Meanwhile, collagen mainly consisting of glycine, proline, and hydroxyproline are structured as a supercoil intertwined with triple helices. Unlike a globular structure, the close association of three chains leaves no room for interior spaces or cavities in the triple helix [30]. It protrudes polar domains/side chains, such as carbonyl (C=O) and amine (N–H) functional groups, to the surface of the fibrous structure and exposes them for interaction. In theory, β-chitin with susceptible structural characteristics could form a complex through extensive hydrogen bonding on the surface of fibrous collagen. The mechanical result of incorporating chitin to collagen supports such a theory. This can be seen in Figure 3b, Col/β-Chi showed a tensile strength of 4.8 MPa that is 14% higher than that of Col/α-Chi.

To determine the effect of α- and β-chitin on the structure of collagen, XRD and thermal analysis were conducted. As presented in Figure 4a, the peak position of collagen at 19.56° shifted to 18.62° and 18.86° corresponding to α- and β-chitin, respectively [31–33]. A decrease in the 2θ value implies that chitin polymorphs are able to penetrate and position themselves in the space between collagen fibers, facilitated by the strong dissolution effect of TFA [34]. However, there was a noticeable shoulder peak at 14.56° in α-chitin, which signifies that there are two distinctive phases in the composite, originating from the lack of any secondary interaction between α-chitin and collagen. It is also interesting to note that the peak intensity of Col/β-Chi is approximately half that of collagen or Col/α-Chi. This means that the structural integrity of collagen has significantly decreased with the addition of β-chitin by the formation of new secondary interactions. This observation supports the result of mechanical properties where the formation of new hydrogen bonds between β-chitin and collagen is stronger than the intermolecular interaction between collagens. Additional evidence can be obtained from the thermal behavior. In the dehydration region, ΔH of Col, Col/α-Chi, and Col/β-Chi corresponds to ~184.54, ~215.02, and ~142.03 J/g, respectively. The energy required for thermal dehydration can imply the hydrogen bonding state of collagen and chitin. As expected, Col/α-Chi shows the highest ΔH since the sites (acceptor and donor) from collagen and α-chitin would not interact and would be occupied by water. A low ΔH value of Col/β-Chi emphasizes that hydrogen bonding sites occupied by water are replaced by a new interaction formed between β-chitin and collagen. The temperatures at which the deconstruction of the crystalline region for Col, Col/α-Chi, and Col/β-Chi begin are ~145 °C, ~139 °C, and ~132 °C, respectively. Since the structural integrity of collagen is heavily affected by the addition of β-chitin, diverse crystalline structures and sizes are present in the system. Thus, the regional area is extended while the starting point for crystal deconstruction shows the lowest value, ~132 °C. Further evidence of new secondary interactions can be observed in the denaturation region of collagen. As indicated with the green arrow at ~229 °C, Col/β-Chi showed a distinctive shoulder in this region followed by a peak at a temperature of ~237 °C, identical to collagen. This shoulder peak is an indication that a new structural interaction between β-chitin and collagen has been formed.

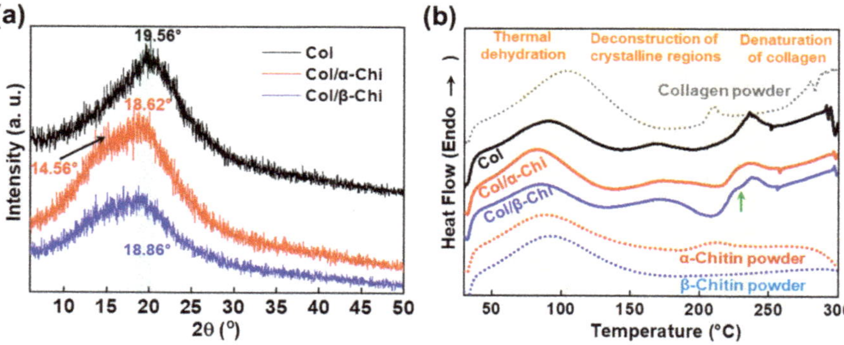

Figure 4. (**a**) Changes in the X-ray diffraction pattern and (**b**) differential scanning calorimetry depending on the corresponding chitin adjuvants (each powder indicates raw materials without electrospinning).

The absence of a secondary interaction by α-chitin and additional hydrogen bonding formation by β-chitin in the collagen composites are visualized using two-dimensional correlation spectroscopy (2DCOS). 2DCOS is one of the most powerful and versatile spectral analysis methods that can highlight the perturbation factors, such as time, temperature, concentration, or pressure. The result of such perturbations applied to the system transforms the behavior of the chemical constituents that can be produced into a simplified result [35]. Synchronous and asynchronous 2DCOS obtained from FT–IR spectra of collagen/α- and β-chitin with increasing chitin contents identify the effect on the collagen structure. Since the intensity of the FT–IR peak is heavily dependent on the concentration of the specific functional group, an increasing or decreasing intensity with increasing chitin content would reveal the presence of a new interaction between them. With the exception of diagonal positive autopeaks (a result of the autocorrelation function of intensity variation) in synchronous 2DCOS, the positive cross peak (red) represents the intensity of the two bands changing in the same direction, either increasing or decreasing together, whereas the negative cross peaks (blue) indicates that one band is increasing as the other is decreasing. When designated cross-peaks from the synchronous 2DCOS match the sign of the asynchronous 2DCOS, the intensity on the x-axis occurs before that of the y-axis and vice versa. Given this information, 2DCOS was conducted and the result is presented in Figure 5a,b with all the peak assignments summarized in Tables S1 and S2. The identical peaks that represent the basic functional groups of chitins and collagens are at 3160–3176, 3045–3050, 1633–1634, 1520–1522, 1370–1372, 1176, and 1110 cm^{-1}, which share identical increases/decreases in intensity [36,37] (Figure 5c). Moreover, C–H related peaks such as 2982 and 2866 cm^{-1}, are not considered due to a lack of information. Without these groups of peaks, the remaining information from the sequence clearly represents the difference in the interactive behavior between α/β-chitin and collagen. Initial impressions of the sequence reveal that there are higher wavenumbers of peaks in collagen/β-chitin 2DCOS sequences compared to collagen/α-chitin. This alone passively informs that collagen is more interactive and sensitive to the concentration of β-chitin than to α-chitin. The peaks at 3442 and 1013 cm^{-1}, corresponding to free O–H and chitin C=O, respectively, function as hydrogen-bonding acceptors and these are only present in collagen/β-chitin 2DCOS sequences [38,39]. The decrease in the intensity indicates that the number of acceptors is decreasing with the formation of new hydrogen bonds with collagen. Additionally, the initial stage of collagen/β-chitin sequence (1280, 3310, and 3176 cm^{-1} representing N–H) are donor-focused and the intensity increases, meaning that the addition of β-chitin creates a donor-friendly environment that increases the chance of new hydrogen bonding formations since characteristically, β-chitin has an abundance of acceptors. Additionally, the peak at 3436 cm^{-1}, which represents intramolecular hydrogen bonding of α-chitin is at the start of the collagen/α-chitin 2DCOS sequence. This means that as the concentration of added chitin increases, α-chitin loses its ability for intramolecular hydrogen bonding.

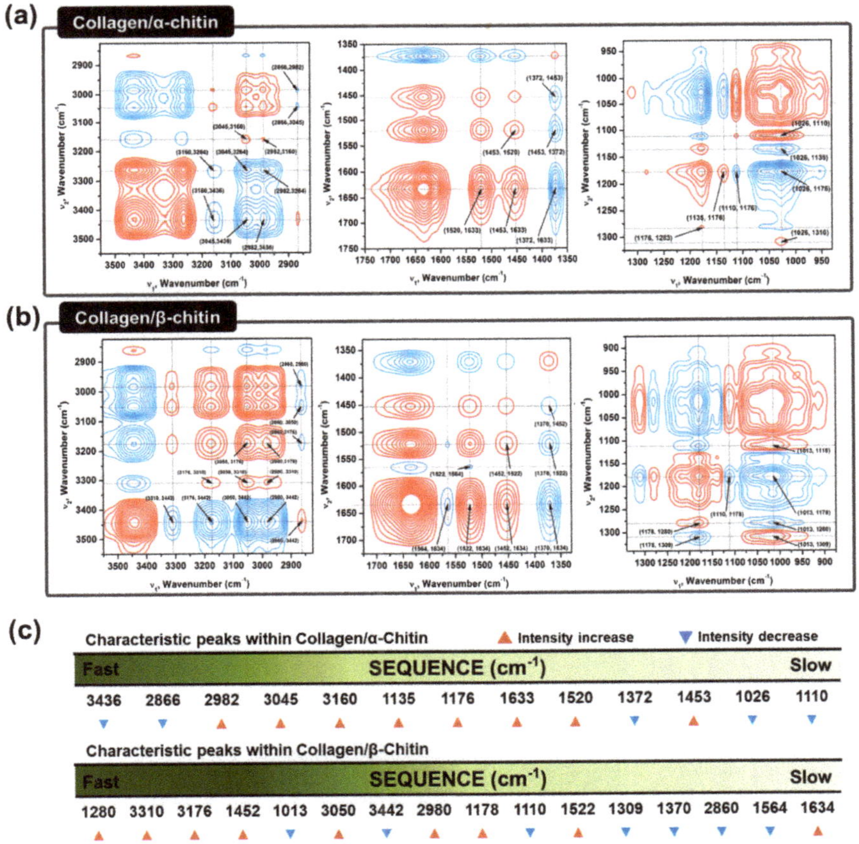

Figure 5. Two-dimensional correlation spectroscopy (2DCOS) analysis to confirm different molecular interactions between collagen and chitins in an HFIP/TFA system. A synchronous contour map from concentration perturbation of (**a**) α-chitin and (**b**) β-chitin in the collagen composites. (**c**) Relative interaction sequence and peak intensity variation of characteristic peaks from concentration perturbation.

3. Conclusions

In summary, we prepared electrospun collagen composites with α-chitin and β-chitin to improve the mechanical properties of the collagen. β-chitin/collagen composites showed better mechanical properties than those of α-chitin/collagen composites. 2DCOS analysis indicates that β-chitin prefers to form intermolecular hydrogen bonds with collagen by rearranging its crystalline regions, which contributes to the increase in the mechanical properties. Consequently, we suggested a means to make the composite through which the chitin phase will achieve a mechanical improvement of collagen.

4. Materials and Methods

4.1. Materials

Type I collagen from porcine skin (PSP-141706, Mw ~30,000) was purchased from SK Bioland Co., Ltd (Cheonan, Korea). High-purity α-chitin (from shrimp, C9752) and β-chitin (from squid pen, ARA-170124FC) were purchased from Sigma-Aldrich and AraBio Co., Ltd. (Seoul, Korea), respectively. The unit cell of α-chitin is a = 4.74 Å, b = 18.86 Å, and c = 10.32 Å, whereas the β-chitin is structurally different, with a = 4.85 Å, b = 9.26 Å, and c = 10.38 Å. In addition, different 2θ values of α- and β-chitin were 9.1 and 7.9 ° for (020); 20 and 19.6 ° for (110), respectively [40,41]. Hexafluoro-2-propanol (HFIP, A1247, Alfa Aesar) and trifluoroacetic acid (TFA, L06374, Alfa Aesar) were used to dissolve collagen and the two types of chitins.

4.2. Electrospinning

Collagen, α-chitin, β-chitin, and their blends were dissolved in HFIP/TFA (85:15, *v*/*v*) solvent at a concentration of 14% (*w*/*v*). The collagen/chitin blend was prepared in a ratio of 13:1. For the complete dissolution of chitin, the corresponding amount of chitin was first dissolved in the solvent in a 40 °C oven for 24 h, followed by the addition of collagen for another 12 h. Pure collagen for use as a control was dissolved in the solvent for 12 h at a concentration of 14% (*w*/*v*). Electrospinning was then performed with a customized electrospinning machine (Nano NC, Seoul, Korea) and syringe pump (KDS100, KD Scientific, Holliston, MA, USA). The solution was placed in a 1 mL syringe with a 26-gauge needle with a clamp connected to serve as an anode with a collector to serve as the cathode, both of which were connected to a high-voltage power supply. The iron block made of 2 × 2 × 1 cm was used as the collector. The distance between the needle edge from the polymer jet and the collector was maintained at 8 cm. The polymer jets generated from the needle by the strong voltage formed ultra-fine nanofibers that accumulated down at the collector in the form of a membrane. The applied voltage and solution feed rate was adjusted to 30 kV and 0.25 mL/h, respectively. All the experiments were carried out at room temperature under 40 ± 2% relative humidity. All the membrane samples were vacuum dried in a 40 °C oven overnight to remove any solvents which had remained prior to characterization.

4.3. Scanning Electron Microscopy

SEM (JSM-6010LV, JEOL, Tokyo, Japan) was used to observe the morphology of the electrospun nanofiber at an accelerating voltage of 10 kV. Sputter coating is performed for 100 s using a gold coating machine (108 Auto Sputter Coater, Cressington Scientific Instruments Co., Ltd., Watford, UK) to observe the nanofibers. Based on the SEM photographs, the average diameter of the nanofibers was analyzed using the Image J software (Wayne Rasband, National Institutes of Health, USA, http://imagej.nih.gov/ij).

4.4. Fourier Transform—Infrared Spectroscopy

A Fourier transform-infrared spectroscopy (FT–IR) spectrophotometer (Nicolet™ iS™ 50 FT–IR Spectrometer, Thermo Scientific Co., Ltd., Waltham, MA, USA) was used for FT–IR analysis and measurements were carried out in the range of 4000 to 400 cm^{-1} by using the absorption mode.

To observe the interaction between collagen and chitin, the concentration of collagen and chitin was adjusted to a 13:1, 12:2, 11:3, 10:4, and 9:5 ratio, and the concentration of blends was adjusted to 14% (*w*/*v*) in a HFIP/TFA (*v*/*v*, 85/15) solution. The polymer solution was poured onto a silicon wafer and cast for more than 24 h. The vibration modes of each specimen were then recorded for 2DCOS.

4.5. 2DCOS Analysis

2DCOS was used to differentiate between the effects of α- and β-chitin on collagen by setting the content of chitin as a perturbation factor. Synchronous and asynchronous 2D correlation spectra were obtained using the 2DShige program (freely downloadable software developed by Prof. Shigeaki Morita (Osaka Electro-Communication University, Japan)), where the red and blue lines in the 2D correlation spectra represent positive and negative cross peaks, respectively.

4.6. Differential Scanning Calorimetry

Differential Scanning Calorimetry (DSC) (DSC 4000, Perkin Elmer, Waltham, MA, USA) was used to observe the thermal behaviors of the electrospun mat. Five milligrams of each specimen were heated at a scan rate of 10 °C/min from 30 to 300 °C under nitrogen gas conditions.

4.7. X-ray Diffraction

Crystal X-ray analysis was taken with Ni-filtered CuKα radiation (λ = 1.5418 Å) using a D/MAX-2500/PC instrument (Rigaku, Tokyo, Japan) under 40 kV/100 mA. The diffractogram was recorded in an angular range of 5° to 60° (2θ) with a step size of 0.02° and a scanning speed of 2° min^{-1}.

4.8. Uniaxial Tensile Test

Mechanical properties of the electrospun collagen/chitin mats were applied to a universal testing machine (UTM, 3344, Instron, Norwood, MA, USA) for confirmation of the reinforced mechanical properties. It was equipped with a 2 kN load cell and a 1 mN resolution with ±0.5% uncertainty. All samples were cut into 5 mm × 20 mm sizes, and the portion held by the jig was 5 mm in the up and down direction, and the length of the extended portion was 10 mm. The tensile speed was adjusted to 10 mm/min. The tensile test was carried out at room temperature with a relative humidity of 40 ± 2%. The thickness was measured using a Digimatic Micrometer (293–240, Mitutoyo, Kawasaki-shi, Japan) using the values averaged by five points for each sample.

4.9. Statistical Analysis

All of the experimental data were presented as the mean ± standard deviation (SD) and were performed at least three independent times. The differences between the experimental data were examined using a student's t-test. A p-value < 0.05 was considered to be statistically significant.

Supplementary Materials: The following are available online at http://www.mdpi.com/1660-3397/17/6/318/s1, Figure S1: Solubility test, Figure S2: Heterogeneous and asynchronous contour map of 2DCOS, Table S1–S2: Results of 2DCOS, Table S3: DSC peak assignment and calculated ΔH values.

Author Contributions: H.M. and S.C. are equally contributed to this work. H.M., S.C., and D.S.H. conceived the idea and planned the research; H.M. and S.C. designed and conducted the experiments; Y.P. and Y.M.J. designed and conducted the FT–IR experiment. S.C., J.M.K., and D.S.H. analyzed the data and drafted the manuscript.

Funding: This research was funded by the Ministry of Education (NRF-2018R1A6A3A03012793), the Ministry of Oceans and Fishers of Korea (D11013214H480000110) and the Ministry of Science, ICT and Future Planning (MSIP) (NRF-2016M1A5A1027594 and 2017R1A2B3006354).

Acknowledgments: J.M.K. acknowledges support from The Basic Science Research Program through the National Research Foundation of Korea (NRF) funded by the Ministry of Education (NRF-2018R1A6A3A03012793). D.S.H. acknowledges the financial support from a Marine Biotechnology program grant (Marine BioMaterials Research Center) funded by the Ministry of Oceans and Fishers of Korea (D11013214H480000110) and the National Research Foundation of Korea Grant funded by the Ministry of Science, ICT and Future Planning (MSIP) (NRF-2016M1A5A1027594 and 2017R1A2B3006354).

Conflicts of Interest: The authors declare no conflict of interest.

References

1. Pham, Q.P.; Sharma, U.; Mikos, A.G. Electrospinning of polymeric nanofibers for tissue engineering applications: A review. *Tissue Eng.* **2006**, *12*, 1197–1211. [CrossRef] [PubMed]
2. Hasan, A.; Memic, A.; Annabi, N.; Hossain, M.; Paul, A.; Dokmeci, M.R.; Dehghani, F.; Khademhosseini, A. Electrospun scaffolds for tissue engineering of vascular grafts. *Acta Biomater.* **2014**, *10*, 11–25. [CrossRef]
3. Meinel, A.J.; Germershaus, O.; Luhmann, T.; Merkle, H.P.; Meinel, L. Electrospun matrices for localized drug delivery: Current technologies and selected biomedical applications. *Eur. J. Pharm. Biopharm.* **2012**, *81*, 1–13. [CrossRef] [PubMed]
4. Rodríguez, M.I.A.; Barroso, L.G.R.; Sánchez, M.L. Collagen: A review on its sources and potential cosmetic applications. *J. Cosmet. Dermatol.* **2018**, *17*, 20–26. [CrossRef] [PubMed]
5. Chieruzzi, M.; Pagano, S.; Moretti, S.; Pinna, R.; Milia, E.; Torre, L.; Eramo, S. Nanomaterials for Tissue Engineering In Dentistry. *Nanomaterials* **2016**, *6*, 134. [CrossRef] [PubMed]
6. Shoulders, M.D.; Raines, R.T. Collagen structure and stability. *Annu. Rev. Biochem.* **2009**, *78*, 929–958. [CrossRef] [PubMed]
7. Di Lullo, G.A.; Sweeney, S.M.; Körkkö, J.; Ala-Kokko, L.; San Antinio, J.D. Mapping the ligand-binding sites and disease-associated mutations on the most abundant protein in the human, type I collagen. *J. Biol. Chem.* **2002**, *277*, 4223–4231. [CrossRef]
8. Ferreira, A.M.; Gentile, P.; Chiono, V.; Ciardelli, G. Collagen for bone tissue regeneration. *Acta Biomater.* **2012**, *8*, 3191–3200. [CrossRef]
9. Dong, C.; Lv, Y. Application of collagen scaffold in tissue engineering: Recent advances and new perspectives. *Polymers* **2016**, *8*, 42. [CrossRef]
10. Duan, X.; Sheardown, H. Dendrimer crosslinked collagen as a corneal tissue engineering scaffold: Mechanical properties and corneal epithelial cell interactions. *Biomaterials* **2006**, *27*, 4608–4617. [CrossRef] [PubMed]
11. Haaparanta, A.M.; Jarvinen, E.; Cengiz, I.F.; Ella, V.; Kokkonen, H.T.; Kiviranta, I.; Kellomaki, M. Preparation and characterization of collagen/PLA, chitosan/PLA, and collagen/chitosan/PLA hybrid scaffolds for cartilage tissue engineering. *J. Mater. Sci. Mater. Med.* **2014**, *25*, 1129–1136. [CrossRef] [PubMed]
12. Chakrapani, V.Y.; Gnanamani, A.; Giridev, V.R.; Madhusoothanan, M.; Sekaran, G. Electrospinning of type I collagen and PCL nanofibers using acetic acid. *J. Appl. Polym. Sci.* **2012**, *125*, 3221–3227. [CrossRef]
13. Niu, X.; Feng, Q.; Wang, M.; Guo, X.; Zheng, Q. Porous nano-HA/collagen/PLLA scaffold containing chitosan microspheres for controlled delivery of synthetic peptide derived from BMP-2. *J. Control. Release* **2009**, *134*, 111–117. [CrossRef] [PubMed]
14. Ma, L.; Gao, C.; Mao, Z.; Zhou, J.; Shen, J.; Hu, X.; Han, C. Collagen/chitosan porous scaffolds with improved biostability for skin tissue engineering. *Biomaterials* **2003**, *24*, 4833–4841. [CrossRef]
15. Zhong, S.; Teo, W.E.; Zhu, X.; Beuerman, R.W.; Ramakrishna, S.; Yung, L.Y.L. An aligned nanofibrous collagen scaffold by electrospinning and its effects on in vitro fibroblast culture. *J. Biomed. Mater. Res. A* **2006**, *79A*, 456–463. [CrossRef] [PubMed]
16. Ghosal, K.; Chandra, A.; Praveen, G.; Snigdha, S.; Roy, S.; Agatemor, C.; Tomas, S.; Provaznik, I. Electrospinning over Solvent Casting: Tuning of Mechanical Properties of Membranes. *Sci. Rep.* **2018**, *8*, 5058. [CrossRef]
17. Younes, I.; Rinaudo, M. Chitin and chitosan preparation from marine sources. Structure, properties and applications. *Mar. Drugs* **2015**, *13*, 1133–1174. [CrossRef] [PubMed]
18. Rinaudo, M. Chitin and chitosan: Properties and applications. *Prog. Polym. Sci.* **2006**, *31*, 603–632. [CrossRef]
19. Lee, S.B.; Kim, Y.H.; Chong, M.S.; Lee, Y.M. Preparation and characteristics of hybrid scaffolds composed of β-chitin and collagen. *Biomaterials* **2004**, *25*, 2309–2317. [CrossRef]
20. Faria, R.R.; Guerra, R.F.; Neto, L.R.D.S.; Motta, L.F.; Franca, E.D.F. Computational study of polymorphic structures of α- and β- chitin and chitosan in aqueous solution. *J. Mol. Graph. Model.* **2016**, *63*, 78–84. [CrossRef]
21. Barber, P.S.; Griggs, C.S.; Ronner, J.R.; Rogers, R.D. Electrospinning of chitin nanofibers directly from an ionic liquid extract of shrimp shells. *Green Chem.* **2013**, *15*, 601–607. [CrossRef]

22. Zavgorodnya, O.; Shamshina, J.L.; Bonner, J.R.; Rogers, R.D. Electrospinning Biopolymers from Ionic Liquids Requires Control of Different Solution Properties than Volatile Organic Solvents. *ACS Sustain. Chem. Eng.* **2017**, *5*, 5512–5519. [CrossRef]
23. Lee, H.; Yamaguchi, K.; Nagaishi, T.; Murai, M.; Kim, M.; Wei, K.; Zhang, K.; Kim, I.S. Enhancement of mechanical properties of polymeric nanofibers by controlling crystallization behavior using a simple freezing/thawing process. *RSC Adv.* **2017**, *7*, 43994–44000. [CrossRef]
24. Baji, A.; Mai, Y.W.; Wong, S.C.; Abtahi, M.; Chen, P. Electrospinning of polymer nanofibers: Effects on oriented morphology, structures and tensile properties. *Compos. Sci. Technol.* **2010**, *70*, 703–718. [CrossRef]
25. Minke, R.; Blackwell, J. The structure of α-chitin. *J. Mol. Biol.* **1978**, *120*, 167–181. [CrossRef]
26. Gardenr, K.H.; Bleckwell, J. Refinement of the structure of β-chitin. *Biopolymers* **1975**, *14*, 1581–1595. [CrossRef] [PubMed]
27. Noishiki, Y.; Nishiyama, Y.; Wada, M.; Okada, S.; Kuga, S. Inclusion complex of β-chitin and aliphatic amines. *Biomacromolecules* **2003**, *4*, 944–949. [CrossRef]
28. Noishiki, Y.; Nishiyama, Y.; Wada, M.; Kuga, S. Complexation of α-chitin with aliphatic amines. *Biomacromolecules* **2005**, *6*, 2362–2364. [CrossRef]
29. Swada, D.; Nishiyama, Y.; Langan, P.; Forsyth, V.T.; Kimura, S.; Wada, M. Direct determination of the hydrogen bonding arrangement in anhydrous β-chitin by neutron fiber diffraction. *Biomacromolecules* **2012**, *13*, 288–291. [CrossRef]
30. Hoppe, H.J.; Barlow, P.N.; Reid, K.B.M. A parallel three stranded alpha-helical bundle at the nucleation site of collagen triple-helix formation. *FEBS Lett.* **1994**, *344*, 191–195. [CrossRef]
31. Chen, Z.; Mo, X.; He, C.; Wang, H. Intermolecular interactions in electrospun collagen–chitosan complex nanofibers. *Carbohydr. Polym.* **2008**, *72*, 410–418. [CrossRef]
32. Chen, Z.G.; Wang, P.W.; Wei, B.; Mo, X.M.; Cui, F.Z. Electrospun collagen–chitosan nanofiber: A biomimetic extracellular matrix for endothelial cell and smooth muscle cell. *Acta Biomater.* **2010**, *6*, 372–382. [CrossRef] [PubMed]
33. Ifuku, S.; Nogi, M.; Abe, K.; Yoshioka, M.; Morimoto, M.; Saimoto, H.; Yano, H. Preparation of Chitin Nanofibers with a Uniform Width as α-Chitin from Crab Shells. *Biomacromolecules* **2009**, *10*, 1584–1588. [CrossRef]
34. Chen, Z.; Mo, X.; Qing, F. Electrospinning of collagen–chitosan complex. *Mater. Lett.* **2007**, *61*, 3490–3494. [CrossRef]
35. Noda, I.; Dowrey, A.E.; Marcott, C.; Story, G.M.; Ozaki, Y. Generalized two-dimensional correlation spectroscopy. *Appl. Spectrosc.* **2000**, *54*, 236A–248A. [CrossRef]
36. Lee, Y.C.; Chiana, C.C.; Huang, P.Y.; Chung, C.Y.; Huang, T.D.; Wang, C.C.; Chen, C.I.; Chang, R.S.; Liao, C.H.; Reisz, R.R. Evidence of preserved collagen in an early jurassic sauropodomorph dinosaur revealed by synchrotron FTIR microspectroscopy. *Nat. Commun.* **2017**, *31*, 14220. [CrossRef] [PubMed]
37. Belbachir, K.; Noreen, R.; Gouspillou, G.; Petibois, C. Collagen types analysis and differentiation by FTIR spectroscopy. *Anal. Bioanal. Chem.* **2009**, *395*, 829–837. [CrossRef]
38. Satio, Y.; Iwata, T. Characterization of hydroxyl groups of highly crystalline β-chitin under static tension detected by FT-IR. *Carbohydr. Polym.* **2012**, *87*, 2154–2159.
39. Shanmugasundaram, N.; Ravichandran, P.; Reddy, P.N.; Ramamurty, N.; Pal, S.; Rao, K.P. Collagen-chitosan polymeric scaffolds for the in vitro culture of human epidermoid carcinoma cells. *Biomaterials* **2001**, *22*, 1943–1951. [CrossRef]
40. Hong, M.S.; Choi, G.M.; Kim, J.; Jang, J.; Choi, B.; Kim, J.K.; Jeong, S.; Leem, S.; Kwon, H.Y.; Hwang, H.B.; et al. Biomimetic Chitin–Silk Hybrids: An Optically Transparent Structural Platform for Wearable Devices and Advanced Electronics. *Adv. Funct. Mater.* **2018**, *28*, 1705480. [CrossRef]
41. Choy, S.; Oh, D.X.; Lee, S.; Lam, D.V.; You, G.; Ahn, J.S.; Lee, S.W.; Jun, S.H.; Lee, S.M.; Hwang, D.S. Tough and Immunosuppressive Titanium-Infiltrated Exoskeleton Matrices for Long-Term Endoskeleton Repair. *ACS Appl. Mater. Interfaces* **2019**, *11*, 9786–9793. [CrossRef] [PubMed]

marine drugs

MDPI

Article

Antifungal and Antioxidant Properties of Chitosan Polymers Obtained from Nontraditional *Polybius henslowii* Sources

Francisco Avelelas [1], André Horta [2], Luís F.V. Pinto [3,4], Sónia Cotrim Marques [2,5], Paulo Marques Nunes [1], Rui Pedrosa [1] and Sérgio Miguel Leandro [1,*]

1 MARE—Marine and Environmental Sciences Centre, ESTM, Instituto Politécnico de Leiria, 2520-641 Peniche, Portugal; franciscoavelelas@gmail.com (F.A.); paulo.nunes@ipleiria.pt (P.M.N.); rpedrosa@ipleiria.pt (R.P.)

2 MARE—Marine and Environmental Sciences Centre, Instituto Politécnico de Leiria, 2520-641 Peniche, Portugal; andre.horta@ipleiria.pt (A.H.); sonia.cotrim@ipleiria.pt (S.C.M.)

3 BioCeramed, S.A., Rua José Gomes Ferreira nº 1 - Armazém D 2660-360 São Julião do Tojal, Portugal; info@bioceramed.com

4 CENIMAT/I3N, Departamento de Ciência dos Materiais, Faculdade de Ciências e Tecnologia FCT, Universidade Nova de Lisboa, Campus da Caparica, 2829-516 Caparica, Portugal

5 Instituto Português do Mar e da Atmosfera (IPMA) Rua Alfredo Magalhães Ramalho, 6, 1449-006 Lisboa, Portugal

* Correspondence: sleandro@ipleiria.pt; Tel.: +351-262-783-607; Fax: +351-262-783-088

Received: 27 January 2019; Accepted: 24 March 2019; Published: 22 April 2019

Abstract: Chitin was extracted from *Polybius henslowii*, a swimming crab, captured in large quantities throughout the Portuguese coast by purse seine vessels as bycatch. After standard chitin extraction procedures, water-soluble chitosan products were obtained via two different methods: (1) *N*-acetylation with the addition of acetic anhydride and (2) a reaction with hydrogen peroxide. The chemical structure and molecular weight of chitosan derivatives, water-soluble chitosan (WSC) and chitooligosaccharides (COS), were confirmed by Fourier Transform Infrared Spectroscopy (FT-IR) and gel permeation chromatography (GPC). Antioxidant and metal chelation activities were evaluated, and the growth inhibition capacity was tested on four phytopatogens. The chitooligosaccharides from pereopods (pCOS) and shell body parts (sCOS) inhibited all fungal species tested, particularly *Cryphonectria parasitica* with 84.7% and 85.5%, respectively. Both radical scavenging and antifungal activities proved to be dose-dependent. Chitooligosaccharides with a low molecular weight (2.7, 7.4, and 10.4 Kg·mol^{-1}) showed the highest activity among all properties tested. These results suggested that chitosan derivatives from *P. henslowii* raw material could potentially be used against phytopathogens or as ingredient in cosmetics and other products related to oxidative stress.

Keywords: *Polybius henslowii*; marine resources; chitosan; chitooligosaccharides; antifungal activity; antioxidant activity

1. Introduction

Fungal pathogens are responsible for huge economic losses worldwide. These pathogens may cause damage to roots, crowns, stems, leaves, and fruits of a large range of economically important plants. In Portugal, several fungi species, such as *Phytophthora cinnamomi*, *Botrytis cinerea*, *Cryphonectria parasitica*, and *Heterobasidion annosum* cause considerable damage in cork oak forests [1], vegetable crops [2], chestnut trees [3], pines, and conifers [4], respectively. Since chemical fungicides such as sulfur dioxide [5] raise health concerns, the agrochemical industry has been searching for less toxic products.

Chitosan, a straight-chain polymer of glucosamine and *N*-acetylglucosamine [6] has emerged as a promising antimicrobial material [7]. As they are obtained from chitin present in crustacean's exoskeleton and fungi cell walls, chitosan products are biocompatible and biodegradable, with a wide range of applications such as in wastewater treatment, food, cosmetics, agrochemicals, cell culture, textiles, and medical devices [8]. Chitosan also exhibits antioxidant activity [9,10] and, therefore, could also be used as a replacement for synthetic antioxidants such as butylated hydroxytoluene (BHT), butylated hydroxy-anisole (BHA), and tert-butylhydroquinone (TBHQ) [11].

In recent years, the valorization of fisheries discards by-products has received much attention due to the increasing awareness of its economic potential and environmental impacts [12]. *Polybius henslowii*, a benthopelagic species is found at depths between 0 and 650 m along the eastern Atlantic coasts from Ireland and Britain to the Alborán Sea [13,14] and Morocco [15]. Despite its benthic habit, it also has periodic pelagic phases when larges swarms move along the surface to coastal waters, gathering at high densities from 0 to 14812 individuals per ha [16], with strong interannual oscillations [17]. Although being an extremely abundant marine resource, it is not presently subject to commercial use, and approximately 1240 tonnes/year (mean values from 2004 to 2009) are discarded annually [18]. In Portugal, it is captured as bycatch during the purse seining of *Sardina pilchardus* [18], having a destructive impact on the fishing nets. As such, it is regarded as a plague by the fisherman and not as a potential source of economic incomes.

The objective of the present study was to determine if this bycatch could be converted into a value-added product by chitin extraction and chitosan production. The products were characterized by gel permeation chromatography (GPC) and FT-IR, and their antioxidant, metal chelation, and antifungal properties were evaluated.

2. Results and Discussion

2.1. *Polybius henslowii* Characterization

The biochemical composition in terms of protein, minerals, lipids, and chitin of the swimming crab *Polybius henslowii* exoskeleton is shown in Table 1.

Table 1. The characterization of dried *P. henslowii* expressed as a percentage of dried weight (% of DW). Mean value (± SD).

Raw Material	Protein (%)	Ash (%)	Lipids (%)	Chitin (%)
Shell	32.1 ± 6.68	44.5 ± 0.57	13.2 ± 0.25	9.7 ± 0.57
Pereopods	16.6 ± 1.21	49.3 ± 5.86	1.6 ± 0.14	11.4 ± 0.19

The shell samples showed a higher percentage of protein and lipids than pereopods. The ash percentage, directly correlated with the calcium carbonate in the exoskeleton, was similar in both body parts. The protein and ash results are in accordance with those reported in previous studies [19], suggesting a higher yield of ash than protein, lipids, or chitin from the crab samples (about 16.6% for protein and 66.6% for ash content). The protein values are in line with the literature [20] for Alaska king crab (from 16.3 to 20.7%) but are lower than those reported for other crab species such as the *Metacarcinus magister* [21], *Callinectes sapidus* [22], and *Carcinus maenas* [23]. Previous studies [23] suggested that differences in the diet of crab at the harvesting site influences their biochemical composition, which could contribute to differences reported in the protein and lipid contents.

Previously published studies on crab species reported values of chitin from 14 to 28% of their total dry weight [24]. The pereopods of the swimming crab showed a higher chitin content than the shells. The chitin values shown in Table 1 are lower than those from other published studies [19,25]; however, authors [25] suggested that differences in chitin yield could be related to such factors as harvest year and/or shell storage duration, which could explain the low yield.

2.2. Chitin Extraction Optimization

The conventional demineralization process of crustacean waste uses strong acids such as hydrochloric acid (HCl). This chemical treatment can result in changes to the physiochemical properties of chitin (the hydrolysis of the chitin chains that reduces the average molecular weight of the biopolymer), produces harmful effluent wastewater, and contributes to the cost of the chitin purification process [26]. A mineral-free chitin with a very low ash content is usually required for applications with a very low impurity tolerance, such as biomedical and nutrition products [8]. Therefore, three different HCl concentrations were tested to minimize chitin chain damage and acid use.

The mineral content in pereopods and shell samples after treatment with HCl was different regarding calcium carbonate removal (Table 2). The lowest ash content was found for the pereopods and shells after treatment with 1 M HCl (Table 2). Nevertheless, all treatments (0.5, 0.75, and 1 M) promoted a high ash removal.

Table 2. The ash and protein contents of segmented body parts of *P. henslowii* after treatment with 1 M, 0.75 M, and 0.5 M HCl and NaOH. Mean value (± SD).

NaOH/HCl	Shells Samples			
	Protein Content (%)	Protein Removal (%)	Ash Content (%)	Ash Removal (%)
1 M	2.0 ± 0.12	96.1 ± 0.25	0.8 ± 0.01	98.2 ± 0.02
0.75 M	2.3 ± 0.14	95.35 ± 0.28	1.0 ± 0.05	97.8 ± 0.11
0.5 M	2.29 ± 0.15	95.39 ± 0.31	1.2 ± 0.17	97.3 ± 0.38
NaOH/HCl	**Pereopods Samples**			
	Protein Content (%)	**Protein Removal (%)**	**Ash Content (%)**	**Ash Removal (%)**
1 M	1.2 ± 0.12	92.2 ± 0.78	0.4 ± 0.19	99.1 ± 0.4
0.75 M	1.5 ± 0.07	90.5 ± 0.48	0.5 ± 0.01	98.9 ± 0.8
0.5 M	1.8 ± 0.06	88.2 ± 0.43	0.7 ± 0.05	98.6 ± 0.1

For an efficient chitin extraction, the associated proteins should be removed at a second stage. Deproteinization carried out with sodium hydroxide (NaOH) at elevated temperatures promoted the removal of protein from crab wastes. Residual protein was determined after each wash in order to evaluate the efficiency of each concentration applied. After treatment with NaOH, the protein values were highest in shells and pereopods treated with 0.5 M NaOH. The residual protein concentration was higher when 0.5 and 0.75 M of NaOH were used, rather than 1 M NaOH (Table 2).

A high-quality chitosan product should have less than 1% protein [27]. Moreover, a complete removal of protein is desirable, since it allows a higher solubility of chitosan after deacetylation [28].

2.3. Chitosan and Water-Soluble Chitosan Characterization

The data for chitosan samples characterization in terms of yield, dynamic viscosity, degree of deacetylation, and molecular weight are shown in Table 3. The degree of deacetylation (DD) of chitosan products was determined by infrared spectroscopy analysis. The ratio A_{1320}/A_{1420} was slightly different between the samples. The degree of deacetylation of chitosan obtained from shell chitin was 95.1 ± 0.01%, while the samples from pereopods were 91 ± 0.04% deacetylated. The difference is probably due to the longer deacetylation process of 7 h, the time needed to allow a complete dissolution in 1% acetic acid. Therefore, chitosan from pereopods resulted in a higher M_w (378 kg.mol^{-1}) and dynamic viscosity (749.2 ± 62.7 cP). Since the average M_w and dynamic viscosity are closely related, the decrease in these values is consistent with a prolonged reaction time. Previous work [29] demonstrated that a longer exposure to NaOH during deacetylation resulted in a decrease in M_w and dynamic viscosity. The yield of chitosan as a percentage of the crab dry weight from both body parts also showed lower values when compared with those from other studies [30], a consequence of the small amount of chitin extracted from the initial raw material.

Table 3. Chitosan yield (%), dynamic viscosity (cP), deacetylation degree (DD%), and molecular weight (kg.mol^{-1}) obtained from *Polybius henslowii* raw material. pWSC—Pereopods water-soluble chitosan; pCOS—pereopods chitooligosaccharides; sWSC—shells water-soluble chitosan; sCOS—shells chitooligosaccharides. Mean value (± SD).

Chitosan Products	Yield (%)	Dynamic Viscosity (cP)	DD (%)	M_w (kg·mol^{-1})
Pereopods chitosan	9.7 ± 0.62	749.2 ± 62.69	94.3 ± 0.04	378.2 ± 78.00
pWSC	-	-	62 ± 0.53	404.0 ± 45.00
pCOS	-	-	93.3 ± 0.04	7.4 ± 1.20
Shells chitosan	8.0 ± 0.24	417.2 ± 94.99	95.1 ± 0.01	247.0 ± 31.20
sWSC	-	-	55.0 ± 3.21	279.0 ± 33.00
sCOS	-	-	95.0 ± 0.62	2.7 ± 0.40
Commercial chitosan	-	-	87.0	780.0
ccWSC	-	-	57.0 ± 0.83	775.0 ± 42.00
ccCOS	-	-	86.0 ± 1.4	10.4 ± 0.70

Chitosan is only soluble in acidic solutions, which limits its applications. The solution viscosity is usually also quite high, which makes it difficult to prepare highly concentrated solutions. In contrast, chitooligosaccharides and other water-soluble chitosan derivatives allow highly concentration solution with low viscosities [31].

In the present study, hydrogen peroxide proved to be an efficient tool for chitosan degradation due to the formation of reactive hydroxyl radicals by the dissociation of hydrogen peroxide [32]. The results in Table 3 show the production of chitooligosaccharides (COS) from both segmented body parts with 7.4 kg.mol^{-1} for pCOS and 2.7 kg.mol^{-1} for sCOS, as well as for commercial chitosan chitooligosaccharides (ccCOS) with 10.4 ± 0.7 kg.mol^{-1}. Due to the decrease in molecular weight and degree of deacetylation, these products showed a good solubility in distilled water as previously observed by other authors [33].

Besides COS, another derivative soluble in water (WSC) was prepared through the *N*-acetylation of degraded chitosan. The water-soluble chitosan (WSC) products had a molecular weight range of 378 to 404 kg.mol^{-1} in pWSC, of 247 to 279 kg.mol^{-1} in sWSC, and of 780.0 to 775 Kg.mol^{-1} in ccWSC. According to previous studies [34], the reason for the increased solubility of chitosan was the destruction of intramacromolecular and interchain hydrogen bonds, which alters the secondary structure of chitosan, decreasing its crystallinity and unfolding its molecular chains. Also, the degree of deacetylation decreased likely due to the acetylation reaction induced by the acetic anhydride acting as a source of acetyl group for the amines.

2.4. DPPH Radical Scavenging Activity

One important mechanism of antioxidation involves scavenging of hydrogen radicals. DPPH (2,2-diphenyl-1-picrylhydrazyl) has a hydrogen-free radical with a characteristic absorption at 517 nm, allowing its detection as the purple color of the DPPH solution fades rapidly when it reacts with proton radical scavengers [35].

The DPPH radical scavenging activity of WSC, COS, and ascorbic acid is shown in Figure 1. At 1 mg·mL^{-1}, all chitosan products exhibited the highest scavenging ability. The scavenging ability proved to be dose-dependent.

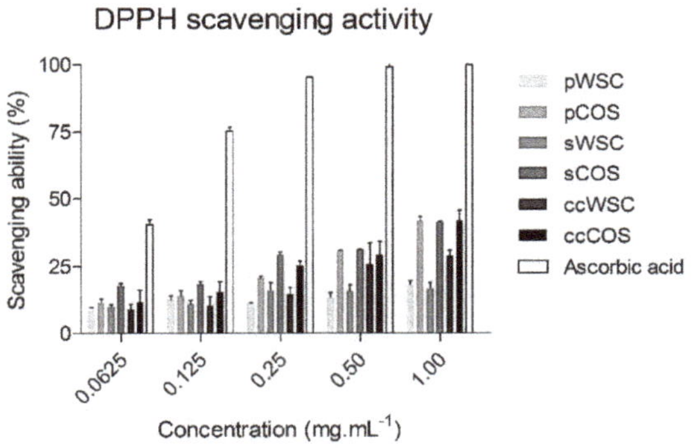

Figure 1. The scavenging ability of water-soluble chitosan (WSC), chitooligosaccharides (COS), and ascorbic acid on 1,1-diphenyl-2-picrylhydrazyl radicals: The values are means of eight replicates ± standard errors.

pCOS, sCOS, and ccCOS showed the highest scavenging activity. The WSC products showed a lower activity than COS at all concentrations tested (Figure 1). Also, no differences were noted between products obtained from *P. henslowii* and the commercial product. However, compared to the scavenging ability of ascorbic acid, all products had lower values.

Previous studies proved that the antioxidant activity of chitosan depends on the molecular weight and the degree of deacetylation [36,37].

Since chitosan chains have active hydroxyl and amino groups that can react with free radicals [38], the scavenging activity of chitosan may be due to the reaction between the free radicals and protonated amino groups [38]. Several researchers suggested that the scavenging mechanism of chitosan was based on the reaction of hydroxyl and superoxide anion radicals with active hydrogen atoms in chitosan to form a stable macromolecule radical. In the chitosan structure, there are three hydrogen sources, at the C−2 (NH_2), C−3 (OH) and C−6 (OH) positions respectively [39]. The present results support this theory, suggesting that the number of free amino groups is definitely important to a good antioxidant performance, since a high degree of deacetylation resulted in chitosans (COS) with better antioxidant properties. Other studies revealed the contribution of a prolonged *N*-deacetylation and its impact on the scavenging activities through the production of highly deacetylated products [40,41]. Once again, this seems to be in line with our findings, when compared the chitooligosaccharides (DD: 86–93%) and water-soluble chitosan (DD: 55–62%), proving that amino groups are a possible major factor for free radical scavenging activity.

In addition, previous investigations have revealed that the DPPH radical scavenging activity of chitosan increased with a decreasing molecular weight (M_W) [36,41]. According to previous studies [36], a high-M_W chitosan (WSC) would have a lower mobility than a low-M_W chitosan (COS). Consequently, this would increase the possibility of inter- and intramolecular bonding of the high-M_W chitosan molecules; thus, the chance of exposure of their amine groups might be restricted. An approximate 20% scavenging ability with 1 mg·mL^{-1} of chitosan from crustaceans has been reported previously [41].

The results obtained in the current study suggest that the degradation of chitosan by hydrogen peroxide enhanced not only the solubility but also its antioxidant activity, supporting the use of *P. henslowii* as raw material for the manufacturing of chitosan products towards antioxidant applications.

2.5. Superoxide Radical (O_2^-) Scavenging Ability

Superoxides are radicals of which unpaired electrons are on oxygen. Despite their limited chemical reactivity, they can form more dangerous species, including singlet oxygen, hydrogen peroxide, and hydroxyl radicals in living organisms [42,43]. Further, superoxides were also known to indirectly initiate lipid peroxidation as a result of H_2O_2 formation, creating precursors of hydroxyl radicals [44].

In the present study a superoxide radical scavenging assay was based on the capacity of water-soluble chitosan (WSC) and chitooligosaccharides (COS) to inhibit the reduction of nitro blue tetrazolium (NBT).

Figure 2 summarizes the scavenging effects of WSCs and COSs produced from *P. henslowii* raw material (pereopods and shells) and commercial chitosan on superoxide radicals within a concentration range from 0.0625 to 1 mg·mL^{-1}. All the products scavenged superoxide in a concentration-dependent manner. The figure showed that chitooligosaccharides (COSs) had the highest scavenging activity towards superoxide anion radicals with concentrations above 0.25 mg·mL^{-1}. Again, no differences were reported between products obtained from *P. henslowii* and commercial samples for both WSCs and COSs. At 0.0625 mg·mL^{-1}, all samples proved a low scavenging activity with values changing from 9.2 ± 1.9% (ccWSC) to 16.1 ± 2.9% (pCOS). On the other hand, EDTA proved much higher superoxide scavenging values (65.1 ± 3.6%) within the same concentrations (0.0625 mg·mL^{-1}). While testing the highest concentration at 1 mg·mL^{-1}, the pCOS, sCOS, and ccCOS samples clearly exhibited a higher scavenging activity (61.9 ± 7%, 60.1 ± 5.2%, and 57.5 ± 4.1%, respectively) when compared to pWSC, sWSC, and ccWSC (28.7 ± 2.7%, 31.9 ± 4.5%, and 28.5 ± 1.5%, respectively)

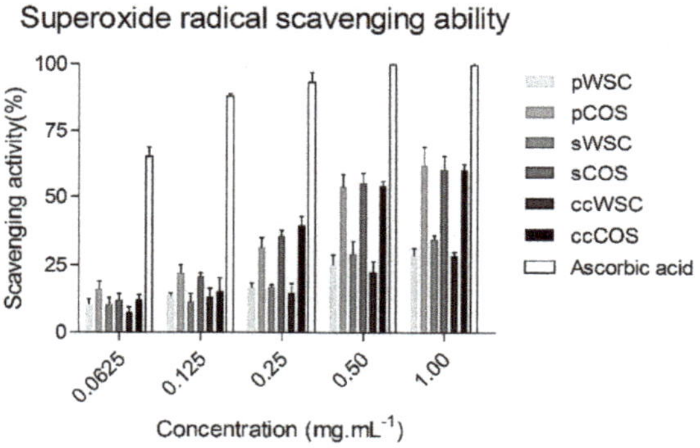

Figure 2. The scavenging ability of water-soluble chitosan (WSC), chitooligosaccharides (COS), and ascorbic acid on superoxide radical: The values are means of eight replicates ± standard errors.

Previously published studies [45–47] suggested a relationship between molecular weight and the ability to scavenge superoxide anions. Compared with chitosan, chitooligosaccharides have very short chains and the ability to form intramolecular hydrogen bonds (O_3–O_5 and N_2–O_6) decreases, which means that the hydroxyl and amino groups are activated, being helpful to the reaction with superoxide anions. This fact may be related once again to the formation of strong intermolecular and intramolecular hydrogen bonds that reduced the reactivity of hydroxyl and amino groups in the polymer chains. Other authors [48] proved the influence of hydroxyl and amino groups in the scavenging process, showing lower scavenging values for chitosan-thiamine pyrophosphate (CS-TPP) and chitosan-hydroxybenzotriazole (CS-HOBt) when compared to chitosan-acetate and chitosan-EDTA. According to the author, it might be due to the higher ability of TPP and HOBt to bond with the hydroxyl and amino groups of chitosan, blocking the reaction with the superoxide.

2.6. Chelating Ability on Ferrous Ions

The generation of radicals can be retarded by chelation of ferrous ions [49], being chitosan and chitosan derivatives reported as significant chelators [50]. This is why chitosan can be considered as a potential natural antioxidant to prolong food shelf life [40].

Figure 3 shows the ferrous-ion chelating ability of WSCs and COSs produced from *P. henslowii* raw material (pereopodes and shells) and from commercial chitosan within a concentration range from 0.0625 to 1 mg·mL^{-1}.

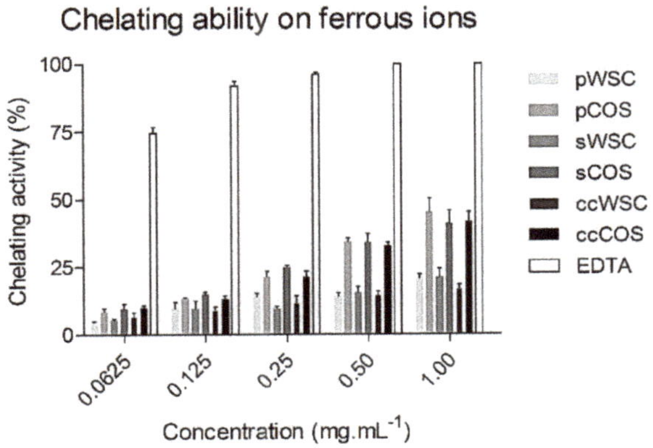

Figure 3. The chelating ability of water-soluble chitosan (WSC), chitooligosaccharides (COS), and ethylenediaminetetraacetic acid (EDTA) on ferrous ions: The values are means of eight replicates ± standard errors.

In general, the chelation ability of all WSCs with concentrations ranging from 0.0625 to 1 mg·mL^{-1} was relatively low. On the contrary, EDTA exhibited an excellent ferrous ion-chelating capacity of approximately 74.6 ± 4.1% at a concentration of 0.0625 mg·mL^{-1}. Nevertheless, all products proved a high chelation ability within 1 mg·mL^{-1}, showing COSs the highest activities, from 40.7 ± 10.1% (sCOS) to 45.2 ± 10% (pCOS). When tested at 0.5 and 1 mg·mL^{-1}, COSs almost presented a two-times-higher chelating power than WCSs. Also, no differences were seen between sCOS, pCOS, and ccCOS. Still, EDTA proved to be much more potent at 1 mg·mL^{-1}, chelating all ferrous ions (100%). Other authors [51] reported similar activities for EDTA when compared to the N-alkylated disaccharide chitosan derivative. Despite the close relation of the chitosan metal ion absorption capability to its amino acid content and their distribution, other factors such as affinity for water, pH, temperature, and crystallinity also affected the ion-chelating activity [52,53].

In addition, the ion-chelating activity of chitosan seems to be strongly affected by the degree of acetylation, with the fully acetylated chitosan showing very little chelating activity [54]. Similar findings were reported in the present study, revealing higher degrees of deacetylation (COSs) and a stronger effect on metal chelation abilities, when compared to low deacetylated products (WSCs).

2.7. Antifungal Assay

The molecular weight of chitosan is known to influence its ability to inhibit the activity of several fungal species [55]. The antifungal activity of WSC and COS products towards the plant pathogens *B. cinerea*, *H. annosum*, *P. cinnamomi*, and *C. parasitica* is shown in Figure 4. The concentrations of chitosan ranged from 0.0125 to 0.1 mg·mL^{-1}. The antifungal activity of all chitosan products proved to be dose-dependent, but despite the observed inhibitory effect, none of the tested fungal species were completely inhibited by COS or WSC at the highest concentrations. However, pCOS and sCOS showed a good inhibition against *Cryphonectria parasitica*. Overall, pCOS exhibited a higher activity against all other tested species than sCOS, pWSC, and sWSC.

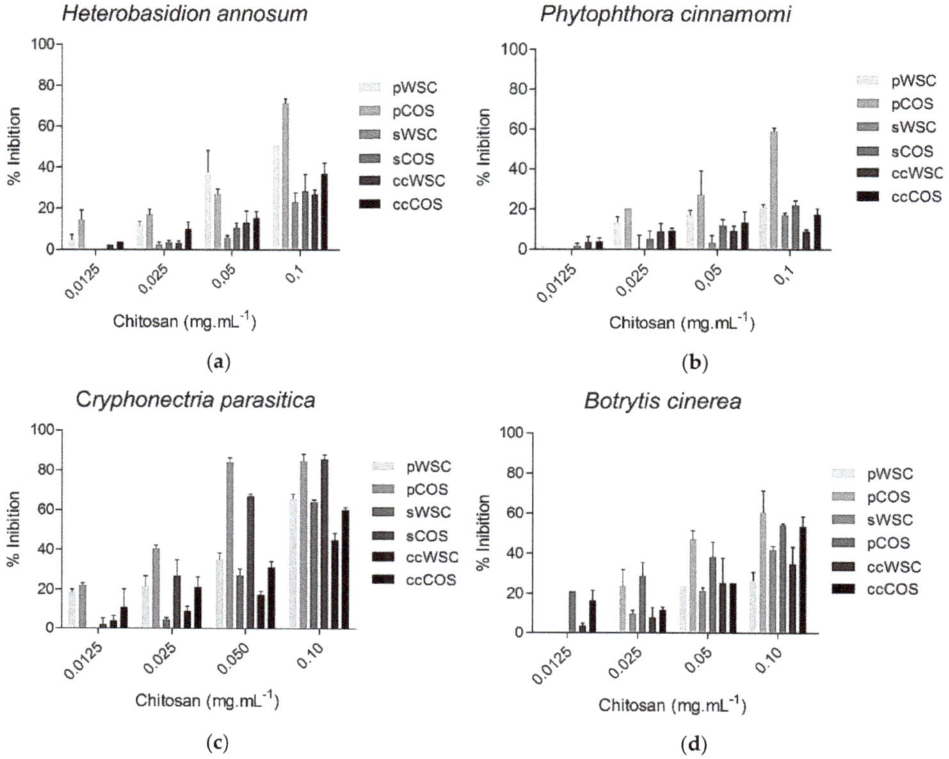

Figure 4. The effect of COS and WSC products (concentration ranging from 0.0125 to 0.1 mg·mL^{-1}) on the growth of *Heterobasidion annosum* (**a**), *Phytophthora cinnamomi* (**b**), *Cryphonectria parasitica* (**c**), and *Botrytis cinerea* (**d**): The values are means of eight replicates ± standard error.

Furthermore, the results showed that the capability to inhibit fungal growth was clearly higher for COS from both segmented body parts, especially the pereopods, than for WSC products. While *P. cinnamomi* exhibited a lower vulnerability towards all chitosans, *B. cinerea* and *C. parasitica* were highly inhibited by COS. *B. cinerea* sensitivity to chitosan has been reported previously [56].

Several mechanisms have been proposed for the antimicrobial action of chitosan. It has been suggested that chitosan may inhibit microbial growth by acting as a chelating agent rendering metals, trace elements, or essential nutrients unavailable for the organism to grow at a normal rate [57]. This could be caused by the accumulation of chitosan precipitates on the membrane surface, as the physiological pH in microbial cells is around neutral [58,59]. On the contrary, water soluble chitosan derivatives, due to their solubility in neutral solutions, would be unable to form such a layer, and therefore, no antimicrobial activity would be expected.

Another hypothesis explains the activity of chitosan as being based on the electrostatic interaction of the protonated amino groups with the negatively charged cell wall surface of the targeted microorganisms, which can lead to the disruption of the cell wall and, therefore, to its death [60]. The importance of protonation has been reported by several studies [61–63], which proved that only positively charged chitosan's are able to inhibit microbial growth.

Moreover, the degree of deacetylation certainly plays an important role not only on the antioxidant activity but also in antifungal activity, since the products with a higher degree of deacetylation (COS), exhibited a higher growth inhibition. Again, the number of free amino groups seems to influence bioactivities. Also, it is possible that chitosan's antifungal activity is caused by its chains, which interact with the cell's membrane and inhibits the intracellular functions [64]. Recently published studies [65] suggested that interactions between low molecular weight chitosans, DNA, RNA, and protein could partly explain the effects of chitosan on translation efficiency. In addition, other studies showed that the effectiveness of chitosan did not depend solely on the chitosan formulation but also on the *type* of fungi [61]. This is in accordance with our findings, since both pathogens from the phylum Ascomycota (*Botrytis cinerea* and *Cryphonectria parasitica*) were highly inhibited at 0.1 mg·mL^{-1} when compared to the remaining species, *Heterobasidion annosum* (phylum Basidiomycota) and *Phytophthora cinnamomi* (phylum Heterokontophyta).

3. Experimental Section

3.1. Biochemical Characterization of Raw Materials

Swimming crab, *Polybius henslowii* was by-catched by fishing vessels when capturing *Sardina pilchardus* along the west coast of Peniche (39°24′22.19′′N, 9°35′50.51′′O), Portugal. Dead organisms were first boiled, then dried in an oven at 100 °C for 2 days, and segmented into shell and pereopods. The raw material was powdered into particles with diameters ranging from 150 to 500 μm. The ash content was determined by initially drying the raw material in an oven at 100 °C for 6h. The dried samples were placed in a furnace at 530 °C for 20 h, and the remaining material was weighed after cooling in a desiccator. The microbiuret method was used for protein assays [66], and the values were compared with a standard curve established with known concentrations of bovine serum albumin (BSA). Free fat was extracted from the raw material by Soxhlet using ether as the solvent [67]. Three replicates were conducted for each sample.

3.2. Chitin Extraction and Deacetylation

Chitin was isolated according to Reference [19] with some modifications. Demineralization was carried out with three different concentrations of HCl in order to optimize the extraction of calcium carbonate: 0.5, 0.75, and 1 M at 21°C for 30 min (ratio of 1:30, *w/v*). After washing with distilled water and drying in an incubator for 24 h at 40 °C, the samples were subjected to different concentrations of sodium hydroxide (0.5 M, 0.75 M, and 1 M of NaOH; ratio of 1:15, *w/v*), thereby removing the organic matter. The shells and pereopods were incubated at 70 °C for 2 h in a water bath and washed with distilled water until a neutral pH was achieved. The demineralization and deproteinization efficiencies were respectively determined through the ash content and microbiuret assay measurements.

The chemical deacetylation of chitin was achieved by subjecting chitin to 12 M of NaOH solution at 120 °C for 3 h (pereopods) and 7 h (shells). After the alkali treatment, chitosan was collected and washed with distilled water to remove NaOH residues until a neutral pH was reached. These conditions yielded chitosan products from both body parts, which exhibited a complete dissolution in acetic acid (1%, *v/v*) at 25 °C.

Three batches were performed in each step, therefore having a minimum of three replicates per sample.

3.3. Chitooligosaccharides and Water-Soluble Chitosan Production

Water-soluble chitosan (WSC) was prepared according to a previously published procedure [34], through *N*-acetylation with acetic anhydride (Ac_2O). One gram of chitosan was dissolved in 25 mL of 2.8 % acetic acid, and 25 mL of ethanol were added. Acetic anhydride was charged after a complete dissolution of chitosan and left shaking for 4 h. The reaction mixture was precipitated with ethanol and dried at 55 °C for 24 h.

The production of chitooligosaccharides (COS) was derived by adding hydrogen peroxide (H_2O_2) [32]. One gram of chitosan was dissolved in 20 mL of 2% (*w/w*) acetic acid. After a complete dissolution, 5.5% H_2O_2 was added to the mixture and incubated at 37 °C for 4 h. Then, chitooligosaccharide products were precipitated with ethanol and dried at 55 °C for 24 h. The same procedure was carried out with the commercial chitosan (cc) product (Altakitin S.A., Portugal) in order to compare its physical and biochemical properties. All samples were performed in triplicate.

3.4. Chitosan Product Characterization

The dynamic viscosity was determined in triplicate with a rotational Haake viscotester 7 plus at (20 ± 1) °C after the samples were dissolved in 1% (*v/v*) acetic acid. The molecular weight (M_w) of chitosan products was determined by gel permeation chromatography (GPC) [68] with some variations. A Varian PL aquagel-OH MIXED bed column (Varian, France) 8-μm column was used. The samples (approx. 5 mg) were dissolved in 1 mL of eluent (AcOH/AcONa buffer pH 4.5, Panreac Spain) and filtered through a microsyringe filter prior to injection. The flow rate was 1 mL/min. A calibration curve was obtained by using Varian pullulan polysaccharides certified standards (Varian, France) at the same chromatographic conditions. FTIR spectroscopy (Bruker FTIR-ATR spectrophotometer) was employed to determine the degree of acetylation (DA) [69]. The spectra of all samples were recorded in KBr pellets (Sigma Aldrich, Steinheim, Germany) by the accumulation a minimum of 64 scans with a resolution of 4 cm^{-1}.

3.5. Scavenging of 1,1-diphenyl-2-picrylhydrazyl Radicals

The chitosan scavenging of 1,1-diphenyl-2-picrylhydrazyl radicals (DPPH) was determined according to a previously described method [70]. DPPH (Sigma Aldrich, Steinheim, Germany) solution was prepared at 0.1 mM with methanol. A volume of 10 μL of each sample was added to 990 μL of a DPPH solution. The sample concentrations varied from 0.0625 to 1 mg·mL^{-1}. The reaction mixture was shaken vigorously and stored in the dark at room temperature for 30 min. The absorbance was read at 517 nm in a microplate reader (Biotek, Vermont, USA). All samples were run in triplicate. Ascorbic acid was used for comparison. The free radical scavenging activity was calculated by the following Equation (1):

$$\text{Scavenging activity (\%)} = (1 - \text{Abs}_{\text{sample}}/\text{Abs}_{\text{control}}) \times 100 \quad (1)$$

3.6. Superoxide Radical (O_2^-) Scavenging Activity

The superoxide scavenging ability of all water-soluble chitosan (WSC) and chitooligosaccharide (COS) samples was assessed by the method of Reference [71]. This assay was based on the reduction of nitro blue tetrazolium (NBT) in the presence of NADH and phenazine methosulphate (PMS) under aerobic condition. The 3.00 mL reaction mixture contained 50 μL of lM NBT, 150 μL of 1 M nicotinamide adenine dinucleotide (NADH), and Trisbuffer (0.02 M, pH 8.0). The samples were added with concentrations ranging from 0.0625 to 1.0 mg·mL^{-1}. The reaction started by adding 15 μL of lM phenazine methosulfate (PMS). After incubation at room temperature for 5 min, 300 μL of each reaction were transferred to a 96-well plate, and the absorbance was recorded at 560 nm against a blank in microplate reader (Biotek, Vermont, USA). EDTA was used as a positive control. The capability of scavenging to superoxide radical was calculated using the following Equation (2):

$$\text{Scavenging effect (\%)} = (1 - A_{\text{sample}}/A_{\text{control}}) \times 100 \quad (2)$$

3.7. Chelating Ability on Ferrous Ions

The ferrous ion-chelating potential of all chitosan products (WSC and COS) was investigated according to the method of Decker and Welch [72]. Each WSC and COS sample (0.0625–1.0 mg·mL^{-1}) in a 0.2% acetic acid solution was mixed with 0.1 mL of $FeCl_2$ (2 mM) and 3.7 mL of methanol. The reaction was initiated by adding 2.0 mL ferrozine (5 mM), shaken vigorously and incubated for 10 min in the dark at room temperature. The ferrous ion-chelating ability was determined by the absorbance at 562 nm against a blank in a microplate reader (Biotek, Vermont, USA). EDTA was used as a positive control. The ability of WSC and COS to chelate ferrous ions was calculated according to the following Equation (3):

$$\text{Chelating activity } (\%) = (1 - \text{Abs}_{\text{sample}}/\text{Abs}_{\text{control}}) \times 100 \quad (3)$$

3.8. Effect of Chitosan on Mycelial Growth

Cryphonectria parasitica (DSMZ 62626), *Phytophthora cinnamomi* (DSMZ 62654), *Botrytis cinerea* (DSMZ 4709), and *Heterobasidion annosum* (DSMZ 1531) were all purchased from the Leibniz Institut DSMZ (German Collection of Microorganisms and Cells Cultures), Germany. The four strains were grown for 5 days at 28 °C on potato dextrose agar (PDA) plates. The antifungal assessment of the chitosan products was conducted through the mycelial radial growth inhibition technique on a PDA medium according to El Ghaouth et al. [73]. Mycelial discs 4 mm in diameter were cut from the margins of the initial colony and placed on PDA plates containing different concentrations of chitosan, ranging from 0.0125 to 0.1 mg·mL^{-1}. Control plates of PDA were prepared without chitosan. The PDA plates were incubated at (23 ± 2) °C for 7 days. The mycelial radial growth was measured when the control colony had grown to the edge of the plate. The diameter of each fungal colony prepared in triplicate was measured in mm. and the activity was expressed as the inhibition of mycelial growth.

4. Conclusions

This study shows that *P. henslowii* captured as bycatch could be applied as a source of chitosan derivatives. The swimming crab characterization clearly showed that, considering its composition, different segments of its body could be applied to several biotechnological applications such as feed supplements, adding value to the raw material. Moreover, the bioavailability of this marine resource, the optimization of chemical processes (through solvent reuse), and, considering all production costs, the final price could be highly competitive compared to the current market offer. The results suggested that the chitosan derivatives, mainly chitooligosaccharides obtained through processing of *P. henslowii* raw material, could be effectively employed as an ingredient in cosmetics or functional products in order to decrease oxidative stress. In general, the chitosan derivatives produced from the raw material of *P. henslowii* remarkably inhibited the tested phytopathogenic fungi, mainly *Cryphonectria parasitica*. In addition, these samples produced an interesting inhibitory activity when compared with commercial chitosan derivatives. However, in order to promote the use of this raw material, extensive research on its characterization (RNM) and other applications (antibacterial activity and allergenic tests) must be addressed.

Author Contributions: R.P., S.M.L., and S.C.M. were responsible for the design of the study. L.F.V.P. and P.M.N. were responsible for the characterization of chitosan samples. A.H. carried out the antifungal assays. F.A. was responsible for the extraction of chitin and the production of chitosan derivatives. S.C.M. evaluated the antioxidant activity. R.P., S.M.L., and F.A. were responsible for the interpretation of the data. F.A. and S.M.L. drafted the article. All authors revised the paper critically for important intellectual content and gave final approval to the version to be published.

Funding: This research was funded by GAC Oeste (PROMAR—European Fisheries Fund) through the project Pilado add value, under the FP7, grant agreement no. 278612 and by Fundação para a Ciência e Tecnologia (FCT), through the strategic project UID/MAR/04292/2019 granted to MARE, the Integrated Programme of SR&TD "Smart Valorization of Endogenous Marine Biological Resources Under a Changing Climate" (Centro-01-0145-FEDER-000018), co-funded by Centro 2020 programme, Portugal 2020, European Union through the European Regional Development Fund and the grant awarded to SCM (SFRH/BPD/110400/2015).

Acknowledgments: The authors would like to thank their colleagues Rui Albuquerque and Pedro Sá (Mare—IP Leiria) for the assistance provided during the preparation of the raw material, as well as Purse seine fishing vessel "Mestre Comboio—Peniche" and Pedro Murraças for providing the swimming crab

Conflicts of Interest: The authors declare no conflict of interest.

References

1. Moreira, A.C.; Caetano, P.; Correia, S.; Brasier, C.M.; Ferraz, J.F.P. Phytophthora species associated with cork oak decline in a Mediterranean forest in in southern Portugal. In Proceedings of the 6th International Congress of Plant Pathology, Montréal, QC, Canada, 28 July–6 August 1993.
2. Droby, S.; Lichter, A. Post-Harvest Botrytis Infection: Etiology, Development and Management. In *Botrytis: Biology, Pathology and Control*; Elad, Y., Williamson, B., Tudzynski, P., Delen, N., Eds.; Springer: Dordrecht, The Netherlands, 2007; pp. 349–367, ISBN 978-1-4020-2626-3.
3. Nuss, D.L. Biological control of chestnut blight: An example of virus-mediated attenuation of fungal pathogenesis. *Microbiol. Rev.* **1992**, *56*, 561–576.
4. Niemelä, T.; Korhonen, K. Taxonomy of the genus Heterobasidion. In *Heterobasidion Annosum: Biology, Ecology, 1988, Impact and Control*; Woodward, S., Stenlid, J., Karjalainen, R., Hu¨ttermann, A., Eds.; CAB International: Wallingford, NY, USA, 2000; pp. 27–33.
5. Smilanick, J.L.; Harvey, J.M.; Hartsell, P.L.; Henson, D.J.; Harris, C.M.; Fouse, D.C.; Assemi, M. Influence of sulfur dioxide fumigant dose on residues and control of postharvest decay of grapes. *Plant Dis. J.* **1990**, *74*, 418–421. [CrossRef]
6. Muzzarelli, R.A.; Rochetti, R.; Stanic, V.; Weckx, M. Methods for the determination of the degree of acetylation of chitin and chitosan. In *Chitin Handbook*; Muzzarelli, R.A.A., Peter, M.G., Eds.; ATEC: College Park, MD, USA, 1997; pp. 109–119.
7. Dutta, P.K.; Tripathi, S.; Mehrotra, G.K.; Dutta, J. Perspectives for chitosan based antimicrobial films in food applications. *Food Chem.* **2009**, *114*, 1173–1182. [CrossRef]
8. Kumar, R.M.N.V. A review of chitin and chitosan applications. Reactive and Functional. *React. Funct. Polym.* **2000**, *46*, 1–27. [CrossRef]
9. Cerdá, C.; Sánchez, C.; Climent, B.; Vázquez, A.; Iradi, A.; El Amrani, F.; Bediaga, A.; Sáez, G.T. Oxidative stress and DNA damage in obesity-related tumorigenesis. *Adv. Exp. Med. Biol.* **2014**, *824*, 5–17. [PubMed]
10. Wölfle, U.; Seelinger, G.; Bauer, G.; Meinke, M.C.; Lademann, J.; Schempp, C.M. Reactive molecule species and antioxidative mechanisms in normal skin and skin aging. *Ski. Pharmacol. Physiol.* **2014**, *27*, 316–332. [CrossRef] [PubMed]
11. Ito, N.; Hirose, M.; Fukushima, H.; Tsuda, T.; Shirai, T.; Tatenatsu, M. Studies on antioxidants: Their carcinogenic and modifying effects on chemical carcinogens. *Food Chem. Toxicol.* **1986**, *24*, 1071–1092. [CrossRef]
12. Ferraro, V.; Cruz, I.B.; Jorge, R.F.; Malcata, F.X.; Pintado, M.E.; Castro, P.M.L. Valorisation of natural extracts from marine source focused on marine by-products: A review. *Food Res. Int.* **2010**, *43*, 2221–2233. [CrossRef]
13. Cartes, J.E.; Abelló, P.; Lloris, D.; Carbonell, A.; Torres, P.; Maynou, F.; Sola, L.G.D. Feeding guilds of western Mediterranean demersal fish and crustaceans: An analysis based on a spring survey. *Sci. Mar.* **2002**, *590*, 209–220. [CrossRef]
14. Serrano, A.; Sánchez, F.; Punzón, A.; Velasco, F.; Olaso, I. Deep sea megafaunal assemblages off the northern Iberian slope related to environmental factors. *Sci. Mar.* **2011**, *75*, 425–437. [CrossRef]
15. Hayward, P.J.; Ryland, J.S. *Handbook of the Marine Fauna of North–West Europe*; Oxford University Press: Oxford, UK, 1995; p. 454.
16. Signa, G.; Cartes, J.E.; Solé, M.; Serrano, A.; Sánchez, F. Trophic ecology of the swimming crab *Polybius henslowii* Leach, 1820 in Galician and Cantabrian Seas: Influences of natural variability and the Prestige oil spill. *Cont. Shelf Res.* **2008**, *28*, 2659–2667. [CrossRef]
17. González-Gurriarán, E. El patexo, Polybius henslowii Leach (Decapoda, Brachyura), en las costas de Galicia (NW de Espanã): I. Distribución espacial y cambios temporales. *Investig. Pesq.* **1987**, *51*, 361–374.
18. Zariquey, R. Crustáceos decápodos ibéricos. *Investig. Pesq.* **1968**, *32*, 83.
19. Abdou, E.S.; Nagy, K.S.A.; Elsabee, M.Z. Extraction and characterization of chitin and chitosan from local sources. *Bioresour. Technol.* **2008**, *99*, 1359–1367. [CrossRef] [PubMed]
20. Krzeczkowski, R.A.; Tenney, R.D.; Kelley, C. Alaska king crab: Fatty acid composition, carotenoid index and proximate analysis. *J. Food Sci.* **2006**, *36*, 604–606. [CrossRef]
21. King, I.; Childs, M.T.; Dorsett, C.; Ostrander, J.G.; Monsen, E.R. Shellfish: Proximate composition, minerals, fatty acids, and sterols. *J. Am. Diet. Assoc.* **1990**, *90*, 677–685.

22. Nalan, G.; Dlua, K.; Yerlikayaa, P. Determination of proximate and mineral contents of blue crab (Callinectes sapidus) and swim crab (*Portunus pelagicus*) caught of the Gulf of Antalya. *Food Chem.* **2003**, *80*, 495–498. [CrossRef]
23. Naczk, M.; Williams, J.; Brennan, K.; Liyanapathirana, C.; Shahidi, F. Compositional characteristics of green crab (*Carcinus maenas*). *Food Chem.* **2004**, *88*, 429–434. [CrossRef]
24. Venugopal, V. *Marine Polysaccharides: Food Applications*; CRC Press Taylor & Francis Group: Boca Raton, FL, USA, 2011; Volume 3, pp. 61–84.
25. Youn, D.K.; No, H.K.; Prinyawiwatkul, W. Physicochemical and functional properties of chitosans prepared from shells of crabs harvested in three different years. *Carbohydr. Polym.* **2009**, *78*, 41–45. [CrossRef]
26. Mahmoud, N.S.; Ghaly, A.E.; Arab, F. Unconventional Approach for Demineralization of Deproteinized Crustacean Shells for Chitin Production. *Am. J. Biochem. Biotechnol.* **2007**, *3*, 1–9. [CrossRef]
27. No, H.K.; Meyers, S.P. Preparation and characterization of chitin and chitosan: A review. *J. Aquat. Food Prod. Technol.* **1995**, *4*, 27–52. [CrossRef]
28. Benhabile, M.S.; Salah, R.; Lounici, H.; Drouiche, N.; Goosen, M.F.A.; Mameri, N. Antibacterial activity of chitin, chitosan and its oligomers prepared from shrimp shell waste. *Food Hydrol.* **2012**, *29*, 48–56. [CrossRef]
29. Yen, M.-T.; Yang, J.-H.; Mau, J.-L. Physicochemical characterization of chitin and chitosan from crab shells. *Carbohydr. Polym.* **2009**, *75*, 15–21. [CrossRef]
30. Al-Sagheer, F.A.; Al-Sughayer, M.A.; Muslim, S.; Elsabee, M.Z. Extraction and characterization of chitin and chitosan from marine sources in Arabian Gulf. Carbohydate. *Polymerst* **2009**, *77*, 410–419.
31. Barroca-Aubry, N.; Pernet-Poil-Chevrier, A.; Domard, A.; Trombotto, S. Towards a modular synthesis of well-defined chitooligosaccharides: Synthesis of the four chitodisaccharides. *Carbohydr. Res.* **2010**, *345*, 1685–1697. [CrossRef]
32. Du, Y.; Zhao, Y.; Dai, S.; Yang, B. Preparation of water-soluble chitosan from shrimp shell and its antibacterial activity. *Innov. Food Sci. Emerg. Technol.* **2009**, *10*, 103–107. [CrossRef]
33. Tian, F.; Liu, Y.; Hu, K.; Zhao, B. Study of the depolymerization behavior of chitosan by hydrogen peroxide. *Carbohydr. Polym.* **2004**, *57*, 31–37. [CrossRef]
34. Lu, S.; Song, X.; Cao, D.; Chen, Y.; Yao, K. Preparation of Water-Soluble Chitosan. *J. Appl. Polym. Sci.* **2004**, *685*, 3497–3503. [CrossRef]
35. Yamaguchi, T.; Takamura, H.; Matoba, T.; Terao, J. HPLC method for evaluation of the free radical-scavenging activity of foods by using 1,1,-diphenyl-2-picrylhydrazyl. *Biosci. Biotechnol. Biochem.* **1998**, *62*, 1201–1204. [CrossRef] [PubMed]
36. Kim, K.W.; Thomas, R.L. Antioxidative activity of chitosan's with varying molecular weight. *Food Chem.* **2007**, *101*, 308–313. [CrossRef]
37. Samar, M.M.; El-Kalyoubi, M.H.; Khalaf, M.M.; El-Razik, M.M.A. Physicochemical, functional, antioxidant and antibacterial properties of chitosan extracted from shrimp wastes by microwave technique. *Ann. Agric. Sci.* **2013**, *58*, 33–41. [CrossRef]
38. Xie, W.; Xu, P.; Liu, Q. Antioxidant activity of water-soluble chitosan derivatives. *Bioorgan. Med. Chem. Lett.* **2001**, *11*, 1699–1701. [CrossRef]
39. Je, J.Y.; Kim, S.K. Reactive oxygen species scavenging activity of aminoderivatized chitosan with different 651 degree of deacetylation. *Bioorgan. Med. Chem.* **2006**, *14*, 5989–5994. [CrossRef]
40. Chien, P.J.; Sheu, F.; Huang, W.T.; Su, M.S. Antioxidant Polymers: Synthesis, Properties, and Applications. *Food Chem.* **2007**, *102*, 1192. [CrossRef]
41. Yen, M.-T.; Yang, J.-H.; Mau, J.-L. Antioxidant properties of chitosan from crab shells. *Carbohydr. Polym.* **2008**, *74*, 840–844. [CrossRef]
42. Korycka-Dahl, M.; Richardson, T. Photogeneration of superoxide anion in serum of bovine milk and in model systems containing riboflavin and amino acids. *J. Dairy Sci.* **1978**, *61*, 400–407. [CrossRef]
43. Bloknina, O.; Virolainen, E.; Fagerstedt, K.V. Antioxidants, oxidative damage and oxygen deprivation stress: A review. *Ann. Bot.* **2003**, *91*, 179–194. [CrossRef]
44. Meyer, A.S.; Isaksen, A. Application of enzymes as food antioxidants. *Trends Food Sci. Technol.* **1995**, *6*, 300. [CrossRef]
45. Feng, T.; Du, Y.M.; Li, J.; Hu, Y.; Kennedy, J.F. Enhancement of antioxidant activity of chitosan by irradiation. *Carbohydr. Polym.* **2008**, *73*, 126–132. [CrossRef]

46. Xing, R.; Liu, S.; Guo, Z.; Yu, H.; Wang, P.; Li, C.; Li, Z.; Li, P. Relevance of molecular weight of chitosan and its derivatives and their antioxidant activities in vitro. *Bioorgan. Med. Chem.* **2005**, *13*, 1573–1577. [CrossRef]
47. Yang, Y.; Shu, R.; Shao, J.; Xu, G.; Gu, X. Radical scavenging activity of chitooligosaccharide with different molecular weights. *Eur. Food Res. Technol.* **2006**, *222*, 36–40. [CrossRef]
48. Charernsriwilaiwat, N.; Opanasopit, P.; Rojanarata, T.; Ngawhirunpat, T. In Vitro Antioxidant Activity of Chitosan Aqueous Solution: Effect of Salt Form. *Trop. J. Pharm. Res.* **2012**, *11*, 235–242. [CrossRef]
49. Halliwell, B.; Aeschbach, R.; Löliger, J.; Aruoma, O.I. The characterization of antioxidants. *Food Chem. Toxicol.* **1995**, *33*, 601–617. [CrossRef]
50. Tikhonov, V.E.; Radigina, L.A.; Yamskov, Y.A. Metal-chelating chitin derivatives via reaction of chitosan with nitrilotriacetic acid. *Carbohydr. Res.* **1996**, *290*, 33–41. [CrossRef]
51. Lin, H.-Y.; Chou, C.-C. Antioxidative activities of water-soluble disaccharide chitosan derivatives. *Food Res. Int.* **2004**, *37*, 883–889. [CrossRef]
52. Milosavljevic, N.B.; Ristica, M.D.; Peric-Grujic, A.A.; Filipovic, J.M.; Strbacb, S.B.; Rakocevic, Z.L.; Krusic, M.T.K. Sorption of zinc by novel pH-sensitive hydrogels based on chitosan, itaconic acid and methacrylic acid. *J. Hazard. Mater.* **2011**, *192*, 846–854. [CrossRef] [PubMed]
53. Kurita, K. Chitin and Chitosan: Functional biopolymers from marine crustaceans. *Mar. Biotechnol.* **2006**, *8*, 203–226. [CrossRef]
54. Qin, Y. The chelating properties of chitosan fibers. *J. Appl. Polym. Sci.* **1993**, *49*, 727–731. [CrossRef]
55. Kong, M.; Chen, X.G.; Xing, K.; Park, H.J. Antimicrobial properties of chitosan and mode of action: A state of the art review. *Int. J. Food Microbiol.* **2010**, *144*, 51–63. [CrossRef]
56. Liu, J.; Tian, S.; Meng, X.; Xu, Y. Effects of chitosan on control of postharvest diseases and physiological responses of tomato fruit. *Postharvest Biol. Technol.* **2007**, *44*, 300–306. [CrossRef]
57. Skjak-Braek, G.; Anthonsen, T.; Sandford, P.A. *Chitin and Chitosan: Sources, Chemistry, Biochemistry, Physical Properties and Applications*; Springer: Dordrecht, The Netherlands, 1989; ISBN 978-1-85166-395-8.
58. Jeon, Y. Antimicrobial effect of chitooligosaccharides produced by bioreactor. *Carbohydr. Polym.* **2001**, *44*, 71–76. [CrossRef]
59. No, H.K.; Young Park, N.; Ho Lee, S.; Meyers, S.P. Antibacterial activity of chitosans and chitosan oligomers with different molecular weights. *Int. J. Food Microbiol.* **2002**, *74*, 65–72. [CrossRef]
60. Singh, T.; Vesentini, D.; Singh, A.P.; Daniel, G. Effect of chitosan on physiological, morphological, and ultrastructural characteristics of wood-degrading fungi. *Int. Biodeterior. Biodegrad.* **2008**, *62*, 116–124. [CrossRef]
61. Ing, L.Y.; Zin, N.M.; Sarwar, A.; Katas, H. Antifungal Activity of Chitosan Nanoparticles and Correlation with Their Physical Properties. *J. Appl. Polym. Sci.* **2012**, *2012*, 632698. [CrossRef] [PubMed]
62. Vallapa, N.; Wiarachai, O.; Thongchul, N.; Pan, J.; Tangpasuthadol, V.; Kiatkamjornwong, S.; Hoven, V.P. Enhancing antibacterial activity of chitosan surface by heterogeneous quaternization. *Carbohydr. Polym.* **2011**, *83*, 868–875. [CrossRef]
63. Wiarachai, O.; Thongchul, N.; Kiatkamjornwong, S.; Hoven, V.P. Surface-quaternized chitosan particles as an alternative and effective organic antibacterial material. *Colloids Surf.* **2012**, *92*, 121–129. [CrossRef]
64. Guo, Z.; Xing, R.; Liu, S.; Zhong, Z.; Ji, X.; Wang, L.; Li, P. Antifungal properties of Schiff bases of chitosan, 629 N-substituted chitosan and quaternized chitosan. *Carbohydr. Res.* **2007**, *342*, 1329–1332. [CrossRef]
65. Galván Márquez, I.; Akuaku, J.; Cruz, I.; Cheetham, J.; Golshani, A.; Smith, M.L. Disruption of protein synthesis as antifungal mode of action by chitosan. *Int. J. Food Microbiol.* **2013**, *164*, 108–112. [CrossRef]
66. Johnson, M.K. Variable Sensitivity in Microbiuret Assay of Protein. *Anal. Biochem.* **1978**, *86*, 320–323. [CrossRef]
67. *ISO 1444 (1996)*; International Organisation for Standardisation: Geneva, Switzerland, 1996.
68. Haastert-Talini, K.; Geuna, S.; Dahlin, L.B.; Meyer, C.; Stenberg, L.; Freier, T.; Heimann, C.; Barwig, C.; Pinto, L.F.V.; Raimondo, S.; et al. Chitosan tubes of varying degrees of acetylation for bridging peripheral nerve defects. *Biomaterials* **2013**, *34*, 9886–9904. [CrossRef]
69. Brugnerotto, J.; Lizardi, J.; Goycoolea, F.M.; Argüelles-Monal, W.; Desbrières, J.; Rinaudo, M. An infrared investigation in relation with chitin and chitosan characterization. *Polymer* **2001**, *42*, 3569–3580. [CrossRef]
70. Shimada, K.; Fujikawa, K.; Yahara, K.; Nakamura, T. Antioxidative properties of xanthan on the autoxidation of soybean oil in cyclodextrin emulsion. *J. Agric. Food Chem.* **1992**, *40*, 945–948. [CrossRef]

71. Nishikimi, M. Oxidation of ascorbic acid with superoxide anion generated by the xanthine-xanthine oxidase system. *Biochem. Biophys. Res. Commun.* **1975**, *63*, 463–468. [CrossRef]
72. Decker, E.A.; Welch, B. Role of ferritin as a lipid oxidation catalyst in muscle food. *J. Agric. Food Chem. (USA)* **1990**, *38*, 674–677. [CrossRef]
73. El Ghaouth, A.; Arul, J.; Grenier, J.; Asselin, A. Antifungal activity of chitosan on two post-harvest 618 pathogens of strawberry fruits. *Phytopathology* **1992**, *82*, 398–402. [CrossRef]

marine drugs

Article

Production of a Thermostable Chitosanase from Shrimp Heads via *Paenibacillus mucilaginosus* TKU032 Conversion and its Application in the Preparation of Bioactive Chitosan Oligosaccharides

Chien Thang Doan [1,2], Thi Ngoc Tran [1,2], Van Bon Nguyen [2], Anh Dzung Nguyen [3] and San-Lang Wang [1,4,*]

1 Department of Chemistry, Tamkang University, New Taipei City 25137, Taiwan; doanthng@gmail.com (C.T.D.); tranngoctnu@gmail.com (T.N.T.)
2 Department of Science and Technology, Tay Nguyen University, Buon Ma Thuot 630000, Vietnam; bondhtn@gmail.com
3 Institute of Biotechnology and Environment, Tay Nguyen University, Buon Ma Thuot 630000, Vietnam; nadzungtaynguyenuni@yahoo.com.vn
4 Life Science Development Center, Tamkang University, New Taipei City 25137, Taiwan
* Correspondence: sabulo@mail.tku.edu.tw; Tel.: +886-2-2621-5656; Fax: +886-2-2620-9924

Received: 19 March 2019; Accepted: 9 April 2019; Published: 10 April 2019

Abstract: Chitosanase has attracted great attention due to its potential applications in medicine, agriculture, and nutraceuticals. In this study, *P. mucilaginosus* TKU032, a bacterial strain isolated from Taiwanese soil, exhibited the highest chitosanase activity (0.53 U/mL) on medium containing shrimp heads as the sole carbon and nitrogen (C/N) source. Using sodium dodecyl sulfate-polyacrylamide gel electrophoresis (SDS-PAGE) analysis, a chitosanase isolated from *P. mucilaginosus* TKU032 cultured on shrimp head medium was determined at approximately 59 kDa. The characterized chitosanase showed interesting properties with optimal temperature and thermal stability up to 70 °C. Three chitosan oligosaccharide (COS) fractions were isolated from hydrolyzed colloidal chitosan that was catalyzed by TKU032 chitosanase. Of these, fraction I showed the highest α-glucosidase inhibitor (aGI) activity (65.86% at 20 mg/mL); its inhibitory mechanism followed the mixed noncompetitive inhibition model. Fractions II and III exhibited strong 2,2-diphenyl1-picrylhydrazyl (DPPH) radical scavenging activity (79.00% at 12 mg/mL and 73.29% at 16 mg/mL, respectively). In summary, the COS fractions obtained by hydrolyzing colloidal chitosan with TKU032 chitosanase may have potential use in medical or nutraceutical fields due to their aGI and antioxidant activities.

Keywords: chitin; chitosan; *Paenibacillus*; chitosanase; chitosan oligomers; α-glucosidase inhibitor; antioxidant

1. Introduction

Chitosan is a polymer composed of β-1,4 linked D-glucosamine with varying amounts (under 50%) of *N*-acetyl-D-glucosamine [1]. Chitosan is of interest to many researchers as it exhibits various biological activities and has many biotechnological uses [2–4]. Unfortunately, chitosan has poor solubility at neutral pH, potentially limiting its application. Chitosan oligosaccharides (COS) are products obtained from hydrolyzed chitosan with an average MW of less than 3900 Da and degrees of polymerization (DP) under 20 [5]. Unlike chitosan, COS possess great solubility in water. Furthermore, COS also demonstrate antidiabetic [6,7], prebiotic [8,9], antioxidant [5,8], anti-inflammatory [5,10], anticancer [10], antitumor [11], and antibacterial biological activities [12,13]. The enzymatic method was recently reported as an efficient and environmentally friendly process for producing bioactive

COS [5,8,9,14–16]. However, the high cost of enzyme production limits its application on a larger scale. As such, an inexpensive and efficient protocol for producing chitinolytic enzymes and converting chitosan into bioactive COS is needed.

Chitosanase (EC 3.2.1.132) is a group of enzymes which hydrolyzes chitosan [17]. It is a useful tool for depolymerizing chitosan into oligosaccharides with various biological activities and degrees of DP [5,9]. Important sources for chitosanase production have primarily been found in bacteria, including *Paenibacillus* [9,18], *Bacillus* [5,19–23], *Serratia* [24], and *Streptomyces* [25]. Until now, the common C/N sources for chitosanase production via bacteria were chitin and chitosan. Commercialized chitin and chitosan products are mostly prepared from fish processing by-products, such as shrimp shells, crab shells, or squid pens, using chemical methods like strong alkaline and acid treatments to remove proteins and mineral salts. To reduce costs, shrimp shells, shrimp heads, crab shells and squid pens have been used as the sole C/N sources for enzyme production via microbial conversion [18–22,26–31].

Recently, several strains of *Paenibacillus* showed excellent ability in producing α-glucosidase inhibitors [32–36], proteases [18], chitosanase [9,18], and exopolysaccharides [37,38] when marine chitinous materials were used as the sole C/N source. In the previous report, *P. mucilaginosus* TKU032, a bacterial strain isolated from Taiwanese soil, produced exopolysaccharides with high antioxidant activity from a medium containing squid pens [37]. Moreover, the culture supernatant also showed chitinolytic, proteolytic and aGI activities [18]. This suggests that *P. mucilaginosus* TKU032 has the potential to produce various biological activities using low-cost chitinous materials. However, an investigation into TKU032's enzyme production was not fully explored.

In this study, chitosanase production of *P. mucilaginosus* TKU032 was tested using four kinds of marine chitinous materials: squid pens powder (SPP), shrimp heads powder (SHP), demineralized shrimp shells powder (deSSP), and demineralized crab shells powder (deCSP) to determine the most suitable C/N source for bioconversion. The isolation and characterization of *P. mucilaginosus* TKU032 chitosanase was performed. Furthermore, the COS obtained by hydrolyzing colloidal chitosan with *P. mucilaginosus* TKU032 chitosanase were fractionated and characterized. The aGI and antioxidant activities of the COS fractions were also estimated and compared to commercial compounds.

2. Results and Discussion

2.1. Screening of Chitinous Materials as Sole C/N Source for Chitosanase Production

To explore chitosanase production by *P. mucilaginosus* TKU032, four chitinous materials from fish processing (SPP, SHP, deCSP, and deSSP) were used as the sole C/N sources during incubation. As shown in Figure 1, TKU032 chitosanase was found to exhibit the highest activity at day 2 of the cultivation on all types of chitinous material sources, in which the maximum enzyme activity was expressed with SHP (0.53 U/mL) higher than SPP (0.42 U/mL, p-value 0.0384), deCSP (0.25 U/mL, p-value 0.0028), and deSSP (0.18 U/mL, p-value 0.0005), respectively. The reason might be related to the difference in protein/chitin/mineral salts ratio of each chitinous material, in which SHP contents had higher amounts of protein and mineral salts but lower amount of chitin than those of the other materials [36,39]. This result was also unlike previous reports, which suggested that chitosanase from *Paenibacillus* strains often show the highest activity on medium containing SPP [9,18].

In the search to find a suitable and cost effective source for producing bioactive compounds via microorganism conversion, shrimp heads, a by-product from shrimp processing, were suggested as potential material as they have been reported as the best sole C/N source for producing chitosanase (*B. cereus* TKU027) [14], aGI (*Staphylococcus* sp. TKU043) [29], nattokinase (*B. subtilis* TKU007) [30], and protease (*B. cereus* TKU022, *B. licheniformis* TKU004) [22,31]. Since TKU032 showed the highest chitosanase activity on medium containing SHP, it was chosen as the sole C/N source.

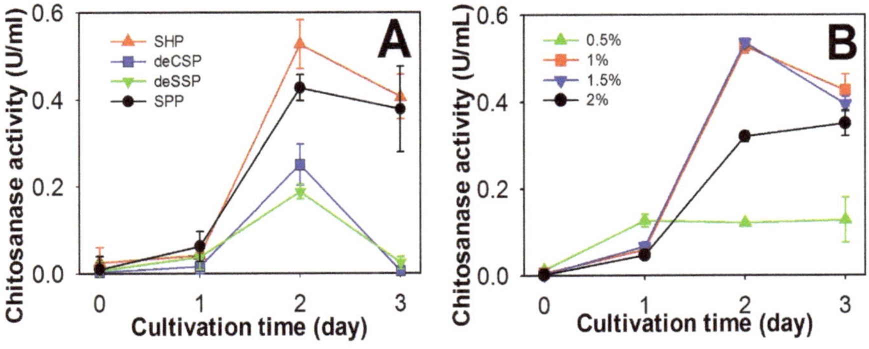

Figure 1. Production of chitosanase by *P. mulaginosus* TKU032; (**A**) using different chitin-containing materials as the C/N source; (**B**) using different concentrations of SHP.

Further experimentation determined the optimal SHP concentration for chitosanase conversion by *P. mulaginosus* TKU032. As shown in Figure 1B, the highest chitosanase activity was found at 1% SHP (0.53 U/mL) and 1.5% SHP (0.54 U/mL). Since there was no significant difference in maximum chitosanase activity (*p*-value 0.5037) and less material loss, 1% SHP was chosen for subsequent experiments.

2.2. Comparison of Chitosanase Production from SHP Using Different Bacteria

Chitinase/chitosanase production by chitinolytic *Paenibacillus* and *Bacillus* strains on SPP and deCSP-containing media were introduced in our previous report [18]. In this study, the potency of SHP in chitinase/chitosanase production via microorganism conversion was also investigated. The results in Table 1 show that all tested species of *Paenibacillus* and *Bacillus* exhibited chitinase and chitosanase activities. The highest chitosanase and chitinase activities were found in *P. mucilaginosus* TKU032 (0.58 U/mL and 0.37 U/mL) and *P. macerans* TKU029 (0.59 U/mL and 0.28 U/mL) with no significant difference in their activities (0.88 and 0.1563 of *p*-value, respectively); the results were better than those of *Paenibacillus* sp. TKU037 (0.05 U/mL and 0.06 U/mL), *Paenibacillus* sp. TKU042 (0.12 U/mL and 0.12 U/mL), *B. subtillis* TKU007 (0.05 U/mL and 0.11 U/mL), and *B. licheniformis* TKU004 (0.01 U/mL and 0.04 U/mL) with a *p*-value range from 0.0004 to 0.0025. By expressing the higher chitinolytic activity on chitosan (0.58 U/mL) than on chitin (0.37 U/mL), *P. mucilaginosus* TKU032 could be considered as a chitosanase-producing bacterium. Similar to the previous study, none of the tested *Paenibacillus* species, including *P. mucilaginosus* TKU032, showed exochitinase activity [18]. Taken together, this result confirmed that SHP was the most suitable C/N source for chitosanase production via *P. mucilaginosus* TKU032 conversion.

Table 1. Comparison of chitosanase, chitinase, and exochitinase production by different *Paenibacillus* and *Bacillus* strains.

Bacterial Strain	Chitosanase Activity (U/mL)	Chitinase Activity (U/mL)	Exochitinase Activity (U/mL)
P. mucilaginosus TKU032	0.58 ± 0.10	0.37 ± 0.04	-
P. macerans TKU029	0.59 ± 0.04	0.28 ± 0.08	-
Paenibacillus sp. TKU037	0.05 ± 0.02	0.06 ± 0.05	-
Paenibacillus sp. TKU042	0.12 ± 0.04	0.12 ± 0.05	-
Bacillus licheniformis TKU004	0.01 ± 0.01	0.04 ± 0.01	10.21 ± 0.89
B. subtillis TKU007	0.05 ± 0.02	0.11 ± 0.01	-

Bacterial strains were cultured in 100 mL of liquid medium in an Erlenmeyer flask (250 mL) containing 1% SHP, 0.1% K_2HPO_4 and 0.05% $MgSO_4 \cdot 7H_2O$ in a shaking incubator for 2 d at 37 °C.

2.3. *Purification and Characterization of Chitosanase*

In order to characterize TKU032 chitosanase, a series of steps was used to purify the enzyme, including $(NH_4)_2SO_4$ precipitation, Macro-prep High S ion exchange chromatography and KW802.5 gel filtration. The chitosanase was eluted by 20 mM Tris-HCl buffer (pH 7) with a linear gradient of 0–1 M NaCl on a Macro-prep High S column. As shown in Figure 2, there was only one peak of chitosanase activity, located at the washing stage of the ion-exchange chromatography separation. This result indicated that pI of TKU032 chitosanase might be $\geq$7. The peak fractions (fraction numbers 5-15) showing chitosanase activity were collected. After Macro-Prep High S chromatography, 15.98 mg of protein was obtained with an increase in the specific activity from 0.7 U/mg to 4.25 U/mg and a slight reduction in the activity yield from 31.69% to 24.06%. The purification was then confirmed by HPLC gel filtration using the KW802.5 column. Similar to the ion-exchange chromatography, only one peak of chitosanase activity was found by the HPLC analysis (data not showed). After purification, one chitosanase was obtained; its profile is summarized in Table 2. In other reports, only one chitinase/chitosanase was isolated from the culture medium of *Paenibacillus* species [1,9,18,40–48]. The specific activity and recovery yield of the purified chitosanase were 5.13 U/mg and 10.94%, respectively. By using SDS-PAGE analysis, the molecular weight (MW) of the TKU032 chitosanase was determined as approximately 59 kDa (Figure 3), which fell within the MW's range (35–85 kDa) of chitinase/chitosanase from most *Paenibacillus* strains [1,9,18,40–48], with an exception from *Paenibacillus* sp. FPU-7 chitinase (150 kDa) [49].

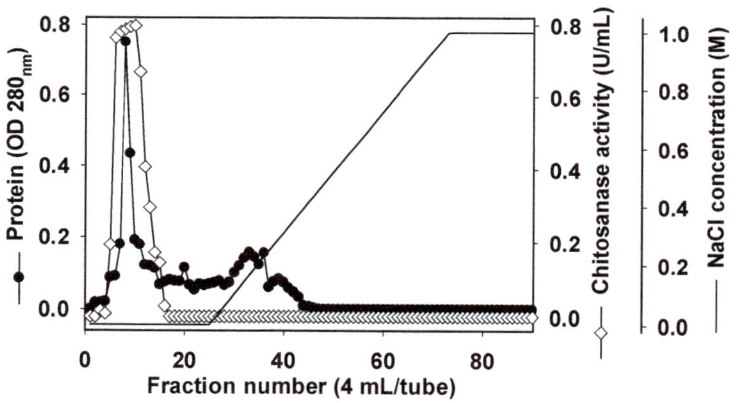

Figure 2. A typical elution profile of chitosanase on Macro-prep High S column.

Table 2. Purification of chitosanase from *P. mucilaginosus* TKU032.

Step	Total Protein (mg)	Total Activity (U)	Specific Activity (U/mg)	Recovery (%)	Purification (Fold)
Cultural supernatant	1499.13	282.28	0.19	100.00	1.00
$(NH_4)_2SO_4$ precipitation	126.97	89.44	0.70	31.69	3.74
Macro-Prep High S	15.98	67.92	4.25	24.06	22.57
KW-802.5	5.13	30.89	6.03	10.94	32.01

P. mucilaginosus TKU032 was cultured in 100 mL of liquid medium in an Erlenmeyer flask (250 mL) containing 1% SHP, 0.1% K_2HPO_4 and 0.05% $MgSO_4{\cdot}7H_2O$ in a shaking incubator for 2 d at 37 °C.

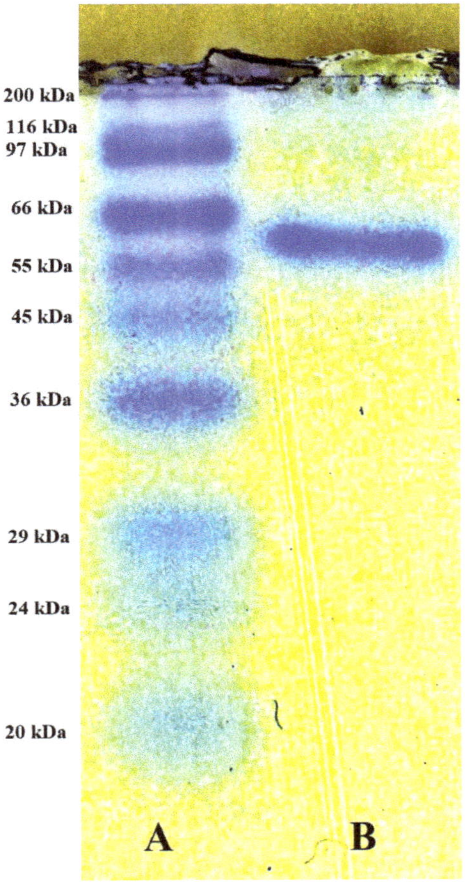

Figure 3. SDS-PAGE analysis of the chitosanase produced by TKU032. A: protein markers; B: Purified chitosanase.

2.4. Effects of pH and Temperature on Activity and Stability of Chitosanase

The effect of pH on *P. mucilaginosus* TKU032 chitosanase is shown in Figure 4A. The optimum pH for the enzyme was 6.0. This result is consistent with most research, which showed chitinase/chitosanase from *Paenibacillus* species expressing the highest activity in acidic conditions [1,41,45–47], with the exceptions of *P. macerans* TKU029 [9], *P. pasadenensis* NCIM5434 [43] and *P. elgii* HOA73 [42]. *P. mucilaginusus* TKU032 was stable over a broad pH range (Figure 4A), with over 80% of activity retained from pH 4 to 8. Once the pH dropped below 4, activity disappeared completely, whereas 50% of activity was retained at pH 9. Several chitinase/chitosanase from *Paenibacillus* showed the same broad pH stability as *P. mucilaginosus* TKU032 [9,46,48,50].

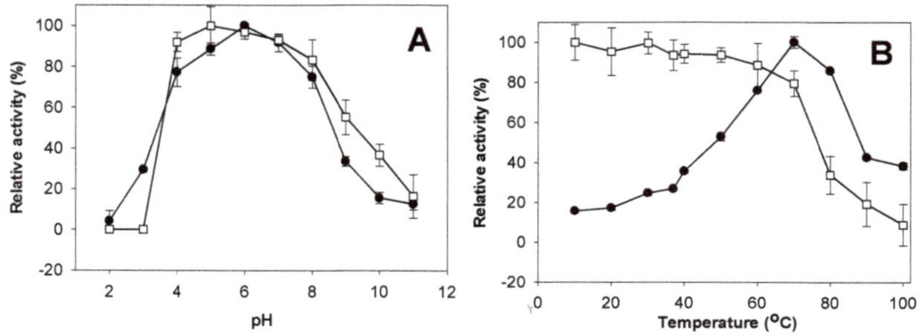

Figure 4. Effect of pH (**A**) and temperature (**B**) on activity (•) and stability (□) of TKU032 chitosanase.

The effect of temperature on the activity and stability of *P. mucilaginosus* TKU032 chitosanase were studied herein (Figure 4B). The optimal temperature was 70 °C, but even at 80 °C, it still showed more than 80% activity. *P. mucilaginosus* TKU032 chitosanase demonstrated thermal stability up to 70 °C, with over 80% of activity retained. This suggests that both the optimal temperature and thermal stability of *P. mucilaginosus* TKU032 chitosanase were higher than most chitinase/chitosanase from other *Paenibacillus* species [9,41–47]; only a chitosanase from *Paenibacillus* sp. 1794 showed similar results [1]. Due to its higher thermal stability, *P. mucilaginosus* TKU032 chitosanase may have potential use in industrial applications.

2.5. Effect of Metal Ions on Activity of Chitosanase

The effects of known divalent metals and enzyme inhibitors on the activity of TKU032 chitosanase were examined; the results are summarized in Table 3. All chemicals reduced the activity of TKU032 chitosanase, a result markedly different from other reports, which showed that the addition of some metal ions, Na^{+} and Fe^{2+} for instance, could enhance the activity of chitosanases from *Paenibacillus* [9,50].

Table 3. Effect of metal ions on the activity of chitosanase

Metal Ion	Relative Activity (%)
Control	100.00 ± 6.39
Cu^{2+}	74.37 ± 3.95
Zn^{2+}	76.78 ± 3.25
Mg^{2+}	84.39 ± 4.51
Na^{+}	91.71 ± 5.21
Ba^{2+}	62.14 ± 12.29
Ca^{2+}	77.07 ± 5.68
Fe^{2+}	65.13 ± 6.77
EDTA	84.39 ± 7.53

2.6. Substrate Specificity of Chitosanase

The activity of the purified *P. mucilaginosus* TKU032 chitosanase on various substrates is shown in Figure 5. Chitosanase activity was expressed in the descending order of colloidal chitosan > cellulose > chitosan > colloidal chitin > water-soluble chitosan > β-chitin > α-chitin. No activity was shown on dextran, starch, or *p*-nitrophenyl-*N*-acetyl-β-D-glucosaminide (*p*NPG). These results suggest that the physical form of the substrate had a strong effect on the rate of hydrolysis. Unlike *P. macerans* TKU029 chitosanase, where the most suitable substrate was water-soluble chitosan [9], *P. mucilaginosus* TKU032 chitosanase demonstrated excellent activity on colloidal chitosan (338.74%), followed by chitosan powder (185.38%). It also showed good activity on chitin substrates, expressing 113.24%, 67.19%, and 27.67% on colloidal chitin, β-chitin, and α-chitin, respectively, as well as on cellulose

(196.84%). These results indicate that *P. mucilaginosus* TKU032 chitosanase could express good activity on various types of substrates, including cellulose, chitin, and chitosan. Since *p*NPG is a specific substrate of exochitinase, it was logical that *P. mucilaginosus* TKU032 chitosanase would not show any exochitinase activity.

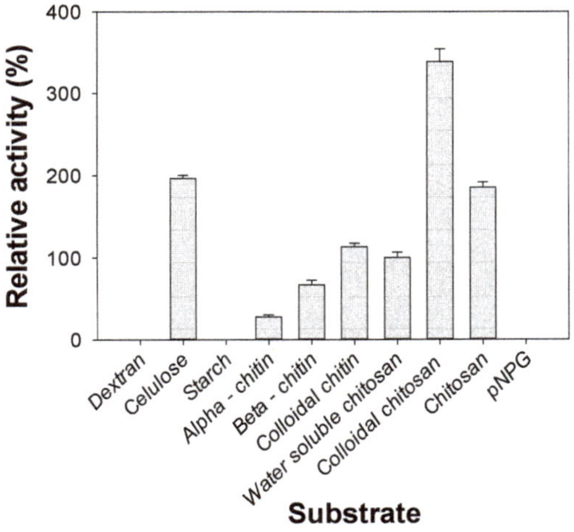

Figure 5. Substrate specificity of *P. mucilaginosus* TKU032 chitosanase.

2.7. COS Production

Since *P. mucilaginosus* TKU032 chitosanase expressed the best activity on colloidal chitosan, this substrate was used to produce COS using the enzyme hydrolysis method. After the reaction finished, a series of steps were used to separate COS from the hydrolyzed solution, including pH neutralization, centrifugation, and dialysis by a 10,000 Da membrane. The obtained COS was then fractionated by MeOH 90% precipitation and gel filtration on a Toyopearl HW-40f column. As shown in Figure 6, 3 COS fractions were collected from the hydrolyzed chitosan solution. The molecular weights of the obtained fractions were determined by HPLC analysis using a KS-802 column (Figure 7). The molecular weights of fractions I, II, and III were approximately 1600-6500 Da, 424-6500 Da, and 221-424 Da, respectively. Fraction I only contained COS with higher MW, while fraction II was a mixture of COS with high and low MW, and fraction III included COS with the lowest MW. Compared to the reference peaks, fraction III mainly contained COS with DP from 1 to 2.

2.8. Evaluation of Antioxidant and aGI Activities of COS Fractions

Free radicals negatively affect living organisms, resulting in DNA mutation, lipid and protein damage, cancer, and cardiovascular or neurodegenerative diseases [51]. The harmful actions of free radicals could be reduced or prevented by antioxidant compounds. In the current study, the DPPH radical scavenging ability was assayed to explore the antioxidant activity of the three obtained COS fractions. As shown in Figure 8A, within a concentration range of 1–20 mg/mL, only fractions II and III showed DPPH radical scavenging activity with a dose-dependent increase. The maximum antioxidant activity of fraction II was 79.00% at a concentration of 12 mg/mL, while fraction III was 73.29% at 16 mg/mL. This suggests that fraction II is the strongest antioxidant among the three fractions. It is well known that COS is a potential candidate for antioxidant activity; however, its antioxidant ability was strongly affected by its MW [5,8]. The obtained results indicated that COS with lower MW could possess higher antioxidant activity. Moreover, this study also showed that low MW COS with DP > 2 expressed higher DPPH radical scavenging activity than COS with DP ≤ 2. Compared to ascorbic acid, a commercial antioxidant compound, fraction II expressed weaker activity. The two compounds generated maximum activity at concentrations of 4 mg/mL and 12 mg/mL, respectively. However, as there was no significant difference (*p*-value 0.404) between the maximum activity of ascorbic acid (82.29%) and fraction II (79.00%), fraction II may have comparable antioxidant activity. As such, COS fraction II could be an acceptable antioxidant compound for use in the medical or food industries.

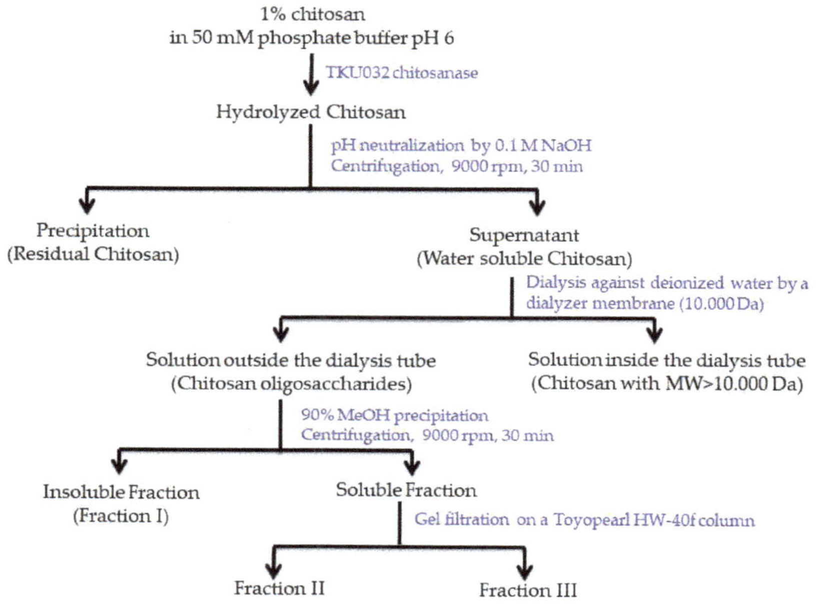

Figure 6. Flow chart for the isolation of COS produced by hydrolyzing chitosan with TKU032 chitosanase

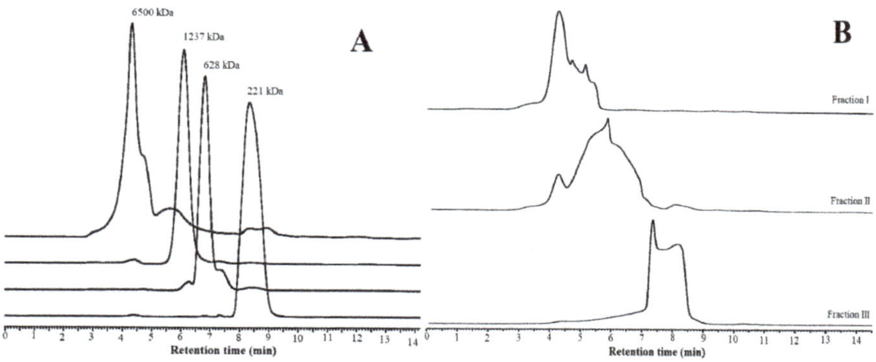

Figure 7. HPLC profiles of chitosan oligosaccharide fractions: (**A**) references; (**B**) chitosan oligosaccharide fractions

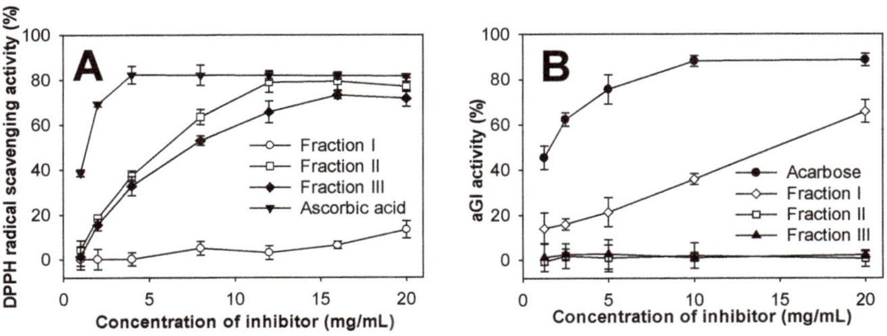

Figure 8. (**A**) antioxidant and (**B**) aGI activities of COS fractions.

As α-glucosidase inhibitors are an important therapy for type 2 diabetes, the COS fractions were also investigated for α-glucosidase inhibitor activity. As shown in Figure 8B, only fraction I expressed dose-dependent aGI activity within a range of 1–20 mg/mL. At 20 mg/mL, fraction I exhibited 65.86% inhibitory activity on yeast α-glucosidase, which was weaker than acarbose (88.21% at 10 mg/mL) with 0.0005 of p-value. Only COS with higher MW showed aGI activity, unlike the results of Jo et al. (2013) who found similar aGI activity in rat α-glucosidase from 3 different molecular weight COS fractions [6]. For further investigation, the inhibition model of fraction I on yeast α-glucosidase was analyzed using a Lineweaver-Burk plot. Figure 9 shows that when the concentration of COS fraction I increased from 0 to 20 mg/mL, $1/V_M$ increased but $-1/K_M$ varied. This suggests that the aGI activity of COS fraction I follows the mixed noncompetitive inhibition model. Although chitosan and COS have been widely studied for treating diabetes [52], there have been few reports on their inhibition of α-glucosidase, a key enzyme in the digestive system that hydrolyzes dietary carbohydrates to increase blood glucose concentration. As such, this result could prove a novel contribution to aGI research.

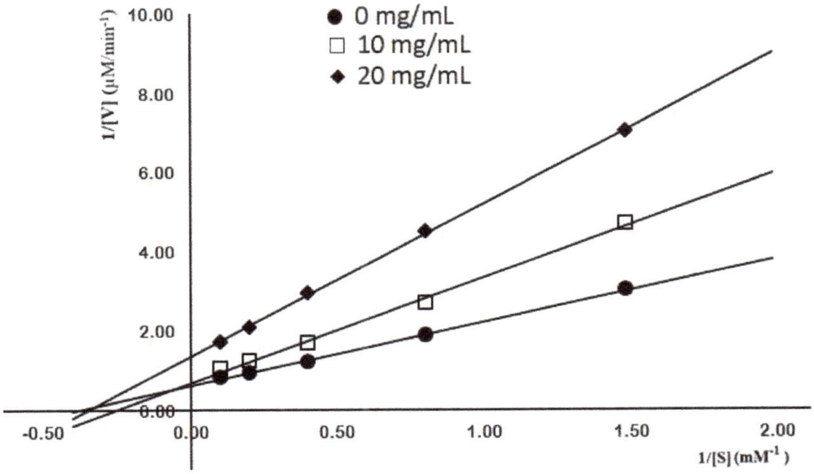

Figure 9. Lineweaver-Burk plot analysis of aGI activity by COS fraction I.

3. Materials and Methods

3.1. Materials

Shrimp shells, squid pens, and crab shells were purchased from Shin-Ma Frozen Food Co. (I-Lan, Taiwan). Shrimp heads was bought from Fwu-Sow Industry (Taichun, Taiwan). Shrimp shells and crab shells were demineralized by acid treatment [8]. All bacterial strains were provided by the Microorganisms and Biochemistry Laboratory, Department of Chemistry, Tamkang University, New Taipei, Taiwan. Chitosan, DPPH, yeast α-glucosidase and 3,5-dinitrosalicylic acid (DNS) reagents were all bought from Sigma-Aldrich Corp. (Singapore). Macro-Prep High S was bought from Bio-Rad (Hercules, CA, USA). All other reagents used were the highest grade available.

3.2. *Measurement of Chitosanase Activity*

The chitosanase activity assay was modified from previously described methods [18]. The substrate solution was prepared by adding water-soluble chitosan into 20 mM Tris-HCl buffer at pH 7 to reach a final concentration of 1% (w/v). The hydrolysis reaction of chitosan was performed with 100 μL of the sample and 100 μl of substrate, and maintained at 37 °C in an incubator for 30 min. The DNS method was used to detect the amount of reducing sugar produced, with D-glucosamine used as the reference. The definition of a unit of chitosanase activity was the amount of enzyme catalyzed to produce 1 μmol of reducing sugar in one min.

3.3. *Screening of Chitinous Materials as Sole C/N Source for Chitosanase Activity*

Four fishery by-products: deCSP, SPP, SHP, and deSSP, were added to 100 mL of basal medium (0.1% K_2HPO_4 and 0.05% $MgSO4{\cdot}7H_2O$) in 250 mL Erlenmeyer flasks at similar concentrations (1%) [9]. Fermentation was performed with 1% of seed culture at 37 °C and a shaking speed of 150 rpm for 3 d. The culture supernatant was measured daily for chitosanase activity.

3.4. *Purification of Chitosanase*

Protein precipitation was performed by adding 480 g of $(NH_4)_2SO_4$ to 600 mL of culture supernatant. The solution was kept at 4 °C overnight. The precipitate was centrifuged at 12,000 x g for 30 min and then dissolved in 50 mL of 20 mM Tris-HCl buffer (pH 7) to produce the crude enzyme solution. The enzyme solution was then loaded onto a Macro-Prep High S column, which had been equilibrated with 20 mM Tris-HCl buffer, and eluted by a linear gradient of 0-1 M NaCl in the same buffer. The obtained fraction, which showed the chitosanase, was then further purified by HPLC analysis using the KW802.5 column following the conditions: mobile phase, 0.3 M NaCl in 20 mM Tris-HCl buffer (pH 7); injection volume, 20 μL; temperature, 20 °C; flowrate, 1mL/min; and detector, ultraviolet 230 nm. The MW of the purified chitosanase was determined using the SDS-PAGE method.

3.5. *Effects of pH and Temperature on Activity and Stability of Chitosanase*

The optimal temperature for the reaction of TKU032 chitosanase was determined over a range of 4–100 °C with 30 min incubation. Thermal stability was determined by treating the enzyme at a range of temperatures for 30 min. The residual activity of the treated enzyme was measured under the standard conditions of the chitosanase activity assay.

The effect of pH on TKU32 chitosanase activity was investigated using the buffer systems, including glycine-HCl, acetate, sodium phosphate, and Na_2CO_3-$NaHCO_3$. The optimal pH of TKU032 chitosanase was tested using a range of 2 to 11. To investigate the pH stability of TKU032 chitosanase, the enzyme was pre-treated from pH 2 to 11 for 30 min; its residual activity was measured at pH 7, as described above.

3.6. *Effect of Metal Ions on Chitosanase Activity*

TKU032 chitosanase was pre-incubated for 30 min at 37 °C with various metal ion salts and an enzyme inhibitor (5 mM), including: Cu^{2+}, Zn^{2+}, Mg^{2+}, Na^{+}, Ba^{2+}, Ca^{2+}, Fe^{2+}, and EDTA. The residual chitosanase activity was then measured, using the methods described above.

3.7. Substrate Specificity of Chitosanase

TKU032 chitosanase was incubated in 20 mM Tris-HCl buffer with numerous substrates at 70 °C for 30 min. These included: dextran, potato starch, cellulose powder, α-chitin powder, β-chitin powder, chitosan powder, colloidal chitin, colloidal chitosan, and *p*NPG. The enzyme activity in water-soluble chitosan was used as a control.

3.8. Antioxidant Activity Assay

DPPH radical scavenging activity was tested as per the previous methods, with modifications [51]. Briefly, 20 μL of sample was mixed with 980 μL DPPH-methanol solution and the mixture was kept in the dark for 20 min. The solution was then measured for optical density at 517 nm. The antioxidant activity was calculated using formula (1):

$$\text{DPPH radical scavenging activity (\%)} = (A_1 - A_2)/A_1 \times 100 \quad (1)$$

where A is the optical density of a blank sample and B is the optical density of the sample solution.

3.9. aGI Activity Assay

The aGI activity test followed the previously described methods [18]. In brief, 10 μL of sample was mixed with an equal amount of yeast α-glucosidase solution (1 U) and 100 μL phosphate buffer (100 mM, pH 6.8). The mixture was immediately incubated at 37 °C for 30 min. The reaction of the enzyme and substrate was started by adding 10 μL *p*-nitrophenyl glucopyranoside to the mixture, and then incubating at 37 °C for a further 30 min. 130 μL Na_2CO_3 solution (1 M) was added to the mixture to stop the reaction. The final solution was measured at 410 nm. The aGI activity was calculated using the following formula (2):

$$\text{aGI activity (\%)} = (B_1 - B_2)/B_1 \times 100 \quad (2)$$

where B_1 is the optical density of the blank sample, and B_2 is the optical density of the sample solution.

4. Conclusions

Chitosan oligosaccharides with various degrees of polymerization and biological activities could be efficiently produced using chitosanase to hydrolyze chitosan. In the current study, *P. mucilaginosus* TKU032 achieved the highest chitosanase production using shrimp head powder, an inexpensive material, as the sole C/N source. The *P. mucilaginosus* TKU032 chitosanase was purified and unlike other *Paenibacillus* strains, had a MW of 59 kDa and a high optimal temperature (70 °C). In order to evaluate the bioactivity of COS, the oligomers obtained by hydrolyzing colloidal chitosan with TKU032 chitosanase were fractionalized and tested for aGI and antioxidant activities. The COS fraction with the highest MW (fraction I) demonstrated aGI activity, whereas the COS fractions with lower MW (fractions II and III) showed antioxidant activity. For the first time, the inhibitory mechanism of COS on yeast α-glucosidase was investigated; the results suggest that it follows the mixed noncompetitive inhibition model. As such, chitosanase from *P. mucilaginosus* TKU032 may have potential applications in bioactive COS production for the food and pharmaceutical industries.

Author Contributions: Conceptualization, S.-L.W. and C.T.D.; Methodology, C.T.D. and T.N.T.; Software, C.T.D.; Validation, S.-L.W. and C.T.D.; Formal Analysis, C.T.D., T.N.T., V.B.N., and A.D.N.; Investigation, C.T.D., T.N.T.; Resources, S.-L.W.; Data Curation, C.T.D.; Writing-Original Draft Preparation, S.-L.W and C.T.D.; Writing, Review & Editing, S.-L.W. and C.T.D.; Visualization, S.-L.W. and C.T.D.; Supervision, S.-L.W.; Project Administration, S.-L.W.; Funding Acquisition, S.-L.W.

Funding: This work was supported in part by a grant from the Ministry of Science and Technology, Taiwan (MOST 106-2320-B-032-001-MY3).

Conflicts of Interest: The authors declare no conflict of interest.

References

1. Zitouni, M.; Fortin, M.; Scheerle, R.K.; Letzel, T.; Matteau, D.; Rodrigue, S.; Brzezinski, R. Biochemical and molecular characterization of a thermostable chitosanase produced by the strain *Paenibacillus* sp. 1794 newly isolated from compost. *Appl. Microbiol. Biotechnol.* **2013**, *97*, 5801–5813. [CrossRef]
2. Kumar, M.N.V.R. A review of chitin and chitosan applications. *React. Funct. Polym.* **2000**, *46*, 1–27. [CrossRef]
3. Wang, S.L.; Liang, T.W. Microbial reclamation of squid pens and shrimp shells. *Res. Chem. Interm.* **2017**, *43*, 3445. [CrossRef]
4. Elieh-Ali-Komi, D.; Hamblin, M.R. Chitin and chitosan: Production and application of versatile biomedical nanomaterials. *Int. J. Adv. Res. (Indore).* **2016**, *4*, 411–427.
5. Liang, T.W.; Chen, W.T.; Lin, Z.H.; Kuo, Y.H.; Nguyen, A.D.; Pan, P.S.; Wang, S.L. An amphiprotic novel chitosanase from *Bacillus mycoides* and its application in the production of chitooligomers with their antioxidant and anti–inflammatory evaluation. *Int. J. Mol. Sci.* **2017**, *17*, 1302. [CrossRef]
6. Jo, S.H.; Ha, K.S.; Moon, K.S.; Kim, J.G.; Oh, C.G.; Kim, Y.C.; Apostolidis, E.; Kwon, Y.I. Molecular weight dependent glucose lowering effect of low molecular weight chitosan oligosaccharide (GO2KA1) on postprandial blood glucose level in SD rats model. *Int. J. Mol. Sci.* **2013**, *14*, 14214–14224. [CrossRef] [PubMed]
7. Lee, H.W.; Park, Y.S.; Choi, J.W.; Yi, S.Y.; Shin, W.S. Antidiabetic effects of chitosan oligosaccharides in neonatal streptozotocin-induced noninsulin-dependent diabetes mellitus in rats. *Biol. Pharm. Bull.* **2003**, *26*, 1100–1103. [CrossRef]
8. Tran, T.N.; Doan, C.T.; Nguyen, V.B.; Nguyen, A.D.; Wang, S.L. The isolation of chitinase from *Streptomyces thermocarboxydus* and its application in the preparation of chitin oligomers. *Res. Chem. Interm.* **2019**, *45*, 727–742. [CrossRef]
9. Doan, C.T.; Tran, T.N.; Nguyen, V.B.; Nguyen, A.D.; Wang, S.L. Reclamation of marine chitinous materials for chitosanase production via microbial conversion by *Paenibacillus macerans*. *Mar. Drugs.* **2018**, *16*, 429. [CrossRef]
10. Azuma, K.; Osaki, T.; Minami, S.; Okamoto, Y. Anticancer and anti–inflammatory properties of chitin and chitosan oligosaccharides. *J. Funct. Biomater.* **2015**, *6*, 33–49. [CrossRef]
11. Liang, T.W.; Chen, Y.J.; Yen, Y.H.; Wang, S.L. The antitumor activity of the hydrolysates of chitinous materials hydrolyzed by crude enzyme from *Bacillus amyloliquefaciens* V656. *Process Biochem.* **2007**, *42*, 527–534. [CrossRef]
12. No, H.K.; Park, N.Y.; Lee, S.H.; Meyers, S.P. Antibacterial activity of chitosans and chitosan oligomers with different molecular weights. *Int. J. Food Microbiol.* **2002**, *74*, 65–72. [CrossRef]
13. Sun, T.; Qin, Y.; Xu, H.; Xie, J.; Hu, D.; Xue, B.; Hua, X. Antibacterial activities and preservative effect of chitosan oligosaccharide Maillard reaction products on *Penaeus vannamei*. *Int. J. Biol. Macromol.* **2017**, *105*, 764–768. [CrossRef]
14. Wang, S.L.; Liu, C.P.; Liang, T.W. Fermented and enzymatic production of chitin/chitosan oligosaccharides by extracellular chitinases from *Bacillus cereus* TKU027. *Carbohydr. Polym.* **2012**, *90*, 1305–1313. [CrossRef]
15. Liang, T.W.; Liu, C.P.; Wu, C.; Wang, S.L. Applied development of crude enzyme from *Bacillus cereus* in prebiotics and microbial community changes in soil. *Carbohydr. Polym.* **2013**, *92*, 2141–2148. [CrossRef]
16. Nguyen, A.D.; Huang, C.C.; Liang, T.W.; Nguyen, V.B.; Pan, P.S.; Wang, S.L. Production and purification of a fungal chitosanase and chitooligomers from *Penicillium janthinellum* D4 and discovery of the enzyme activators. *Carbohydr. Polym.* **2014**, *108*, 331–337. [CrossRef]
17. Park, J.K.; Shimono, K.; Ochiai, N.; Shigeru, K.; Kurita, M.; Ohta, Y.; Tanaka, K.; Matsuda, H.; Kawamukai, M. Purification, characterization, and gene analysis of a chitosanase (ChoA) from *Matsuebacter chitosanotabidus* 3001. *J. Bacteriol.* **1999**, *181*, 6642–6649.
18. Doan, C.T.; Tran, T.N.; Nguyen, V.B.; Nguyen, A.D.; Wang, S.L. Conversion of squid pens to chitosanases and proteases via *Paenibacillus* sp. TKU042. *Mar. Drugs* **2018**, *16*, 83. [CrossRef]
19. Wang, S.L.; Yu, H.T.; Tsai, M.H.; Doan, C.T.; Nguyen, V.B.; Do, V.C.; Nguyen, A.D. Conversion of squid pens to chitosanases and dye adsorbents via *Bacillus cereus*. *Res. Chem. Interm.* **2018**, *44*, 4903–4911. [CrossRef]
20. Wang, C.L.; Su, J.W.; Liang, T.W.; Nguyen, A.D.; Wang, S.L. Production, purification and characterization of a chitosanase from *Bacillus cereus*. *Res. Chem. Interm.* **2014**, *40*, 2237–2248. [CrossRef]

21. Liang, T.W.; Chen, Y.Y.; Pan, P.S.; Wang, S.L. Purification of chitinase/chitosanase from *Bacillus cereus* and discovery of an enzyme inhibitor. *Int. J. Biol. Macromol.* **2014**, *63*, 8–14. [CrossRef]
22. Liang, T.W.; Hsieh, J.L.; Wang, S.L. Production and purification of a protease, a chitosanase and chitin oligosaccharides by Bacillus cereus TKU022 fermentation. *Carbohyd. Res.* **2012**, *362*, 38–46. [CrossRef]
23. Wang, S.L.; Chen, T.R.; Liang, T.W.; Wu, P.C. Conversion and degradation of shellfish wastes by *Bacillus cereus* TKU018 fermentation for the production of chitosanase and bioactive materials. *Biochem. Eng. J.* **2009**, *48*, 111–117. [CrossRef]
24. Liang, T.W.; Kuo, Y.H.; Wu, P.C.; Wang, C.L.; Nguyen, A.D.; Wang, S.L. Purification and characterization of a chitosanase and a protease by conversion of shrimp shell wastes fermented by *Serratia marcescens* subsp. *sakuensis* TKU019. *J. Chin. Chem. Soc–Taip.* **2010**, *57*, 857–863. [CrossRef]
25. Boucher, I.; Dupuy, A.; Vidal, P.; Neugebauer, W.A.; Brzezinski, R. Purification and characterization of a chitosanase from *Streptomyces* N174. *Appl. Microbiol. Biotechnol.* **1992**, *38*, 188–193. [CrossRef]
26. Liang, T.W.; Lo, B.C.; Wang, S.L. Chitinolytic bacteria-assisted conversion of squid pen and its effect on dyes and adsorption. *Mar. Drugs* **2015**, *13*, 4576–4593. [CrossRef]
27. Wang, S.L.; Wu, P.C.; Liang, T.W. Utilization of squid pen for the efficient production of chitosanase and antioxidants through prolonged autoclave treatment. *Carbohydr. Res.* **2009**, *244*, 979–984. [CrossRef]
28. Wang, S.L.; Chen, S.J.; Liang, T.W.; Lin, Y.D. A novel nattokinase produced by *Pseudomonas* sp. TKU015 using shrimp shells as substrate. *Process Biochem.* **2009**, *44*, 70–76. [CrossRef]
29. Wang, S.L.; Su, Y.C.; Nguyen, V.B.; Nguyen, A.D. Reclamation of shrimp heads for the production of α–glucosidase inhibitors by *Staphylococcus* sp. TKU043. *Res. Chem. Intermed.* **2018**, *44*, 4929–4937. [CrossRef]
30. Wang, S.L.; Wu, Y.Y.; Liang, T.W. Purification and biochemical characterization of a nattokinase by conversion of shrimp shell with *Bacillus subtilis* TKU007. *New Biotechnol.* **2011**, *28*, 196–202. [CrossRef]
31. Doan, C.T.; Tran, T.N.; Nguyen, M.T.; Nguyen, V.B.; Nguyen, A.D.; Wang, S.L. Anti-α-glucosidase activity by a protease from *Bacillus licheniformis*. *Molecules* **2019**, *24*, 691. [CrossRef]
32. Nguyen, V.B.; Wang, S.L. New novel α–glucosidase inhibitors produced by microbial conversion. *Process Biochem.* **2018**, *65*, 228–232. [CrossRef]
33. Nguyen, V.B.; Nguyen, T.H.; Doan, C.T.; Tran, T.N.; Nguyen, A.D.; Kuo, Y.H.; Wang, S.L. Production and bioactivity-guided isolation of antioxidants with α–glucosidase inhibitory and anti-NO properties from marine chitinous material. *Molecules* **2018**, *23*, 1124. [CrossRef]
34. Nguyen, V.B.; Wang, S.L. Production of potent antidiabetic compounds from shrimp head powder via *Paenibacillus* conversion. *Process Biochem.* **2019**, *76*, 18–24. [CrossRef]
35. Nguyen, V.B.; Nguyen, A.D.; Wang, S.L. Utilization of fishery processing byproduct squid pens for *Paenibacillus* sp. fermentation on producing potent α–glucosidase inhibitors. *Mar. Drugs.* **2017**, *15*, 274. [CrossRef]
36. Nguyen, V.B.; Wang, S.L. Reclamation of marine chitinous materials for the production of α–glucosidase inhibitors via microbial conversion. *Mar. Drugs.* **2017**, *15*, 350. [CrossRef]
37. Liang, T.W.; Tseng, S.C.; Wang, S.L. Production and characterization of antioxidant properties of exopolysaccharides from *Paenibacillus mucilaginosus* TKU032. *Mar. Drugs.* **2016**, *12*, 40. [CrossRef]
38. Liang, T.W.; Wu, C.C.; Cheng, W.T.; Chen, Y.C.; Wang, C.L.; Wang, I.L.; Wang, S.L. Exopolysaccharides and antimicrobial biosurfactants produced by *Paenibacillus macerans* TKU029. *Appl. Biochem. Biotech.* **2014**, *172*, 933–950. [CrossRef]
39. Doan, C.T.; Tran, T.N.; Nguyen, V.B.; Vo, T.P.K.; Nguyen, A.D.; Wang, S.L. Chitin extraction from shrimp waste by liquid fermentation using an alkaline protease–producing strain, *Brevibacillus parabrevis*. *Int. J. Biol. Macromol.* **2019**, *131*, 706–715. [CrossRef]
40. Garcia–Gonzalez, E.; Poppinga, L.; Fünfhaus, A.; Hertlein, G.; Hedtke, K.; Jakubowska, A.; Genersch, E. *Paenibacillus larvae* chitin-degrading protein PlCBP49 is a key virulence factor in American foulbrood of honey bees. *PLoS Pathogen.* **2014**, *10*, e1004284. [CrossRef]
41. Singh, A.K.; Chhatpar, H.S. Purification and characterization of chitinase from *Paenibacillus* sp. D1. *Appl. Biochem. Biotechnol.* **2011**, *164*, 77–88. [CrossRef]
42. Kim, Y.H.; Park, S.K.; Hur, J.Y.; Kim, Y.C. Purification and characterization of a major extracellular chitinase from a biocontrol bacterium, *Paenibacillus elgii* HOA73. *Plant Pathol. J.* **2017**, *33*, 318–328. [CrossRef]
43. Loni, P.P.; Patil, J.U.; Phugare, S.S.; Bajekal, S.S. Purification and characterization of alkaline chitinase from *Paenibacillus pasadenensis* NCIM 5434. J. *Basic Microbiol.* **2014**, *54*, 1080–1089. [CrossRef]

44. Ueda, J.; Kurosawa, N. Characterization of an extracellular thermophilic chitinase from *Paenibacillus thermoaerophilus* strain TC22-2b isolated from compost. *World J. Microbiol. Biotechnol.* **2015**, *31*, 135–143. [CrossRef]
45. Jung, W.J.; Kuk, J.K.; Kim, K.Y.; Kim, T.H.; Park, R.D. Purification and characterization of chitinase from *Paenibacillus illinoisensis* KJA-424. J. *Microbiol. Biotechnol.* **2005**, *15*, 274–280.
46. Fu, X.; Yan, Q.; Wang, J.; Yang, S.; Jiang, Z. Purification and biochemical characterization of novel acidic chitinase from *Paenibacillus barengoltzii*. *Int. J. Biol. Macromol.* **2016**, *91*, 973–979. [CrossRef]
47. Guo, X.; Xu, P.; Zong, M.; Lou, W. Purification and characterization of alkaline chitinase from *Paenibacillus pasadenensis* CS0611. *Chin. J. Catalys.* **2017**, *38*, 665–672. [CrossRef]
48. Kimoto, H.; Kusaoke, H.; Yamamoto, I.; Fujii, Y.; Onodera, T.; Taketo, A. Biochemical and genetic properties of *Paenibacillus* glycosyl hydrolase having chitosanase activity and discoidin domain. *J. Biol. Chem.* **2002**, *277*, 14695–14702. [CrossRef]
49. Itoh, T.; Sugimoto, I.; Hibi, T.; Suzuki, F.; Matsuo, K.; Fujii, Y.; Taketo, A.; Kimoto, H. Overexpression, purification, and characterization of *Paenibacillus* cell surface expressed chitinase ChiW with two catalytic domains. *Biosci. Biotechnol. Biochem.* **2014**, *78*, 624–634. [CrossRef]
50. Meena, S.; Gothwal, R.K.; Saxena, J.; Nehra, S.; Mohan, M.K.; Ghosh, P. Effect of metal ions and chemical compounds on chitinase produced by a newly isolated thermotolerant *Paenibacillus* sp. BISR-047 and its shelf-life. *Int. J. Curr. Microbiol. Appl. Sci.* **2015**, *4*, 872–881.
51. Nguyen, V.B.; Wang, S.L.; Nguyen, A.D.; Lin, Z.H.; Doan, C.T.; Tran, T.N.; Huang, H.T.; Kuo, Y.H. Bioactivity-Gùded purification of novel herbal antioxidant and anti-NO compounds from *Euonymus laxiflorus* Champ. *Molecules* **2019**, *24*, 120. [CrossRef]
52. Naveed, M.; Phil, L.; Sohail, M.; Hasnat, M.; Baig, M.M.F.A.; Ihsan, A.U.; Shumzaid, M.; Kakar, M.U.; Khan, T.M.; Akabar, M.D.; Hussain, M.I.; Zhou, Q.G. Chitosan oligosaccharide (COS): An overview. *Int. J. Biol. Macromol.* **2019**, *129*, 827–843. [CrossRef]

marine drugs

MDPI

Article

Express Method for Isolation of Ready-to-Use 3D Chitin Scaffolds from *Aplysina archeri* (Aplysineidae: Verongiida) Demosponge

Christine Klinger [1], Sonia Żółtowska-Aksamitowska [2,3], Marcin Wysokowski [2,3,*], Mikhail V. Tsurkan [4], Roberta Galli [5], Iaroslav Petrenko [3], Tomasz Machałowski [2], Alexander Ereskovsky [6,7], Rajko Martinović [8], Lyubov Muzychka [9], Oleg B. Smolii [9], Nicole Bechmann [10], Viatcheslav Ivanenko [11,12], Peter J. Schupp [13], Teofil Jesionowski [2], Marco Giovine [14], Yvonne Joseph [3], Stefan R. Bornstein [15,16], Alona Voronkina [17] and Hermann Ehrlich [3,*]

1 Institute of Physical Chemistry, TU Bergakademie-Freiberg, Leipziger str. 29, 09559 Freiberg, Germany; cjtk1991@web.de
2 Institute of Chemical Technology and Engineering, Faculty of Chemical Technology, Poznan University of Technology, Berdychowo 4, 61131 Poznan, Poland; soniazolaks@gmail.com (S.Ż.-A.); tomasz.g.machalowski@doctorate.put.poznan.pl (T.M.); teofil.jesionowski@put.poznan.pl (T.J.)
3 Institute of Electronics and Sensor Materials, TU Bergakademie Freiberg, Gustav Zeuner Str. 3, 09599 Freiberg, Germany; iaroslavpetrenko@gmail.com (I.P.); yvonne.joseph@esm.tu-freiberg.de (Y.J.)
4 Leibnitz Institute of Polymer Research Dresden, 01069 Dresden, Germany; tsurkan@ipfdd.de
5 Clinical Sensoring and Monitoring, Department of Anesthesiology and Intensive Care Medicine, Faculty of Medicine, Technische Universität Dresden, 01307 Dresden, Germany; roberta.galli@tu-dresden.de
6 Institut Méditerranéen de Biodiversité et d'Ecologie (IMBE), CNRS, IRD, Aix Marseille Université, Avignon Université, Station Marine d'Endoume, 13003 Marseille, France; alexander.ereskovsky@imbe.fr
7 Department of Embryology, Faculty of Biology, Saint-Petersburg State University, 19992 Saint-Petersburg, Russia
8 Institute of Marine Biology, University of Montenegro, 85330 Kotor, Montenegro; rajko.mar@ucg.ac.me
9 Institute of Bioorganic Chemistry and Petrochemistry, National Academy of Science of Ukraine, Murmanska Str., 1, 02094 Kyiv, Ukraine; smolii@bpci.kiev.ua (O.B.S.); lmuzychka@rambler.ru (L.M.)
10 Institute of Clinical Chemistry and Laboratory Medicine, University Hospital Carl Gustav Carus, Faculty of Medicine Carl Gustav Carus, Technische Universität Dresden, 01307 Dresden, Germany; Nicole.bechmann@uniklinikum-dresden.de
11 Department of Invertebrate Zoology, Biological Faculty, Lomonosov Moscow State University, 119992 Moscow, Russia; ivanenko.slava@gmail.com
12 Naturalis Biodiversity Center, 2332 Leiden, The Netherlands
13 Institute for Chemistry and Biology of the Marine Environment, University of Oldenburg, Carl-von-Ossietzky-Straße 9-11, 26111 Oldenburg, Germany; peter.schupp@uni-oldenburg.de
14 Department of Sciences of Earth, Environment and Life, University of Genoa, Corso Europa 26, 16132 Genova, Italy; mgiovine@unige.it
15 Department of Internal Medicine III, University Hospital Carl Gustav Carus, Technische Universität Dresden, 01307 Dresden, Germany; Stefan.bornstein@uniklinikum-dresden.de
16 Diabetes and Nutritional Sciences Division, King's College London, London WC2R 2LS, UK
17 National Pirogov Memorial Medical University, Vinnytsya, Department of Pharmacy, Pirogov str. 56, 21018, Vinnytsia, Ukraine; algol2808@gmail.com
* Correspondence: marcin.wysokowski@put.poznan.pl (M.W.); hermann.ehrlich@esm.tu-freiberg.de (H.E.)

Received: 26 January 2019; Accepted: 19 February 2019; Published: 22 February 2019

Abstract: Sponges are a valuable source of natural compounds and biomaterials for many biotechnological applications. Marine sponges belonging to the order Verongiida are known to contain both chitin and biologically active bromotyrosines. *Aplysina archeri* (Aplysineidae: Verongiida) is well known to contain bromotyrosines with relevant bioactivity against human and animal diseases. The aim of this study was to develop an express method for the production of naturally prefabricated 3D chitin and bromotyrosine-containing extracts simultaneously. This new method is based on microwave irradiation (MWI) together with stepwise treatment using 1% sodium hydroxide, 20% acetic acid, and 30% hydrogen peroxide. This approach, which takes up to 1 h, made it possible to isolate chitin from the tube-like skeleton of *A. archeri* and to demonstrate the presence of this biopolymer in this sponge for the first time. Additionally, this procedure does not deacetylate chitin to chitosan and enables the recovery of ready-to-use 3D chitin scaffolds without destruction of the unique tube-like fibrous interconnected structure of the isolated biomaterial. Furthermore, these mechanically stressed fibers still have the capacity for saturation with water, methylene blue dye, crude oil, and blood, which is necessary for the application of such renewable 3D chitinous centimeter-sized scaffolds in diverse technological and biomedical fields.

Keywords: chitin; marine sponges; scaffolds; *Aplysina archeri*; express method; bromotyrosines; crude oil; blood; methylene blue

---

1. Introduction

Chitin is composed of β(1,4)-linked N-acetyl-glucosamine units and represents the most abundant structural polysaccharide of invertebrates, including such marine phyla as sponges, corals, annelid worms, mollusks, and arthropods [1]. This biopolymer is mostly found in the skeletal structures of invertebrates, and plays a crucial role in their rigidity, stiffness, and other mechanical properties. Chitin is recognized as one of the universal templates in biomineralization, with respect to both biocalcification and biosilicification [2]. Chitin has been found in diverse organisms as layers—in mollusks' shells [3], glass sponges' skeletal frameworks [4], and spicules [5]—or as three-dimensional (3D) constructs: cuticles of crustaceans [6], skeletons of certain demosponges [7–10], and especially within mineralized tissues [11]. Very often, chitin is found in association with such organic compounds as proteins, lipids, pigments, and other polysaccharides [12]. Thus, the efficient extraction of pure chitin from the marine sources listed above is strongly dependent on methodological progress, which, however, is usually limited by the presence of corresponding mineral and foreign organic phases. Consequently, the industrial methods of chitin isolation most used in this case are based on chemical treatments that enable depigmentation [13], hydrolysis of proteins, and demineralization of inorganic matter [14–19].

Industrial deproteinization is carried out using a base solution of KOH or NaOH (for review, see [20,21]). The effectiveness of this treatment depends on the ratio of shells to solution, the temperature and duration of the process, as well as the concentration of the base. Industrial methods also include a depigmentation (decolorization) step, which improves the color of the chitin. For this purpose, hydrogen peroxide or sodium hypochlorite solutions are commonly used [22].

Demineralization can be achieved using chelators (ethylenediamine tetraacetic acid-EDTA [23]), or various acids, most commonly diluted hydrochloric acid, acetic acid, or sulfuric acid (for examples, see [22,24,25]). To achieve complete dissolution of all the inorganic salts, the acid intake should be greater than the stoichiometric quantity of the corresponding mineral phases [26,27]. Furthermore, the penetration of solvent into the chitin-based matrix is strongly dependent on the particle size [28]. In the case of crustacean shells, due to the heterogeneity of the solid matrix and difficulties in removing calcium debris, larger volumes, or more concentrated acid solutions, have traditionally been used [24,29]. Demineralization at higher temperatures has also been reported [30]. Methods based on long-term demineralization (even up to several days) may cause degradation of the biopolymer [31]. Alternatively, deproteinization and demineralization can also be carried out using microorganisms and corresponding enzymatic treatment. It has been reported [32] that biological treatment leads to better results than chemical methods, as it preserves the structure of chitin. New data on methods for chitin isolation, including applications of ionic liquids and eutectic solvents, have recently been published by

Berton et al. [33], El Knidri et al. [34], Tokatlı & Demirdöven [35], Dun et al. [36], Saravana et al. [37], Castro et al. [38], Huang et al. [39], and Hong et al. [40].

A schematic overview of biological and chemical methods of chitin isolation for obtaining chitosan, following the example of crustacean sources based on the literature reports cited above, is presented in Figure 1.

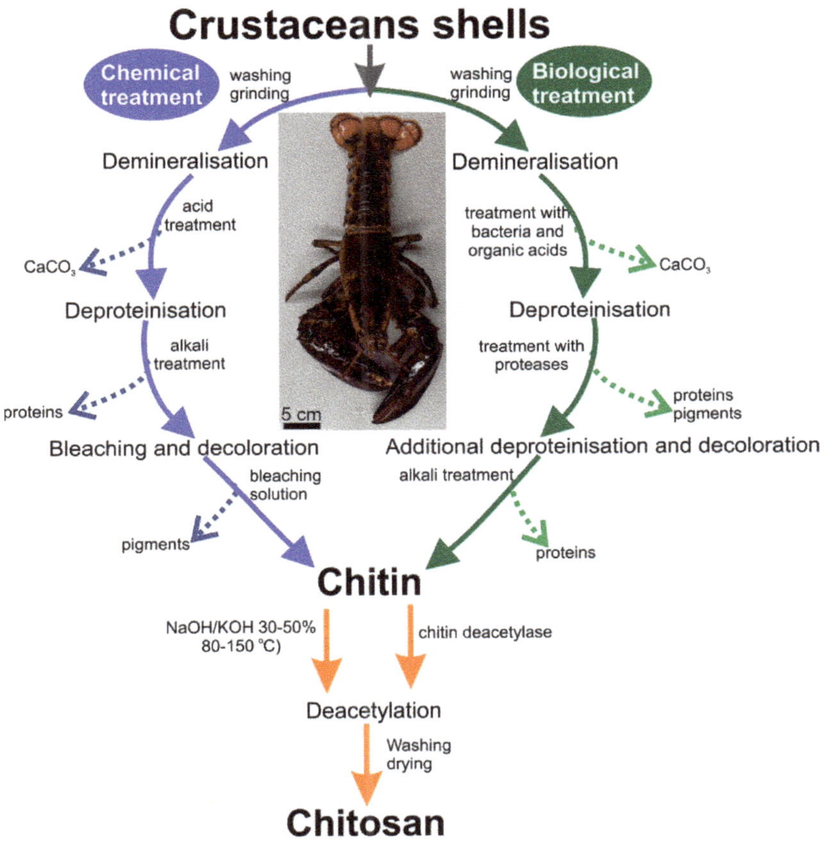

Figure 1. Schematic view of the standard biological and chemical approaches to the isolation of chitin-based biomaterials of crustacean origin.

Unlike chitin of crustacean origin, poriferan chitin has never been used as a source for chitosan. Besides spongin [41], chitin is one of the main structural biopolymers in demosponges with a 3D architecture, whose porous, fibrous network supports the sponges' cells. Moreover, chitin is a key biological material for the stabilization of the sponges' skeletons in marine habitats with strong ocean currents.

Since 2007, when chitin in the form of 3D scaffolds was isolated from selected demosponges for the first time [4], chitin has been verified in 17 marine species, mostly representing the order Verongiida [42,43].

For the isolation of chitin from demosponges, a well-established method based on alternating alkaline (NaOH) and acidic (HF, HCl, CH_3COOH) extraction steps, enabling the desilicification and decalcification of the mineralized sponge skeleton, has been used (for review, see [42,43]). Pigments, lipids and proteins are removed at the same time. In view of the large quantities of chemicals used and the time required by the individual extraction steps (up to 7 days), the method needs to be improved. In this study, we decided to use, for the first time, a complex approach that includes microwave irradiation (MWI) together with stepwise treatment using 1% sodium hydroxide, 20% acetic acid, and 30% hydrogen peroxide to isolate chitin from the tube-like skeleton of *Aplysina archeri* (Higgin, 1875) (phylum Porifera, class Demospongiae, Aplysineidae: order Verongiida, family Aplysinellidae) (Figure 2) [44]. An additional goal of the study was to develop an express isolation method (Figure 3), enabling the production of (i) crude extracts containing the pigments and (ii) ready-to-use 3D chitin scaffolds for practical applications in technology and biomedicine.

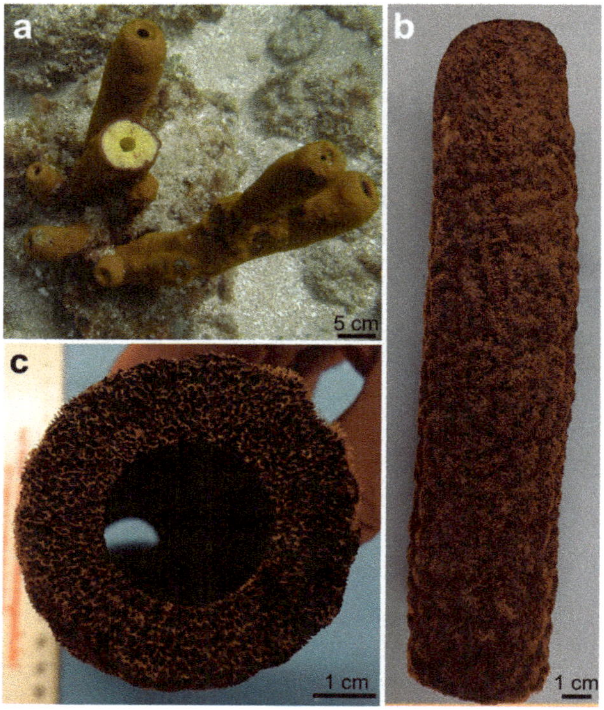

Figure 2. Underwater image (**a**) of the demosponge *A. archeri* shows the typical apical growth form of tube-like sponge bodies measuring up to 50 cm (or in some cases more than 2 m). A dried fragment of the sponge (**b**) remains pigmented and is hard enough to be cut using a metal saw (**c**). See also Figure 3a.

2. Results

2.1. Isolation and Identification of Chitin

The investigated sponge belongs to the family Aplysinellidae (order Verongiida), and hence is reported as a renewable source of chitin (for review, see [42,43]) as well as of the pharmaceutically relevant bromotyrosines [45]. The methodology is described in Figure 3. For comparative purposes, we carried out preliminary experiments on the isolation of chitin from the sponge fragments using the standard alkaline-based procedure, which takes up to 7 days (for details, see [9,10]). Using this approach, the naturally occurring mineralized skeletons of *A. archeri* became completely soft, colorless, and demineralized in a time of 114 h. However, the application of microwaves (750 W and 2450 MHz), as reported here, decreased the treatment time to only 55 min. The most time (33 min) was taken by the water rinsing procedures. The estimated chitin content in the skeletons of *A. archeri* is ~5% by weight.

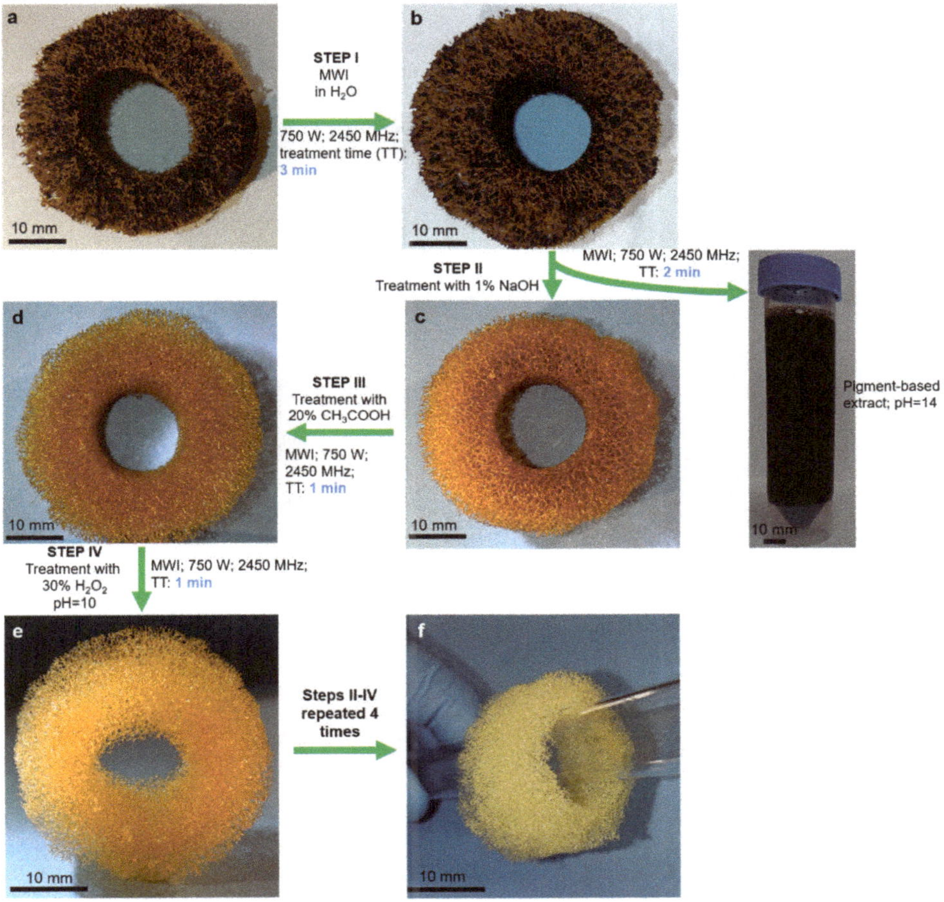

Figure 3. Schematic view of the microwave-assisted extraction of 3D chitin scaffold from a selected skeleton fragment (**a**) of the demosponge *A. archeri*. In step I, residual water soluble salts were removed by pretreatment of the sponge skeleton in distilled water under microwave irradiation (MWI) for 3 min. Afterwards, in step II (**b**), the sample was treated with 1% NaOH and irradiated with microwaves for 2 min. This procedure obtained both a 3D scaffold and a dark red-brownish pigment-containing extract (**c**). The 3D scaffold was carefully isolated and rinsed three times with distilled water to remove residual pigments. In step III, the 3D scaffolds were treated with 20% acetic acid under MWI for 1 min, and afterwards were washed in distilled water up to pH 6.8. In step IV (**d**,**e**), the sample was completely decolorized using 30% H_2O_2 at pH~10 under MWI for 1 min and washed with distilled water up to neutral pH. Steps II–IV were repeated four times to obtain a pure, colorless, ready-to-use 3D chitinous scaffold (**f**).

The microstructure of the demosponge skeletal fibers before (Figure 4a,b) and after isolation of the chitin scaffold (Figure 5a,b) was investigated using scanning electron microscopy (SEM). The recorded microphotographs display no visible changes in the microwave-stressed structure of the isolated material. Similar to the standard alkaline-based method for chitin isolation from demosponges using

5% NaOH at 37 °C [4,9,10], the new approaches lead to the preservation of the generic fibrous structure. The microphotographs of the fibers isolated from *A. archeri*, with the microwave approach also displaying the typical fibrous structure with concentric layers typical for microtubular chitin, previously reported in other representatives of the family Aplysinellidae [9,46]. The typical wrinkled structure (Figure 5a) due to the alkaline treatment occurs in chitinous fibers independent of microwave treatment, probably due to the very short time of microwave irradiation. EDX analysis of the naturally occurring skeletal structures of *A. archeri* (Figure 4c) and of the isolated chitin (Figure 5c) confirms the purity of the isolated biological material. The lack of characteristic elements in the isolated sample confirms that this proposed method is effective with respect to both demineralization and deproteinization.

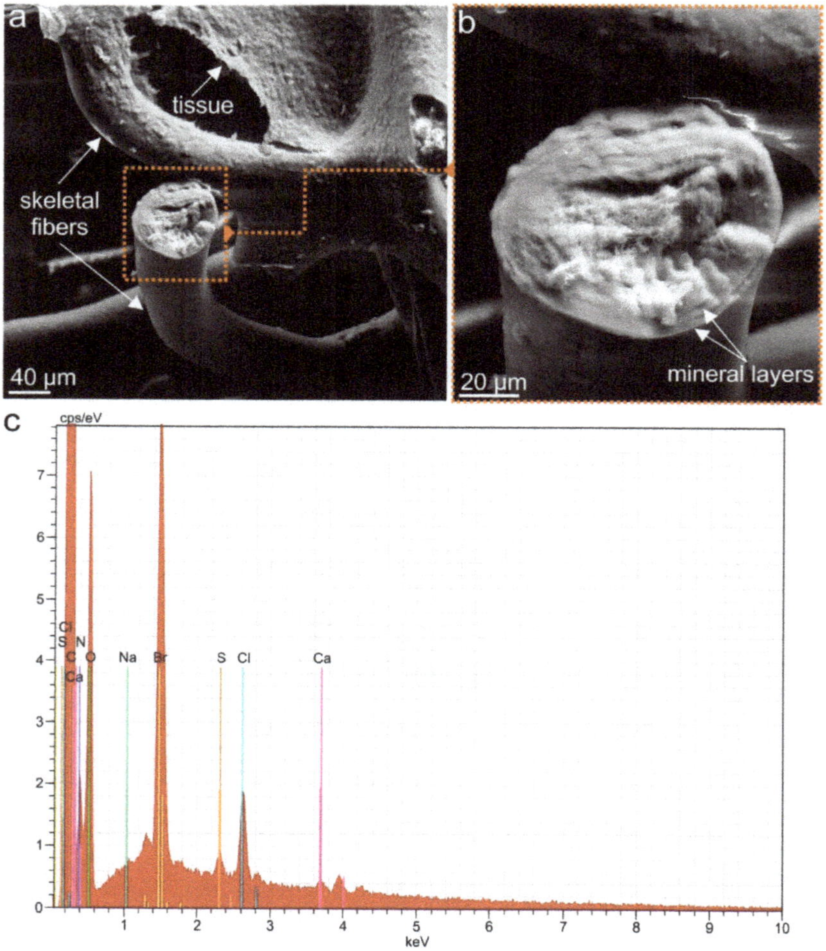

Figure 4. SEM microphotographs of the *A. archeri* skeletal fibers as collected (see Figure 3a,b) in different magnifications (**a**,**b**). EDX analysis of the fiber cross-section (**b**) reveals the presence of Ca, Cl, S and Br (**c**). This is similar to EDX data reported previously for naturally occurring skeletons of other verongiid demosponges (see [11]). The presence of bromine is likely determined by the localization of bromotyrosines within the chitinous layers of the skeletal fibers.

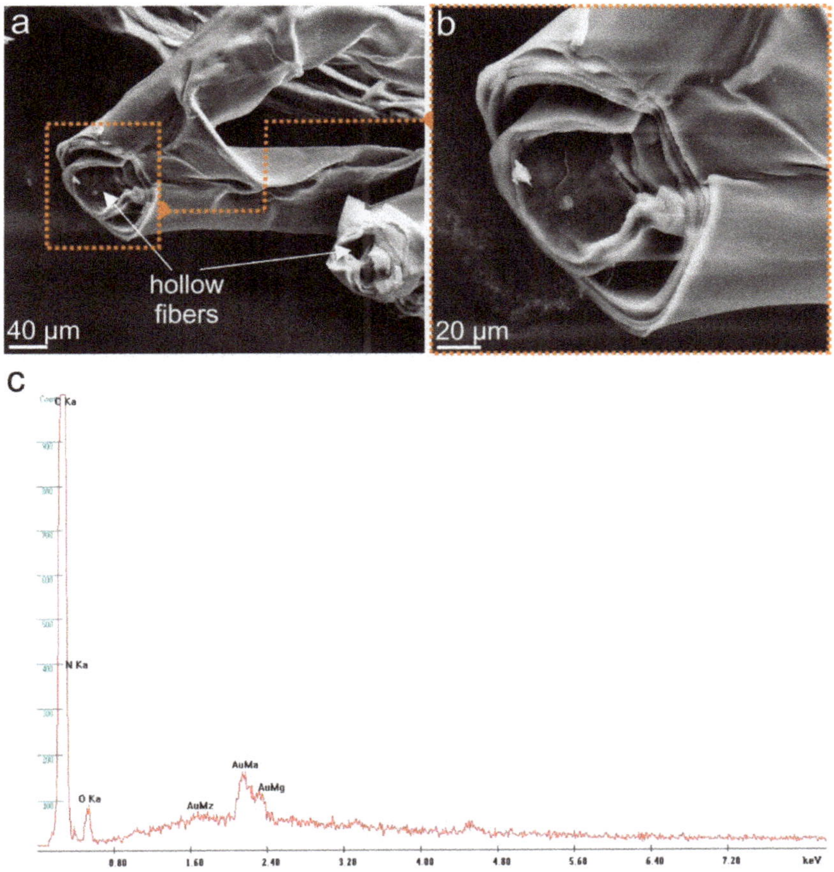

Figure 5. SEM imagery of the demineralized and depigmented tube-like skeletal fibers (see Figure 3f) obtained after microwave treatment (**a**,**b**). EDX analysis of these hollow structures (initially sputtered with Au) reveals the presence of C, N, and O only (**c**).

After isolating completely colorless and mineral-free 3D scaffolds from selected fragments of the *A. archeri* skeleton (Figure 3f), we continued experiments in order to identify if either chitin or chitosan (due to the harsh treatment conditions with pH 14 and 95 °C) were present.

The first step in identifying the isolated biological material as chitin or chitosan was calcofluor white (CFW) staining. On binding to polysaccharides, such as chitin, this fluorochrome emits a blue light. The microfibers of the scaffold isolated from *A. archeri* with the microwave-assisted method (Figure 3) show characteristic enhanced fluorescence after CFW staining (Figure 6). This result is similar to CFW-based poriferan chitin identification, as reported previously [4,8–10,42,43,46].

Chitinase digestion is a well-recognized and highly specialized test to determine the chitinous nature of isolated scaffolds from diverse sponges. The enzyme catalyzes the endo-hydrolysis of *N*-acetyl-β-D-glucosamine-β-(1→4)-linkages. The activity of chitinase against microfibers isolated from the scaffolds being studied is shown in Figure 7.

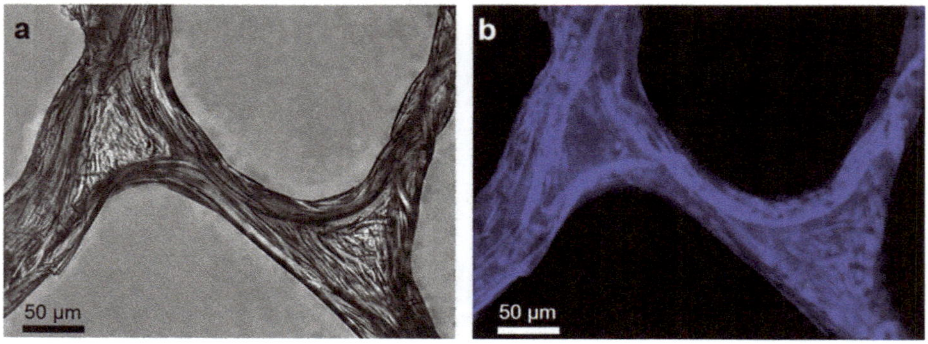

Figure 6. Light microscopy (**a**) and fluorescence microscopy (**b**) images of the selected fragment of a *A. archeri* scaffold after calcofluor white (CFW) staining. Intensive blue fluorescence remains measurable under a light exposure time of 1/3700 s.

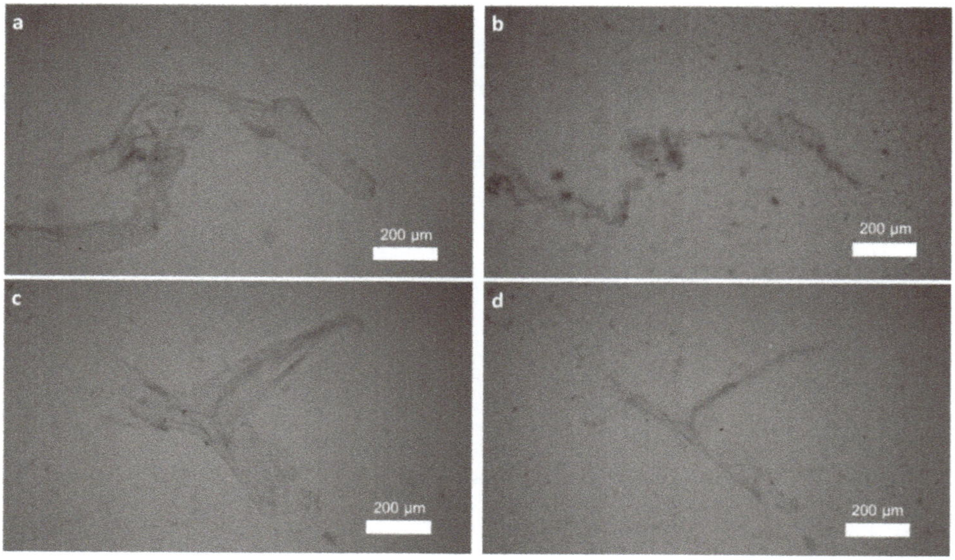

Figure 7. Chitinase test with chitin isolated from *A. archeri* using the standard method (see for details [9]) (**a**,**b**) and the microwave-based method (**c**,**d**). Images (**b**) and (**d**) were obtained after 4 h of incubation in chitinase solution.

Additionally, we used electrospray ionisation mass spectrometry (ESI-MS) for identification of *N*-acetylglucosamine as a characteristic marker of the presence of chitin in unknown biological samples. Acetic hydrolysis of chitin by strong acids resulted in the formation of D-glucosamine (dGlcN), which can be easily visualized in ESI-MS spectroscopy. This method is a standard for chitin identification and has been used to identify chitin in various organisms [5,47] and fossil remains [48]. The ESI-MS spectrum of the *A. archeri* hydrolyzed scaffold, shown in Figure 8a, has five main ion peaks at m/z 130.16, 162.08, 180.09, 202.07 and 381.15. Four of the main peaks at m/z 162.08, 180.09, 202.07, and 381.15 are similar to those on the spectrum of the dGlcN standard (Figure 8b). These peaks correspond to dGlcN species of molecular ion (m/z 180.09), the specie with the loss of one H_2O molecule $[M - H_2O + H]^+$ (m/z 162.08), the specie of sodium ion bound dGlcN monomer $[M + Na]^+$ (m/z 202.07), and the noncovalent dimer [2M + Na]$^+$ (m/z 381.15). A similar proton-bound GlcN covalent dimer with m/z = 359.17 was observed in the spectra. Together, these data indicate the high purity of the chitin in the *A. archeri* scaffold.

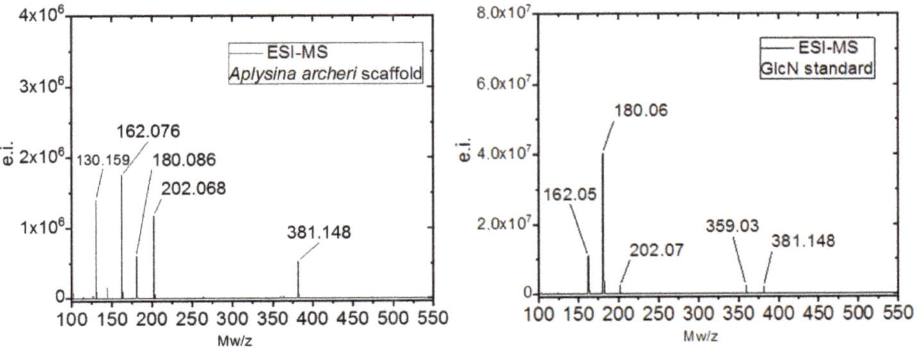

(**a**) (**b**)

Figure 8. Electrospray-ionization mass spectroscopy (ESI-MS) spectra of (**a**) chitin from the scaffold of *A. archeri;* (**b**) a commercial (dGlcN) standard for comparison.

However, the analytical methods described above cannot provide an answer as to the possible transformation of chitin from *A. archeri* into chitosan under the conditions applied. Consequently, we decided to use both ATR-FTIR and Raman spectroscopy as highly sensitive methods to investigate this possibility. To exclude the possibility of deacetylation during the isolation of chitin with the microwave approach (see Figure 3), ATR-FTIR (Figure 9) and Raman spectra (Figure 10) of the scaffolds isolated from *A. archeri* are compared with the spectra of a chitosan standard and the α-chitin standard (Figure 9).

The ATR-FTIR spectrum, obtained for the scaffold isolated from *A. archeri*, shows a characteristically split amide I band at the positions 1651 and 1628 cm^{-1}, associated with the stretching vibrations of the C=O bonds (Figure 9). This splitting of the amide I band is observed in the spectrum recorded for the α-chitin standard and is representative of this polymorph. It is observed due to the presence of stretching vibrations from intermolecular (C=O· · · HN) and intramolecular (C=O· · · HO(C6); C=O· · · HN) hydrogen bonds in the α-chitin chain [46,49,50]). These peaks are not visible in the spectrum of chitosan, because chitosan is a deacetylated derivative of chitin. Differences between the spectra recorded for the isolated scaffold, α-chitin standard and chitosan standard are also visible in the amide II band. For the isolated scaffold and α-chitin, the amide II band (N–H stretching vibrations) is recorded at the positions 1551 cm^{-1} and 1556 cm^{-1}, whereas for chitosan it is shifted to the higher wavenumber, 1587 cm^{-1} (Figure 9). Another distinctive feature is the position of the amide III band (C–N stretching and N–H bending vibrations). In the spectra of *A. archeri* and α-chitin, this band is present at 1308 cm^{-1} and 1306 cm^{-1} respectively, while for chitosan the amide III band is shifted to a higher value (1318 cm^{-1}), and its intensity is significantly lower. As an additional feature, the characteristic intense bands at 945 cm^{-1} and 950 cm^{-1}, attributed to wagging vibrations of CH_x, are observed only in the isolated scaffold and the α-chitin standard, respectively (Figure 9). Detailed analysis of the bands indicates that the spectra of the isolated scaffolds are very similar to those of the α-chitin standard. It can be concluded that the proposed microwave-assisted extraction, despite the very high temperature and alkaline pH, does not lead to the deacetylation of chitin, likely due to the very short time of microwave irradiation. Further studies should be carried out to optimize the isolation procedure based on microwave-assisted controlled surface deacetylation of tubular chitin scaffolds of poriferan origin.

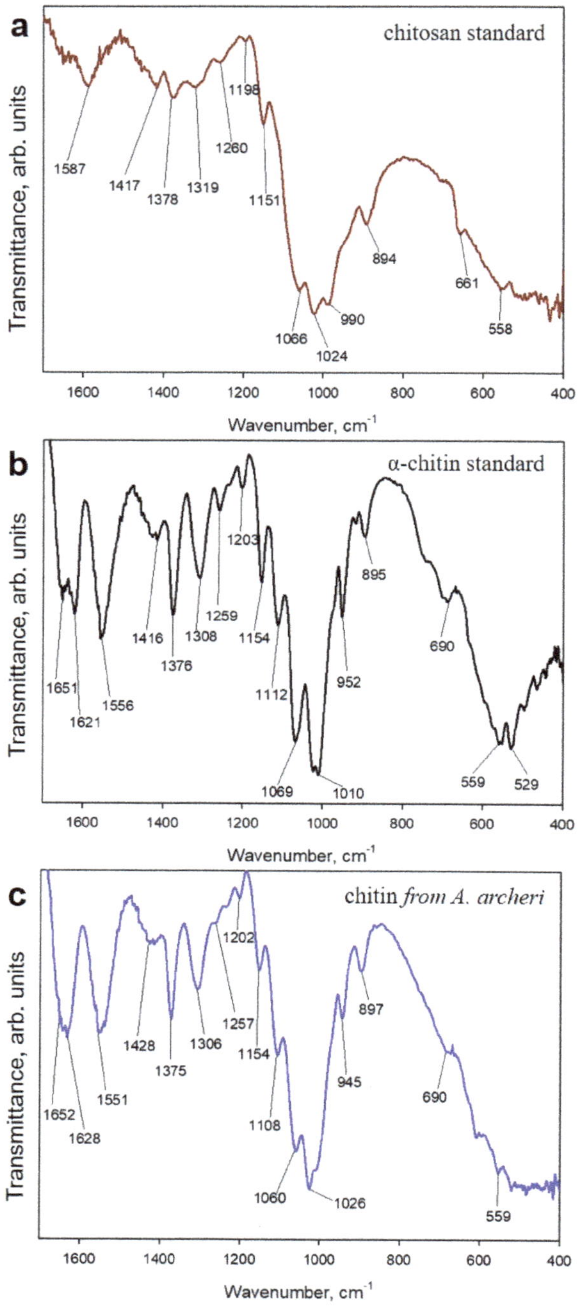

Figure 9. ATR-FTIR spectra of (**a**) chitosan, (**b**) α-chitin and (**c**) chitin isolated from *A. archeri* using the microwave-assisted approach (see Figure 3).

The results of Raman analysis confirm those of ATR-FTIR. The Raman spectra of the scaffolds of *A. archeri* isolated using the microwave-assisted method exhibit good equivalence with the spectrum of α-chitin, and not with that of chitosan (Figure 10). The main differences are clearly visible in the amide I, amide II, and amide III regions.

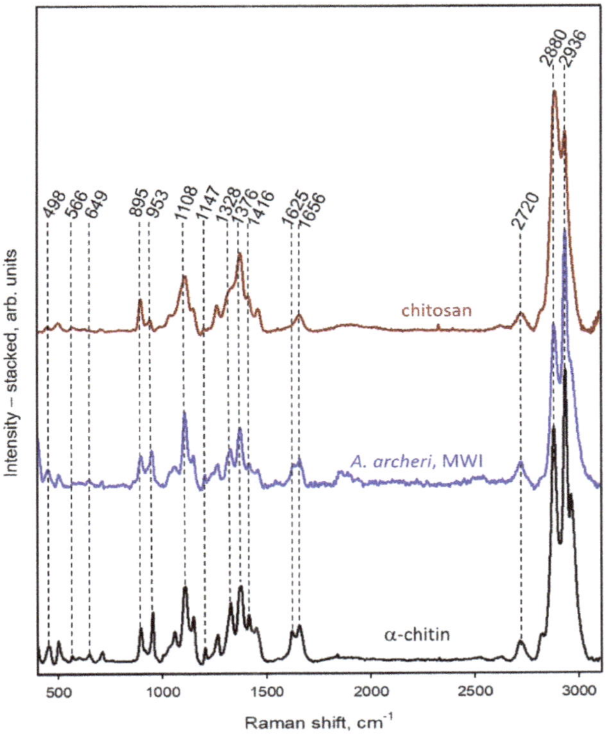

Figure 10. Raman spectra of chitosan standard (red line), α-chitin standard (black line), and chitin isolated from *A. archeri* demosponge using the microwave-assisted approach (blue line).

2.2. Capillary Effect of 3D Chitin Scaffolds

We also investigated the properties of 3D microtubular sponge chitin, related to its function as a capillary system. Previously, we reported that due to their tubular structure, chitinous scaffolds from the demosponge *Aplysina aerophoba* swelled with zirconyl salt solution and could be used as liquid delivery constructs [51]. Here, we chose to use several different model liquids, such as crude oil, pig blood, and methylene blue dye, particularly due to the differences in their physicochemical properties.

In spite, of the hydrophilic nature of the purified (lipid- and wax-free) 3D chitin scaffold isolated from *A. archeri*, the chitin reacts immediately on coming into contact with the surface of the tested crude oil (Figure 11). The same effect was observed by the team of Bo Duan when comparing an artificial chitin sponge synthesized by a freeze-drying method with a modified hydrophobic surface [52]. It has also been reported that chitin has a low oil absorbance capacity, if there is competition between water and oil absorption [53,54]. The rapid uptake of oil may result from the capillary action of the 3D tubular network and the presence of van der Waals forces.

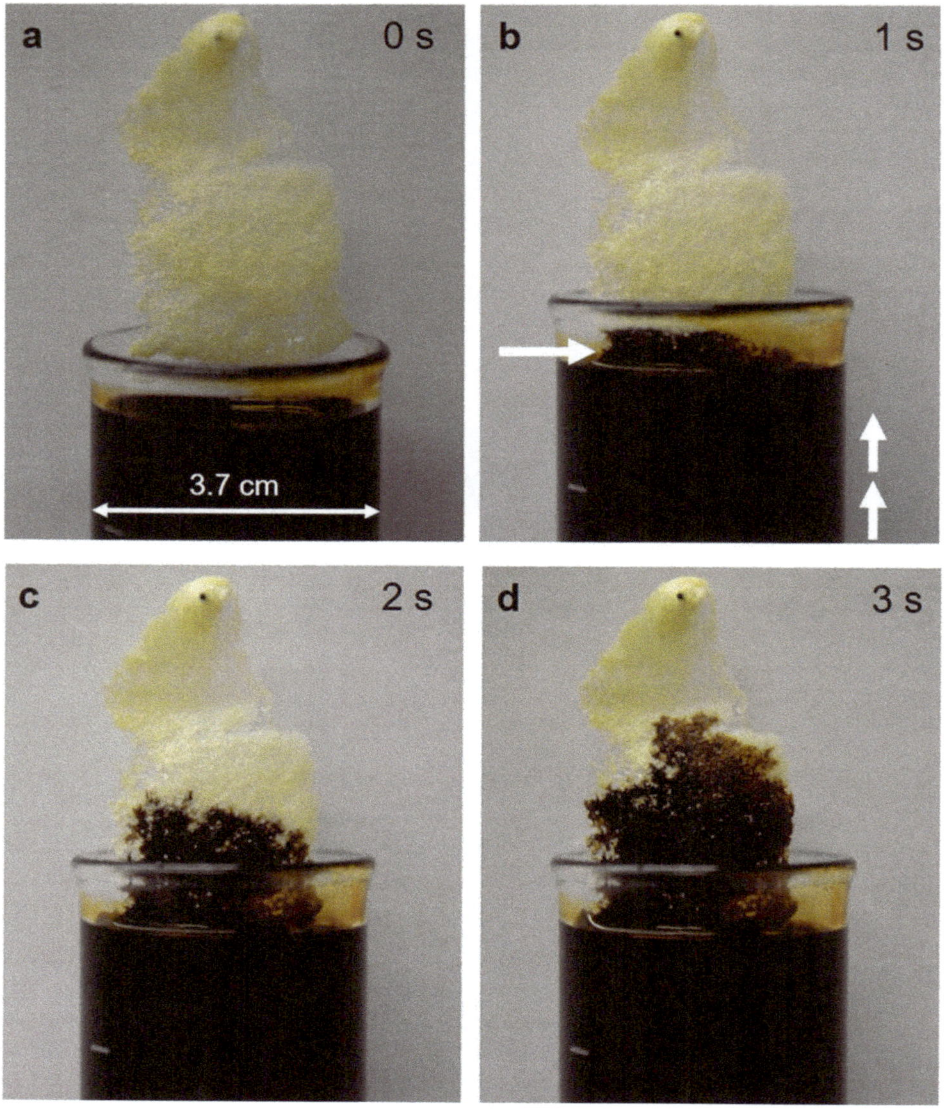

Figure 11. Capillary effect of the 3D chitinous microtubular scaffold isolated from *A. archeri* with respect to crude oil (**a**). On contact of the chitin with the surface of the oil (arrow, **b**), the latter is promptly distributed through the microtubular network (**b**,**c**,**d**). See also Figure 12.

Rinsing the scaffold contaminated with crude oil (Figure 11d) in a soap solution at 40 °C removes the oil from the scaffold's surface (Figure 12a). However, light microscopy observation of the inner surface of the microtubes of the chitinous scaffolds shows a significant presence of oil within those tubular structures (Figure 12b).

We observed a similar effect when pig blood was used (Figure 13). Due to its red color, this blood, located within the axial channels of the anastomosing microtubes of the *A. archeri* chitin microfibers, is very visible (Figure 13e).

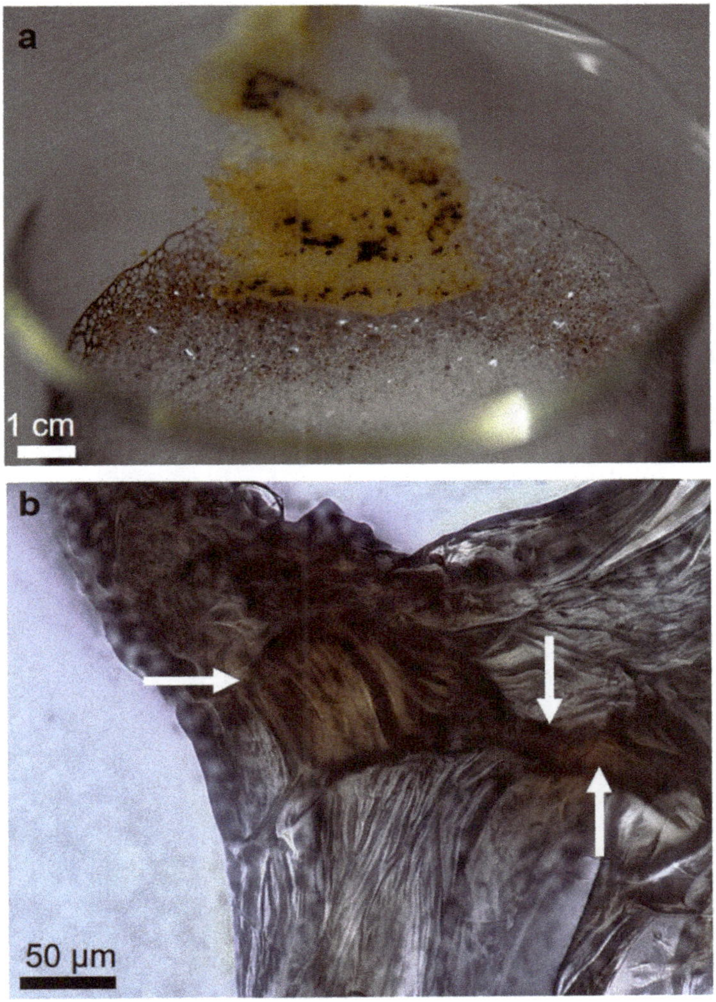

Figure 12. Rinsing of the chitin scaffold initially contaminated with crude oil (see Figure 11d) in soap solution promotes its removal from the surface of the scaffold (**a**). Nevertheless, residual oil is observable within the chitinous microtubes (arrows, **b**).

One possible application of 3D structured sponge-like hemostatic biomaterials could be as a compress during uncontrolled hemorrhaging (open wounds). It has been recognized that chitin of crustacean origin induces blood coagulation by adhering to platelets, forming a chitin/platelet complex that accelerates the polymerization of the fibrin monomer to form a blood clot (for review, see [55]). Consequently, several studies on chitin in the form of nanocrystals [56] or powders [55] as a potential hemostatic biomaterial have been carried out. However, for example, a hydrosol containing nanocrystalline particles showed no effect on the aggregation of human platelets and the clotting time of platelet-poor plasma in corresponding coagulation tests [56]. Therefore, we propose that experiments using 3D structured sponge chitins, including those from *A. archeri*, should be carried out to evaluate their hemostatic properties in future clinical settings.

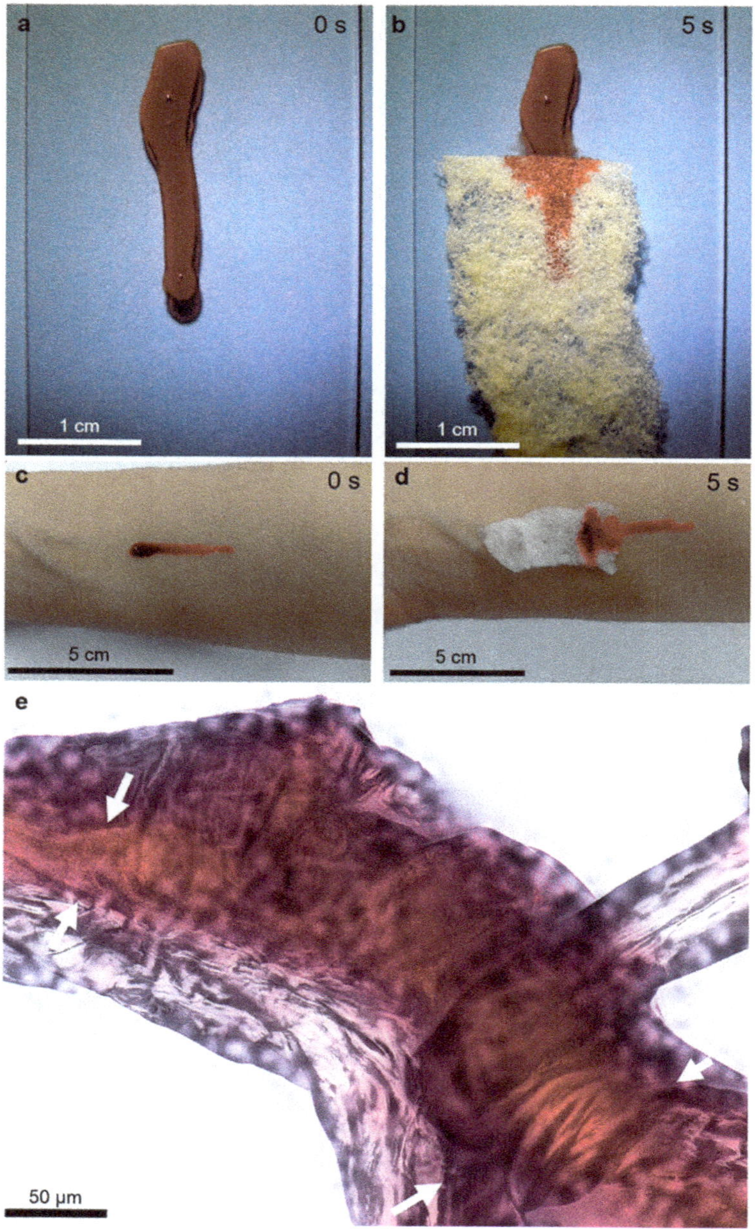

Figure 13. Pig blood as a model liquid is adsorbed by chitinous scaffold isolated from the *A. archeri* demosponge both from glass (**a**,**b**) and from a human skin surface (**c**,**d**). The blood remains confined within the axial channels (arrows) of the microtubular sponge chitin, even after rinsing with distilled water at room temperature (**e**).

Chitin has been considered recently as a biopolymer, which can be used as a low-cost and eco-friendly material for dye adsorption. Dotto et al. [57] reported ultrasonically-modified chitin as an effective sorbent for the removal of methylene blue (MB) from aqueous solutions by adsorption. Correspondingly, we have proven that 3D chitinous tubular scaffolds from *A. archeri*, obtained by the microwave-assisted method, can be used as a potential sorbent for MB. The swelling capacity of these scaffolds, with respect to water, was measured at 255 ± 8%. It should be noted that adsorption of the dye occurs on the surface as well as within the chitinous microtubes, and the dye could not be removed from the chitin by simply washing the chitin in hot distilled water (Figure 14). This confirms that the dye is chemically bonded to the chitin through electrostatic interactions with the chitin's OH and *N*-acetyl groups [57]. The unique 3D morphology and open cell structure of the isolated chitin scaffold and its observed affinity to MB open the way to use such scaffolds as a new type of renewable filling for fixed bed reactors used for the purification of dye-contaminated wastewater.

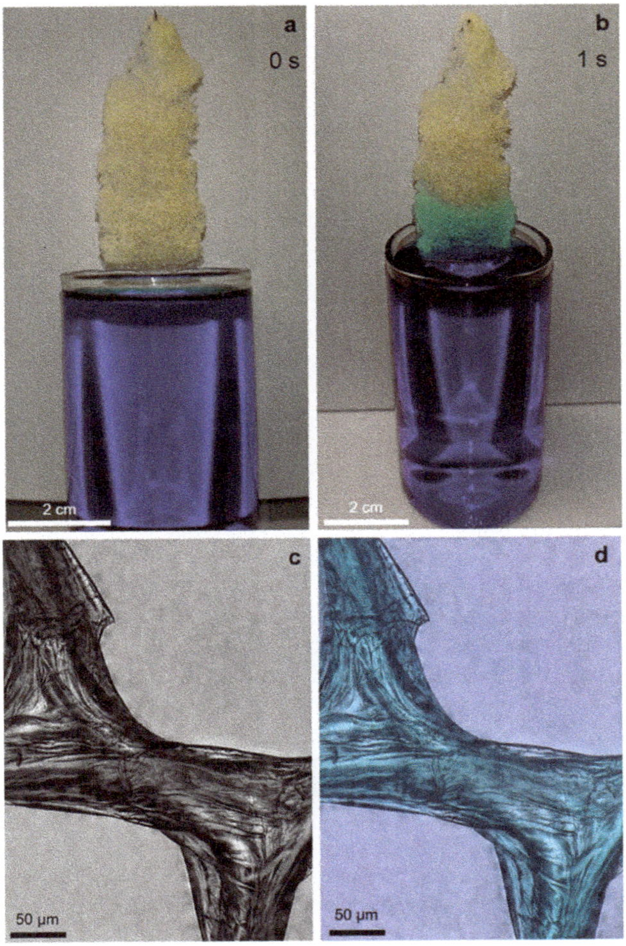

Figure 14. Image illustrating the adsorption of methylene blue (MB) on isolated 3D chitin scaffolds (**a**,**b**). The MB solution clearly reveals the tubular nature of the chitinous fiber in the scaffolds, resulting in the rising of liquid due to capillary forces. Light microscopy images of chitin after MB adsorption (**c**,**d**) clearly indicate that this dye is chemically adsorbed on the chitin surface as well as inside the chitinous microtubes, and cannot be removed from chitin by washing in hot distilled water.

3. Discussion

Microwave radiation has recently been shown to be a useful tool in modern green chemistry, with potential applications in a wide range of chemical processes [58,59]. Microwave-assisted extraction (MAE) is a green technique that offers numerous advantages, including the reduction of both extraction time and solvent consumption [60]. This method allows the acceleration of energy transfer, facilitating the solvation reaction and promoting the disruption of weak hydrogen bonds. It is currently considered a very attractive alternative to conventional extraction approaches (e.g., the Soxhlet method). Recently, microwave irradiation has been shown to be a promising technique for the extraction and modification of polysaccharides from natural sources [61], including chitin chemistry. This method is mostly used as an alternative for the preparation of chitosan from various chitinous sources [62–65]. It has been confirmed that microwave-assisted chitin processing reduces the time of deacetylation from ~8 h [64] to 5.5 min [65]. The application of microwave irradiation reduces not only process duration, but also the quantities of energy and chemicals used for highly deacetylated chitosan production from crustacean shell waste from the food industry. Microwave-assisted chitin activation was patented by Peniston and Johnson in 1979 [66]. Those authors claimed that exposure to microwave energy for a period from about 1 to 30 min, for example, can result in greatly increased reactivity of the chitin. They selected a preferred microwave frequency of about 2450 MHz. While this is a frequency at which water is absorptive, it is far removed from frequencies causing resonance for water molecules. It thus appears that effects other than agitation of water molecules are responsible for the pronounced activation of the chitin. On this basis, we used a similar microwave frequency in our experiments with *A. archeri*. Interestingly, Wongpanit et al. [67] reported microwave treatment as an effective method for activation of carboxymethyl chitin and carboxymethyl chitosan. They showed that human fibroblasts adhered on the surface of microwave-treated CM-chitosan films much better than on the surface of microwave-treated CM-chitin films. Our contribution to this area of research is that both (i) morphologically defined chitinous scaffolds with highly organized architecture and (ii) pigments can be effectively isolated using microwave-assisted extraction after only 55 min of treatment, including rinsing procedures.

The obtained pigment-based extracts (see Figure 3) will be studied in our future work with regard to the identification of bromotyrosines typical for *A. archeri*. For example, Fistularin 3 and 11-ketofistularin 3, isolated previously from this sponge species, showed antiviral activity against feline leukemia [68]. Another bromotyrosine, known as *archerine*, exhibited antihistamine activity on the isolated guinea pig ileum at concentrations as low as 1 μM [69]. Because of the dark color of the isolated pigments it is possible that the extract may also contain uranidine [70]. Interestingly, the influence of alkaline treatment on the yield and molecular structure of bromotyrosines remains unknown.

Practical applications of demosponge chitinous scaffolds for uranium adsorption [71] for the development of supercapacitors [72] and hybrid composites [73,74], including extreme biomimetics approaches [75,76], as well as in tissue engineering [10,77–79], have previously been reported. Here, we describe, for the first time, the ability of 3D chitinous constructs isolated from *A. archeri* using an express method to swell with such substances as crude oil, pig blood, and MB dye in a few seconds, due to a capillary effect. This property may open the way to key applications of the unique and renewable sponge chitin in remediation, biomedicine, and wastewater treatment. One of the advantages of such chitin is that it can be quickly isolated as a ready-to-use microtubular scaffold.

Furthermore, a corresponding paper about mechanical properties of selected chitinous scaffolds isolated from diverse verongiid sponges using different methodological approaches is currently in preparation. In that work, we will also present data concerning crystallinity index, degree of acetylation, specific surface area (BET), Young modulus, etc. Obviously, we will present these data in comparison with chitin of crustacean and fungal origins.

One of the most promising applications of ready-to-use chitinous microtubular scaffolds of sponge origin is biomedicine. However, it should be noted that both natural as well synthetic biopolymer-based three-dimensional, open pore scaffolds have evolved as gold standards for biomedicine in recent applications, owing to their superior role in tissue regeneration [80]. Three-dimensional polymer networks have attracted significant attention owing to their "soft-and-wet" nature, which is similar to biological tissues. The major drawback of such scaffolds is their relatively poor mechanical strength [81]. However, several possible solutions can be used to overcome this drawback. Among them, we highlight the controlled remineralization of biopolymers with selected inorganic compounds (i.e., hydroxyapatite) [82] or silica [83,84]. The infiltration and crystallization of the mentioned inorganic phases on all three levels of the chitin's hierarchical organization will definitively lead to the formation of a mechanically robust scaffold with superior performance in such advanced applications. Alternatively, to increase mechanical properties, biopolymeric scaffolds are often crosslinked. Inspired by the sclerotization of an insect cuticle, Chen et al. [85] reported a quinone crosslinking reaction for chitin hydrogels to increase their mechanical properties. The obtained crosslinked product shown a tenfold higher mechanical strength. Nevertheless, this is a topic for further studies. We believe that the present article will trigger scientific interest on the application of naturally pre-structured 3D scaffolds of sponge origin in biomedicine, and we believe that mechanical reinforcement of such scaffolds will soon be reported.

However, if the large-scale testing and application of chitin scaffolds is to be promoted, it will be necessary to secure the supply of such sponges via aquaculture [86], as wild harvest of these organisms will be not sustainable. Rohde and Schupp [87] have already demonstrated in a study of another Verongid sponge, *Ianthella basta*, that growth and regeneration rates in this sponge were sufficient to secure a supply for potential biomedical application. Further studies with other Verongiid sponges will be needed to establish this order of sponges as a viable source of chitin scaffolds and to enable the use of these naturally prefabricated constructs in biomedical applications.

4. Materials and Methods

4.1. Sample Collection

Samples of the demosponge, *Aplysina archeri* (Higgin 1875), were collected at depths of 10–25 m by scuba divers around the Caribbean islands of Saint Vincent and Curaçao in May 2015 and June 2017, during the Pacotilles expedition. All permits that were required for the described study were obtained during this expedition and complied with all relevant regulations. The species was identified by A. Ereskovsky.

4.2. Isolation of Chitin

4.2.1. Modified Standard Method

The isolation of the chitin scaffold from *A. archeri* was performed by a modification of the well-known standard method [4]. Firstly, the organic material was extracted with 2.5 M NaOH (Th. Geyer GmbH & Co. KG, Renningen, Germany,) at 37 °C for 6 h. Next, the resulting mineral skeletons of the sponges were treated with 2.5 M NaOH at 37 °C for 18 h. They were then washed with distilled water. The neutralized skeleton was then treated with 20% acetic acid (Th. Geyer GmbH & Co. KG, Renningen, Germany) at 37 °C for 6 h and neutralized by washing with distilled water. Alkaline and acidic extraction was repeated until the skeleton was completely demineralized, transparent, and soft (114 h).

4.2.2. Microwave-Assisted Approach for Chitin Isolation

The sample material of *A. archeri* was cut into pieces 5 cm × 2 cm in size and used for chitin isolation. The isolation procedure is presented schematically in Figure 3. Briefly, in step I the residual water-soluble salts were removed by pretreatment of sponge skeletons in distilled water using microwave irradiation (MWI) for 3 min. In step II, the sample was treated with 1% NaOH and irradiated with microwaves for 2 min. The 3D scaffolds were then carefully isolated and rinsed three times with distilled water to remove and separate residual red-brownish pigments. In step III, the 3D scaffolds were treated with 20% acetic acid under MWI for 1 min and were then washed in distilled water (up to pH 6.8). In step IV, samples were decolorized using H_2O_2 treatment at pH~10 under MWI for 1 min and then washed with distilled water until a neutral pH was reached.

Hydrogen peroxide was chosen for bleaching because it is reported that hydrogen peroxide in a microwave field, under the conditions of the experiment, does not cause significant changes in the chemical structure of the polymer [88]). Steps II–IV were repeated four times to obtain pure, colorless, 3D chitinous scaffolds.

4.2.3. Fluorescent Microscopy Analysis

The isolated chitin fibers were observed using a BZ-9000 instrument (Keyence, Osaka, Japan) in fluorescent and light microscopy mode.

4.2.4. Calcofluor White Staining

Upon binding with polysaccharides, calcofluor white (CFW) enhanced their fluorescence. The isolated fibers from the selected *A. archeri* skeletons were investigated with light and fluorescent microscopy before and after staining with CFW (Fluorescent Brightener M2R, Sigma-Aldrich). For staining, 20 µL of a solution of 10 g glycerin and 10 g NaOH in 90 mL water was applied. After 15 s, the CFW was added and kept for 30 min in darkness at room temperature. The fibers were washed with distilled water to remove unattached CFW and then dried at room temperature.

4.2.5. Chitinase Digestion Test

To observe the chitinase digestion process of the fibers isolated from sponge skeletons, the BZ-9000 instrument was used in light and fluorescent microscopy mode. Single fibers were rinsed with 50 mL phosphate buffer (pH 6.0). After the removal of the phosphate buffer, chitinase from *Streptomyces griseus* (EC 3.2.1.14, No. C-6137, Sigma-Aldrich) was added. In the following 10 h, the microscope documented the digestion of the fibers by taking light field and fluorescent images every 30 min.

4.2.6. ATR-FTIR Spectroscopy

Infrared spectroscopy was used for qualitative analysis of the isolated fibers. ATR-FTIR (attenuated total reflectance Fourier transformation infrared spectroscopy) spectra were recorded with the Nicolet 380 FTIR spectrometer (Thermo Scientific, Inc., Madison, WA, USA). The spectra were analyzed with appropriate software (OMNIC Lite Software, Madison, WA, USA). In addition to the spectra of the fiber material, spectra of the *α*-chitin standard (INTIB GmbH, Freiberg, Germany) and a chitosan standard (Sigma-Aldrich) were recorded. Postprocessing of the recorded spectra was performed with OriginLab 2015.

4.2.7. Raman Spectroscopy

Raman spectra were recorded with a Raman spectrometer (Raman Rxn1^{TM}, Kaiser Optical Systems Inc., Ann Arbor, MI, USA) coupled with a light microscope (DM2500 P, Leica Microsystems GmbH, Wetzlar, Germany). The laser beam had a power of 400 mW, which resulted in 110 mW at the sample due to the transmission of the microscope optics. The spectral range was from 200 to 3250 cm^{-1}, with a set resolution of 4 cm^{-1}. For improvement of the signal-to-noise ratio, the integration time was set to 1 s and an addition of 50 spectra was performed. The baseline was implemented with MATLAB (MathWorks Inc., Natick, MA, USA) and further postprocessing was carried out with OriginPro 2015.

4.2.8. Scanning Electron Microscopy

Scanning electron microscopy was performed using an XL 30 ESEM Philips-Scanning Electron Microscope (FEI Company, Peabody, MA, USA). Samples were fixed on a sample holder with carbon patches, and these were then covered with carbon or with a 5–10 µm gold layer using an Edwards Sputter Coater S150B (BOC Edwards, Wilmington, MA, USA).

4.2.9. EDX

The elements were analyzed by energy dispersive X-ray spectroscopy in the EDX analysis system from EDAX (Mahwah, NJ, USA) and XL 30 ESEM Philips-Scanning Electron Microscope (FEI Company, Peabody, MA, USA).

4.2.10. Electrospray Ionisation Mass Spectrometry (ESI-MS)

Samples were prepared for ESI-MS as follows. The isolated chitin scaffold was hydrolyzed in 6M HCl for 24 h at 90 °C. The resulting solution was filtered with a 0.4-micron filter, and the filtrate was freeze-dried to remove excess HCl. The solid residue was dissolved in water for ESI-MS analysis. Standard d-glucosamine, used as a control, was purchased from Sigma (Sigma-Aldrich, Taufkirchen, Germany). All ESI-MS measurements were performed on an Agilent Technologies 6230 TOF LC/MS spectrometer (Applied Biosystems, Foster City, CA, USA). Nitrogen was used as a nebulizing and desolvation gas. Graphs were generated using Origin 8.5 for PC.

4.2.11. Sorption Experiments

For the sorption experiments, crude oil (collected using sterile glass bottles from the oilfield located in Borislav, Ukraine), pig blood (Südost-Fleisch GmbH, Altenburg, Germany) and methylene blue (Sigma-Aldrich) were used.

4.2.12. Swelling Capacity Measurements

The swelling capacity (water) of isolated 3D chitinous scaffolds was calculated using the following formula [89]:

$$Swelling\ capacity\ (\%) = \frac{m_S - m_d}{m_d} \cdot 100\%$$

where, m_S is the mass of the swollen sponge chitin and m_d is the mass of the dry sponge chitin.

5. Conclusions

In this study, the presence of chitin in the skeleton of *A. archeri* has been proven for the first time. Furthermore, microwave-assisted demineralization and deproteinization have been established as new and rapid methods for both chitin and pigment extraction from verongiid demosponges. It has been demonstrated, beyond a doubt, that the new approaches enable a significant improvement in the time efficiency of chitin isolation from Verongiida sponges without destruction of the unique fibrous interconnected structure of the isolated biological material. Furthermore, these mechanically stressed fibers still have the capacity for saturation with water, methylene blue dye, crude oil, and blood, which will be crucial for future applications of such naturally prefabricated 3D chitinous centimeter-sized scaffolds in diverse technological and biomedical fields. As the analysis of the isolated scaffolds has shown, under the conditions studied here, the microwaves do not deacetylate the chitin to chitosan. The method proposed in this study both reduced the consumption of the aggressive chemicals as well as drastically reduced the time of chitin extraction. Therefore, microwave assisted extraction is a viable, cost efficient, and fast method for the production of chitin scaffolds from marine sources.

Author Contributions: H.E., M.W., Y.J., S.R.B. and M.G. designed the study protocol and wrote the manuscript; A.E., R.M., V.I., P.J.S. collected the sponge materials and carried out species identification; C.K., S.Ż.A., T.M., M.V.T., R.G., I.P., L.M., O.B.S., A.V., Y.J. and N.B. prepared samples, performed detailed physico-chemical characterization of obtained chitin as well as carried out saturation tests. T.J., P.S. and N.B. edited the manuscript. All the authors critically reviewed and approved the final version of the manuscript.

Funding: This work was partially supported by the DFG Project HE 394/3 (Germany); SMWK Project 2018 no. 02010311 (Germany); DAAD-Italy Project "Marine Sponges as Sources for Bioinspired Materials Science" (No. 57397326). The Temminck Fellowship from Naturalis Biodiversity and CARMABI Marine Research Center (Curaçao) provided financial and logistical support of V.I., respectively. Samples from Curaçao were processed with support of the Russian Foundation for Basic Research (grant 18-54-34007). Marcin Wysokowski was supported by DAAD (No 91528917). There was no additional external funding received for this study. This research was partially funded by the Ministry of Science and Higher Education (Poland) through a financial subsidy to PUT (S.Ż.-A., M.W., T.M. & T.J.).

Acknowledgments: Special thanks for technical assistance and discussions are given to BromMarin GmbH and INTIB GmbH (Germany).

Conflicts of Interest: The authors declare no conflict of interest.

References

1. Wysokowski, M.; Petrenko, I.; Stelling, A.L.; Stawski, D.; Jesionowski, T.; Ehrlich, H. Chitin as a versatile template for extreme biomimetics. *Polymers* **2015**, *7*, 235–265. [CrossRef]
2. Ehrlich, H. Chitin and collagen as universal and alternative templates in biomineralization. *Int. Geo. Rev.* **2010**, *52*, 661–699. [CrossRef]
3. Agbaje, O.B.A.; Ben, S.I.; Zax, D.B.; Schmidt, A.; Jacob, D.E. Biomacromolecules within bivalve shells: Is chitin abundant? *Acta Biomater.* **2018**, *80*, 176–187. [CrossRef] [PubMed]
4. Ehrlich, H.; Maldonado, M.; Spindler, K.D.; Eckert, C.; Hanke, T.; Born, R.; Goebel, C.; Simon, P.; Heinemann, S.; Worch, H. First evidence of chitin as a component of the skeletal fibers of marine sponges. Part I. Verongidae (demospongia: Porifera). *J. Exp. Zool. B Mol. Dev. Evol.* **2007**, *308B*, 347–356. [CrossRef] [PubMed]
5. Ehrlich, H.; Maldonado, M.; Parker, A.R.; Kulchin, Y.N.; Schilling, J.; Köhler, B.; Skrzypczak, U.; Simon, P.; Reiswig, H.M.; Tsurkan, M.V.; et al. Supercontinuum generation in naturally occurring glass sponges spicules. *Adv. Opt. Mater.* **2016**, *4*, 1608–1613. [CrossRef]
6. Nikolov, S.; Petrov, M.; Lymperakis, L.; Friak, M.; Sachs, C.; Fabritius, H.O.; Raabe, D.; Neugebauer, J. Revealing the design principles of high-performance biological composites using Ab initio and multiscale simulations: The example of lobster cuticle. *Adv. Mater.* **2010**, *22*, 519–526. [CrossRef]
7. Brunner, E.; Ehrlich, H.; Schupp, P.; Hedrich, R.; Hunoldt, S.; Kammer, M.; Machill, S.; Paasch, S.; Bazhenov, V.V.; Kurek, D.V.; et al. Chitin-based scaffolds are an integral part of the skeleton of the marine demosponge *Ianthella basta*. *J. Struct. Biol.* **2009**, *168*, 539–547. [CrossRef]
8. Ehrlich, H.; Krautter, M.; Hanke, T.; Simon, P.; Knieb, C.; Heinemann, S.; Worch, H. First evidence of the presence of chitin in skeletons of marine sponges. Part II. Glass sponges (Hexactinellida: Porifera). *J. Exp. Zool.* **2007**, *308B*, 473–483. [CrossRef]
9. Ehrlich, H.; Ilan, M.; Maldonado, M.; Muricy, G.; Bavestrello, G.; Kljajic, Z.; Carballo, J.L.; Schiaparelli, S.; Ereskovsky, A.; Schupp, P.; et al. Three-dimensional chitin-based scaffolds from Verongida sponges (Demospongiae: Porifera). Part I. Isolation and identification of chitin. *Int. J. Biol. Macromol.* **2010**, *47*, 132–140. [CrossRef]
10. Ehrlich, H.; Steck, E.; Ilan, M.; Maldonado, M.; Muricy, G.; Bavestrello, G.; Kljajic, Z.; Carballo, J.L.; Schiaparelli, S.; Ereskovsky, A.; et al. Three-dimensional chitin-based scaffolds from Verongida sponges (Demospongiae: Porifera). Part II: Biomimetic potential and applications. *Int. J. Biol. Macromol.* **2010**, *47*, 141–145. [CrossRef]
11. Ehrlich, H.; Simon, P.; Carrillo-Cabrera, W.; Bazhenov, V.V.; Botting, J.P.; Ilan, M.; Ereskovsky, A.V.; Muricy, G.; Worch, H.; Mensch, A.; et al. Insights into chemistry of biological materials: Newly discovered silica-aragonite-chitin biocomposites in demosponges. *Chem. Mater.* **2010**, *22*, 1462–1471. [CrossRef]
12. Roberts, G.A.F. *Chitin Chemistry*, 1st ed.; MacMillian: London, UK, 1992.
13. Cahú, T.B.; Santos, S.D.; Mendes, A.; Córdula, C.R.; Chavante, S.F.; Carvalho, L.B.; Nader, H.B.; Bezerra, R.S. Recovery of protein, chitin, carotenoids and glycosaminoglycans from Pacific white shrimp (*Litopenaeus vannamei*) processing waste. *Process Biochem.* **2012**, *47*, 570–577. [CrossRef]
14. Hackman, R.H. Studies on chitin V. The action of mineral acids on chitin. *Aust. J. Biol. Sci.* **1962**, *15*, 526–537. [CrossRef]

15. Brine, C.J.; Austin, P.R. Chitin variability with species and method of preparation. *Comp. Biochem. Physiol.* **1981**, *69B*, 283–286. [CrossRef]
16. Hayes, M.; Carney, B.; Slater, J.; Brück, W. Mining marine shellfish wastes for bioactive molecules: Chitin and chitosan – Part B: Applications. *Biotechnol. J.* **2008**, *3*, 878–889. [CrossRef] [PubMed]
17. Rasti, H.; Parivar, K.; Baharara, J.; Iranshahi, M.; Namvar, F. Chitin from the Mollusc chiton: extraction, characterization and chitosan preparation. *Iran J. Pharm. Res.* **2017**, *16*, 366–379. [PubMed]
18. Bulut, E.; Sargin, I.; Arslan, O.; Odabasi, M.; Akyuz, B.; Kaya, M. In situ chitin isolation from body parts of a centipede and lysozyme adsorption studies. *Mater. Sci. Eng. C* **2017**, *70*, 552–563. [CrossRef] [PubMed]
19. Ibitoye, E.B.; Lokman, I.H.; Hezmee, M.N.M.; Goh, Y.M.; Zuki, A.B.Z.; Jimoh, A.A. Extraction and physicochemical characterization of chitin and chitosan isolated from house cricket. *Biomed. Mater.* **2018**, *13*, 025009. [CrossRef] [PubMed]
20. Soon, C.Y.; Tee, Y.B.; Tan, C.H.; Rosnita, A.T.; Khalina, A. Extraction and physicochemical characterization of chitin and chitosan from *Zophobas morio* larvae in varying sodium hydroxide concentration. *Int. J. Biol. Macromol.* **2018**, *108*, 135–142. [CrossRef] [PubMed]
21. Rinaudo, M. Chitin and chitosan: properties and applications. *Prog. Polym. Sci.* **2006**, *31*, 603–632. [CrossRef]
22. Younes, I.; Rinaudo, M. Chitin and chitosan preparation from marine sources. Structure, properties and applications. *Mar. Drugs* **2015**, *13*, 1133–1174. [CrossRef] [PubMed]
23. Foster, A.B.; Hackman, R.H. Application of ethylenediaminetetraacetic acid in the isolation of crustacean chitin. *Nature* **1957**, *180*, 40–41. [CrossRef]
24. Arbia, W.; Arbia, L.; Adour, L.; Amrane, A. Chitin extraction from crustacean shells using biological methods - A review. *Food Technol. Biotechnol.* **2013**, *51*, 12–25.
25. Kaya, M.; Karaarslan, M.; Baran, T.; Can, E.; Ekemen, G.; Bitim, B.; Duman, F. The quick extraction of chitin from an epizoic crustacean species (*Chelonibia patula*). *Nat. Prod. Res.* **2014**, *28*, 2186–2190. [CrossRef] [PubMed]
26. Shahidi, F.; Synowiecki, J. Isolation and characterization of nutrients and value-added products from snow crab (*Chionoecetes opilio*) and shrimp (*Pandalus borealis*) processing discards. *J. Agric. Food Chem.* **1991**, *39*, 1527–1532. [CrossRef]
27. Martin, R.E.; Flick, G.J.; Hebard, C.E.; Ward, D.R. *Chemistry & Biochemistry of Marine Food Products;* AVI Publishing Co.: Westport, CT, USA, 1982.
28. Marquis-Duval, F.O. Isolation et valorisation des constituants de la carapace de la crevette nordique. Ph.D. Thesis, Laval University, Quebec, QC, Canada, 2008.
29. Kaur, S.; Dhillon, G.S. Recent trends in biological extraction of chitin from marine shell wastes: A review. *Crit. Rev. Biotechnol.* **2015**, *35*, 44–61. [CrossRef] [PubMed]
30. Truong, T.O.; Hausler, R.; Monette, F.; Niquette, P. Valorisation des residus industriels de peches pour la transformation de chitosane par technique hydrothermo-chimique. *Rev. Sci. Eau.* **2007**, *20*, 253–262.
31. Okafor, V. Isolation of chitin from the shell of the cuttlefish, *Sepia officinalis* L. *BBA* **1965**, *101*, 193–200. [CrossRef]
32. Khanafari, A.; Marandi, R.; Sanatei, S. Recovery of chitin and chitosan from shrimp waste by chemical and microbial methods. *Iran J. Env. Heal. Sci. Eng.* **2008**, *5*, 1–24.
33. Berton, P.; Shamshina, J.L.; Ostadjoo, S.; King, C.A.; Rogers, R.D. Enzymatic hydrolysis of ionic liquid-extracted chitin. *Carbohydr. Polym.* **2018**, *199*, 228–235. [CrossRef]
34. Knidri, H.E.; Belaabed, R.; Addaou, A.; Laajeb, A.; Lahsini, A. Extraction, chemical modification and characterization of chitin and chitosan. *Int. J. Biol. Macromol.* **2018**, *120*, 1181–1189. [CrossRef] [PubMed]
35. Tokatli, K.; Demirdöven, A. Optimization of chitin and chitosan production from shrimp wastes and characterization. *J. Food. Process. Preserv.* **2017**, *42*, e13494. [CrossRef]
36. Dun, Y.; Li, Y.; Xu, J.; Hu, Y.; Zhang, C.; Liang, Y.; Zhao, S. Simultaneous fermentation and hydrolysis to extract chitin from crayfish shell waste. *Int. J. Biol. Macromol.* **2018**, *123*, 420–426. [CrossRef] [PubMed]
37. Saravana, P.S.; Ho, T.C.; Chae, S.J.; Cho, Y.J.; Park, J.S.; Lee, H.J.; Chun, B.S. Deep eutectic solvent-based extraction and fabrication of chitin films from crustacean waste. *Carbohydr. Polym.* **2018**, *195*, 622–630. [CrossRef] [PubMed]
38. Castro, R.; Guerrero-Legarreta, I.; Bórquez, R. Chitin extraction from *Allopetrolisthes punctatus* crab using lactic fermentation. *Biotechnol. Rep.* **2018**, *20*, e00287. [CrossRef] [PubMed]

39. Huang, W.C.; Zhao, D.; Guo, N.; Xue, C.; Mao, X. Green and facile production of chitin from crustacean shells using a natural deep eutectic solvent. *J. Agric. Food Chem.* **2018**, *66*, 11897–11901. [CrossRef]
40. Hong, S.; Yang, Q.; Yuan, Y.; Chen, L.; Song, Y.; Lian, H. Sustainable co-solvent induced one step extraction of low molecular weight chitin with high purity from raw lobster shell. *Carbohydr. Polym.* **2019**, *205*, 236–243. [CrossRef]
41. Jesionowski, T.; Norman, M.; Żółtowska-Aksamitowska, S.; Petrenko, I.; Joseph, Y.; Ehrlich, H. Marine spongin: naturally prefabricated 3D scaffold-based biomaterial. *Mar. Drugs* **2018**, *16*, 88. [CrossRef]
42. Żółtowska-Aksamitowska, S.; Shaala, L.A.; Youssef, D.T.A.; Elhady, S.S.; Tsurkan, M.V.; Petrenko, I.; Wysokowski, M.; Tabachnick, K.; Meissner, H.; Ivanenko, V.N.; et al. First report on chitin in a non-Verongiid marine Demosponge: *the Mycale euplectellioides* case. *Mar. Drugs* **2018**, *16*, 68. [CrossRef]
43. Żółtowska-Aksamitowska, S.; Tsurkan, M.V.; Lim, S.C.; Meissner, H.; Tabachnick, K.; Shaala, L.A.; Youssef, D.T.A.; Ivanenko, V.N.; Petrenko, I.; Wysokowski, M.; et al. The demosponge *Pseudoceratina purpurea* as a new source of fibrous chitin. *Int. J. Biol. Macromol.* **2018**, *112*, 1021–1028. [CrossRef]
44. Van Soest, R.W.M.; Boury-Esnault, N.; Hooper, J.N.A.; Rützler, K.; de Voogd, N.J.; Alvarez, B.; Hajdu, E.; Pisera, A.B.; Manconi, R.; Schönberg, C.; et al. World Porifera database. *Aplysina Archeri* **1875**. Available online: http://www.marinespecies.org/porifera/porifera.php?p=taxdetails&id=169636 (accessed on 22 February 2019).
45. Bechmann, N.; Ehrlich, H.; Eisenhofer, G.; Ehrlich, A.; Meschke, S.; Ziegler, C.G.; Bornstein, S.R. Anti-tumorigenic and anti-metastatic activity of the sponge-derived marine drugs Aeroplysinin-1 and Isofistularin-3 against Pheochromocytoma in vitro. *Mar. Drugs* **2018**, *16*, 172. [CrossRef] [PubMed]
46. Wysokowski, M.; Bazhenov, V.V.; Tsurkan, M.V.; Galli, R.; Stelling, A.L.; Stöcker, H.; Kaiser, S.; Niederschlag, E.; Gärtner, G.; Behm, T.; et al. Isolation and identification of chitin in three-dimensional skeleton of *Aplysina fistularis* marine sponge. *Int. J. Biol. Macromol.* **2013**, *62*, 94–100. [CrossRef] [PubMed]
47. Nickerl, J.; Tsurkan, M.; Hensel, R.; Neinhuis, C.; Werner, C. The multi-layered protective cuticle of Collembola: a chemical analysis. *J. R. Soc. Interface* **2014**, *11*, 6–19. [CrossRef]
48. Ehrlich, H.; Rigby, J.K.; Botting, J.P.; Tsurkan, M.; Werner, C.; Schwille, P.; Petrasek, Z.; Pisera, A.; Simon, P.; Sivkov, V.; et al. Discovery of 505-million-year old chitin in the basal demosponge *Vauxia gracilenta*. *Sci. Rep.* **2013**, *3*, 3497. [CrossRef] [PubMed]
49. Focher, B.; Naggi, T.; Cosani, A.; Terbojevich, M. Structural differences between chitin polymorphs and their precipitates from solutions—evidence from CP-MAS 13C-NMR, FT-IR and FT-Raman spectroscopy. *Carbohydr. Polym.* **1992**, *17*, 97–102. [CrossRef]
50. Kumirska, J.; Czerwicka, M.; Kaczyński, Z.; Bychowska, A.; Brzozowski, K.; Thöming, J.; Stepnowski, P. Application of spectroscopic methods for structural analysis of chitin and chitosan. *Mar. Drugs* **2010**, *8*, 1567–1636. [CrossRef]
51. Wysokowski, M.; Motylenko, M.; Bazhenov, V.V.; Stawski, D.; Petrenko, I.; Ehrlich, A.; Behm, T.; Kljajic, Z.; Stelling, A.L.; Jesionowski, T.; et al. Poriferan chitin as template for hydrotermal zirconia deposition. *Front. Mater. Sci.* **2013**, *7*, 248–260.
52. Duan, B.; Gao, H.; He, M.; Zhang, L. Hydrophobic Modification on surface of chitin sponges for highly effective separation of oil. *Appl. Mater. Interfaces* **2014**, *6*, 19933–19942. [CrossRef]
53. Setti, L.; Mazzieri, S.; Pifferi, P.G. Enhanced degradation of heavy oil in an aqueous system by a *Pseudomonas sp.* in the presence of natural and synthetic sorbents. *Biores. Technology* **1999**, *67*, 191–199. [CrossRef]
54. De Freitas Barros, F.C.; Grombone Vasconcellos, L.C.; Vieira Carvalho, T.; Ferreira do Nascimento, R. Removal of petroleum spill in water by chitin and chitosan. *Electron. J. Chem.* **2014**, *6*, 70–74.
55. Lv, L.; Tang, F.; Lan, G. Preparation and characterization of a chitin/platelet-poor plasma composite as a hemostatic material. *RSC Advances* **2016**, *6*, 95358–95368. [CrossRef]
56. Drozd, N.N.; Torlopov, M.A.; Udoratina, E.V.; Logvinova, Y.S. Effect of nanocrystalline particles of chitin on blood components in humans and experimental animals. *Bull Exp. Biol. Med.* **2018**, *164*, 766–769. [CrossRef] [PubMed]
57. Dotto, G.L. Adsorption of Methylene Blue by ultrasonic surface modified chitin. *J. Colloid Interface Sci.* **2015**, *446*, 133–140. [CrossRef] [PubMed]
58. Ravichandran, S.; Karthikeyan, E. Microwave synthesis-a potential tool for green chemistry. *Int. J. Chem. Tech. Res.* **2011**, *3*, 466–470.

59. Nüchter, M.; Ondruschka, B.; Bonrath, W.; Gum, A. Microwave assisted synthesis–a critical technology overview. *Green Chem.* **2004**, *6*, 128–141. [CrossRef]
60. Duarte, K.; Justino, C.I.L.; Gomes, A.M.; Rocha-Santos, T.; Duarte, A.C. Green analytical methodologies for preparation of extracts and analysis of bioactive compounds. *Compr. Anal. Chem.* **2014**, *65*, 59–78.
61. Soria, A.C.; Ruiz-Aceituno, L.; Ramos, L.; Sanz, L.M. Microwave-assisted extraction of polysaccharides. In *Polysaccharides*; Ramawat, K., Mérillon, J.M., Eds.; Springer: Cham, Germany, 2014; pp. 1–18.
62. Apriyanti, D.T.; Susanto, H.; Rokhati, N. Influence of microwave irradiation on extraction of chitosan from shrimp shell waste. *Reaktor* **2018**, *18*, 45–50. [CrossRef]
63. Al Sagheer, F.A.; Al-Sughayer, M.A.; Muslim, S.; Elsabee, M.Z. Extraction and characterization of chitin and chitosan from marine sources in Arabian Gulf. *Cabohydr. Polym.* **2009**, *77*, 410–419. [CrossRef]
64. Sahu, A.; Goswami, P.; Bora, U. Microwave mediated rapid synthesis of chitosan. *J. Mater Sci. Mater Med.* **2009**, *20*, 171–175. [CrossRef]
65. Lertwattanaseri, T.; Ichikawa, N.; Mizoguchi, T.; Tanaka, Y.; Chirachanchai, S. Microwave technique for efficient deacetylation of chitin nanowhiskers to a chitosan nanoscaffold. *Carbohydr. Res.* **2009**, *344*, 331–335. [CrossRef] [PubMed]
66. Peniston, Q.P.; Johnson, E.L. Process for activating chitin by microwave treatment and improved activated chitin product. US4159932, 7 March 1979.
67. Wongpanit, P.; Sanchavanakit, N.; Pavasant, P.; Supaphol, P.; Tokura, S.; Rujiravanit, R. Preparation and characterization of microwave-treated carboxymethyl chitin and carboxymethyl chitosan films for potential use in wound care application. *Macromol Biosci.* **2005**, *5*, 1001–1012. [CrossRef]
68. Gunasekera, S.P.; Cross, S.S. Fistularin 3 and 11-ketofistularin 3. Feline leukemia virus active bromotyrosine metabolites from the marine sponge *Aplysina archeri*. *J. Nat. Prod.* **1992**, *55*, 509–512. [CrossRef] [PubMed]
69. Ciminiello, P.; Dell'Aversano, C.; Fattorusso, E.; Magno, S. Archerine, A novel anti-histaminic bromotyrosine-derived compound from the caribbean marine sponge *Aplysina archeri*. *Eur. J. Org. Chem.* **2001**, *1*, 55–60. [CrossRef]
70. Cimino, G.; De Rosa, S.; De Stefano, S.; Sodano, G. The zoochrome of the sponge *Verongia aerophoba* ("Uranidine"). *Tetrahedron Lett.* **1984**, *25*, 2925–2928. [CrossRef]
71. Schleuter, D.; Günther, A.; Paasch, S.; Ehrlich, H.; Kljajic, Z.; Hanke, T.; Bernhard, G.; Brunner, E. Chitin-based renewable materials from marine sponges for uranium adsorption. *Carbohydr. Polym.* **2013**, *92*, 712–718. [CrossRef] [PubMed]
72. Stepniak, I.; Galinski, M.; Nowacki, K.; Wysokowski, M.; Jakubowska, P.; Bazhenov, V.V.; Leisegang, T.; Ehrlich, H.; Jesionowski, T. A novel chitosan/sponge chitin origin material as a membrane for supercapacitors – preparation and characterization. *RSC Advances* **2016**, *6*, 4007–4013. [CrossRef]
73. Wysokowski, M.; Behm, T.; Born, R.; Bazhenov, V.V.; Meissner, H.; Richter, G.; Szwarc–Rzepka, K.; Makarova, A.; Vyalikh, D.; Schupp, P.; et al. Preparation of chitin–silica composites by in vitro silicification of two–dimensional *Ianthella basta* demosponge chitinous scaffolds under modified Stöber conditions. *Mater. Sci. Eng.* **2013**, *33*, 3935–3941. [CrossRef]
74. Ehrlich, H. Biomimetic potential of chitin–based composite biomaterials of poriferan origin. In *Biomimetic Biomaterials: Structure and Applications*; Ruys, A.J., Ed.; Woodhead Publishing: Cambridge, UK, 2013; pp. 47–67.
75. Wysokowski, M.; Motylenko, M.; Beyer, J.; Makarova, A.; Stöcker, H.; Walter, J.; Galli, R.; Kaiser, S.; Vyalikh, D.; Bazhenov, V.V.; et al. Extreme biomimetic approach for development of novel chitin–GeO2 nanocomposites with photoluminescent properties. *Nano Res.* **2015**, *8*, 2288–2301. [CrossRef]
76. Petrenko, I.; Bazhenov, V.V.; Galli, R.; Wysokowski, M.; Fromont, J.; Schupp, P.J.; Stelling, A.L.; Niederschlag, E.; Stöcker, H.; Kutsova, V.Z.; et al. Chitin of poriferan origin and the bioelectrometallurgy of copper/copper oxide. *Int. J. Biol. Macromol.* **2017**, *104*, 1626–1632. [CrossRef]
77. Steck, E.; Burkhardt, M.; Ehrlich, H.; Richter, W. Discrimination between cells of murine and human origin in xenotransplants by species specific genomic in situ hybridization. *Xenotransplantation* **2010**, *17*, 153–159. [CrossRef] [PubMed]
78. Mutsenko, V.V.; Bazhenov, V.V.; Rogulska, O.; Tarusin, D.N.; Schütz, K.; Brüggemeier, S.; Gossla, E.; Akkineni, A.R.; Meissner, H.; Lode, A.; et al. 3D chitinous scaffolds derived from cultivated marine demosponge *Aplysina aerophoba* for tissue engineering approaches based on human mesenchymal stromal cells. *Int. J. Biol. Macromol.* **2017**, *104*, 1966–1974. [CrossRef] [PubMed]

79. Mutsenko, V.V.; Gryshkov, O.; Lauterboeck, L.; Rogulska, O.; Tarusin, D.N.; Bazhenov, V.V.; Schütz, K.; Brüggemeier, S.; Gossla, E.; Akkineni, A.R.; et al. Novel chitin scaffolds derived from marine sponge *Ianthella basta* for tissue engineering approaches based on human mesenchymal stromal cells: biocompatibility and cryopreservation. *Int. J. Biol. Macromol.* **2017**, *104*, 1955–1965. [CrossRef] [PubMed]
80. Okamoto, M.; John, B. Synthetic biopolymer nanocomposites for tissue engineering scaffolds. *Prog. Polym. Sci.* **2013**, *38*, 1487–1503. [CrossRef]
81. Prasadh, S.; Wong, R.C.W. Unraveling the mechanical strength of biomaterials used as a bone scaffold in oral and maxillofacial defects. *Oral Sci. Int.* **2018**, *15*, 48–55. [CrossRef]
82. Chang, C.; Peng, N.; He, M.; Teramoto, Y.; Nishio, Y.; Zhang, L. Fabrication and properties of chitin/hydroxyapatite hybrid hydrogels as scaffold nano-materials. *Carbohydr.Polym.* **2013**, *91*, 7–13. [CrossRef] [PubMed]
83. Niu, L.N.; Jiao, K.; Qi, Y.; Yiu, C.K.Y.; Ryou, H.; Arola, D.D.; Chen, J.; Breschi, L.; Pashley, D.H.; Tay, F.R. Infiltration of Silica Inside Fibrillar Collagen. *Angew. Chem. Int. Ed.* **2011**, *50*, 11688–11691. [CrossRef] [PubMed]
84. Smolyakov, G.; Pruvost, S.; Cardoso, L.; Alonso, B.; Belamie, E.; Duchet-Rumeau, J. AFM PeakForce QNM mode: Evidencing nanometre-scale mechanical properties of chitin-silica hybrid nanocomposites. *Carbohydr. Polym.* **2016**, *151*, 373–380. [CrossRef] [PubMed]
85. Chen, C.; Li, D.; Yano, H.; Abe, K. Bioinspired hydrogels: Quinone crosslinking reaction for chitin nanofibers with enhanced mechanical strength via surface deacetylation. *Carbohydr. Polym.* **2019**, *207*, 411–417. [CrossRef]
86. Shaala, L.A.; Asfour, H.Z.; Youssef, D.T.A.; Żółtowska-Aksamitowska, S.; Wysokowski, M.; Tsurkan, M.; Galli, R.; Meissner, H.; Petrenko, I.; Tabachnick, K.; et al. New source of 3D chitin scaffolds: the Red Sea demosponge *Pseudoceratina arabica* (Pseudoceratinidae, Verongiida). *Mar. Drugs* **2019**, *17*, 92. [CrossRef]
87. Rohde, S.; Schupp, P.J. Growth and regeneration of the elephant ear sponge *Ianthella basta* (Porifera). *Hydrobiologia* **2012**, *687*, 219–226. [CrossRef]
88. Wojtasz-Pająk, A.; Szumilewicz, J. Degradation of chitin with hydrogen peroxide in microwave fields. In *Progress on Chemistry of Chitin and Its Derivatives*; Jaworska, M., Ed.; Polish Chitin Society: Łódź, Poland, 2007; Volume 12, pp. 13–24.
89. Felinto, M.C.F.C.; Parra, D.F.; da Silva, C.C.; Angerami, J.; Oliveira, M.J.A.; Lugao, A.B. The swelling behavior of chitosan hydrogels membranes obtained by UV- and γ-radiation. *Nucl. Instrum. Methods Phys. Res. B* **2007**, *265*, 418–424. [CrossRef]

marine drugs

MDPI

Article

Synthesis and Evaluation of a Chitosan Oligosaccharide-Streptomycin Conjugate against *Pseudomonas aeruginosa* Biofilms

Ruilian Li [1,2], Xianghua Yuan [3], Jinhua Wei [2], Xiafei Zhang [3], Gong Cheng [2], Zhuo A. Wang [2,*] and Yuguang Du [2,*]

1 University of Chinese Academy of Sciences, Beijing 100049, China; rlli@ipe.ac.cn
2 Key Laboratory of Biopharmaceutical Production & Formulation Engineering, PLA and State Key Laboratory of Biochemical Engineering, Institute of Process Engineering, Chinese Academy of Sciences, Beijing 100190, China; jhwei@ipe.ac.cn (J.W.); gcheng@ipe.ac.cn (G.C.)
3 College of Life Science, Sichuan Normal University, Chengdu 610101, China; lemonlyty@sohu.com (X.Y.); feifei_2016@126.com (X.Z.)
* Correspondence: wangzhuo@ipe.ac.cn (Z.A.W.); ygdu@ipe.ac.cn (Y.D.); Tel./Fax: +86-10-8254-5070 (Z.A.W. & Y.D.)

Received: 28 November 2018; Accepted: 7 January 2019; Published: 10 January 2019

Abstract: Microbial biofilms are considerably more resistant to antibiotics than planktonic cells. It has been reported that chitosan coupling with the aminoglycoside antibiotic streptomycin dramatically disrupted biofilms of several Gram-positive bacteria. This finding suggested the application of the covalent conjugate of antimicrobial natural polysaccharides and antibiotics on anti-infection therapy. However, the underlying molecular mechanism of the chitosan-streptomycin conjugate (CS-Strep) remains unclear and the poor water-solubility of the conjugate might restrict its applications for anti-infection therapy. In this study, we conjugated streptomycin with water-soluble chitosan oligosaccharides (COS). Unlike CS-Strep, the COS-streptomycin conjugate (COS-Strep) barely affected biofilms of tested Gram-positive bacteria. However, COS-Strep efficiently eradicated established biofilms of the Gram-negative pathogen *Pseudomonas aeruginosa*. This activity of COS-Strep was influenced by the degree of polymerization of chitosan oligosaccharide. The increased susceptibility of *P. aeruginosa* biofilms to antibiotics after conjugating might be related to the following: Suppression of the activation of MexX-MexY drug efflux pump system induced by streptomycin treatment; and down-regulation of the biosynthesis of biofilm exopolysaccharides. Thus, this work indicated that covalently linking antibiotics to chitosan oligosaccharides was a possible approach for the development of antimicrobial drugs against biofilm-related infections.

Keywords: chitosan oligosaccharides; streptomycin; *Pseudomonas aeruginosa*; biofilms; conjugation

1. Introduction

Biofilms are a form of existence of microorganisms encapsulated in an extracellular matrix that holds cells together and forms a three-dimensional structure against environmental challenges [1]. Recent studies indicated the antimicrobial resistance in bacteria was closely related to the formation of biofilms, which is associated with about 75% of human bacterial infections [2–5]. The drug-resistance of bacteria in biofilms raised 10–1000 times compared to their planktonic counterparts [6–8]. Several factors have been attributed to the resistance, including hampered penetration of antimicrobials through the biofilm matrix, upregulation of the drug efflux pump system, etc. [9,10]. There are limited drugs specifically targeting the biofilms of bacteria. The development of biofilm-specific drugs to treat biofilm-related infections is urged.

Chitosan coupled with streptomycin (CS-Strep) could efficiently disrupted the pre-formed bacterial biofilms. However, the anti-biofilm specificity of CS-Strep was likely restricted to Gram-positive organisms such as *Staphylococcus aureus*, *Listeria monocytogenes*, *Enterococcus faecalis*, but not Gram-negative bacteria *Pseudomonas aeruginosa* [11,12]. These findings suggested an innovative strategy to combat biofilm-related infections by conjugating antibiotics with natural polysaccharides. However, the mechanism behind this intriguing activity is still unclear. The low water solubility and high viscosity of chitosan and CS-Strep might restrict their applications on anti-biofilm therapies.

Chitosan oligosaccharides (COS), composed of β-(1-4)-linked D-glucosamine and *N*-acetyl-D-glucosamine with the degree of polymerization (DP) 2–10, were prepared from degradation of chitosan. Compared to chitosan, COS have a much lower average molecular weight (MW) and better water-solubility [13]. COS also possess versatile biological activities, such as antimicrobial, antioxidant, anticancer, and immune-stimulant effects [14]. In this study, we coupled streptomycin with COS. The anti-biofilm activities of the COS-streptomycin conjugate (COS-Strep) against bacterial biofilms were evaluated. The structure and function relationships of the anti-biofilm activities were preliminarily explored.

2. Materials and Methods

2.1. Reagents and Bacteria Strains

COS (DP 2~8, average MW: 835) and COS2 (DP 2~20, average MW: 1419) were purchased from GlycoBio (GlycoBio, Dalian, China). The average MW and DP of COS was determined by HPLC and LC-MS [15] (Figure S1). Chitosan with MW of 50–190 kD was purchased from Sigma (Sigma-Aldrich, St. Louis, MO, USA). Streptomycin (Strep) was purchased from Solarbio (Solarbio, Beijing, China). The *P. aeruginosa* (PAO1) strain used in the experiment was generously granted by Prof. Ma Lvyan. The *S. aureus* strain (CGMCC1.2910) was purchased from China General Microbiological Culture Collection Center (CGMCC). *L. monocytogenes* (CVCC1597) was purchased from China Veterinary Culture Collection Center (CVCC). *P. aeruginosa* and *L. monocytogenes* were cultured with LB medium at 28 or 37 °C respectively. *S. aureus* was cultured with TSB medium at 37 °C.

2.2. Synthesis of Chitosan Oligosaccharide–Streptomycin Conjugates

The synthesis of the conjugates was based on the oxidation-reduction reaction between COS and streptomycin. The COS-Strep conjugates were prepared as previously described [16]. Briefly, 100 mg COS was first dissolved in 2 mL deionized water, then the pH was adjusted to 4.0 with 0.2 M acetic acid. Then, 525 mg streptomycin was mixed with COS solution at 35 °C with stirring for 1 h in the dark. The synthesis reaction was initialized by the addition of 1 mL 113 mg/mL $NaCNBH_3$ with stirring for 24 h and terminated with 2 M NaOH. The solution was then dialyzed (molecular weight cut off: 500–1000 Da) with deionized water for 48 h. A total of 120 mg of COS-Strep conjugates was collected after lyophilization.

2.3. Matrix-Assisted Laser Desorption/Ionization Time of Flight (MALDI-TOF) Mass Spectrometry and Nuclear Magnetic Resonance (NMR) Analysis

Samples were prepared in 2 mg/mL water solution and filtered with a 0.22 μm syringe filter (Pall, Ann Albor, MI, USA). Then, 1 μL of sample was mixed with the same volume of 2,5-dihydroxybenzoic acid (Sigma-Aldrich, St. Louis, MO, USA) as a sample matrix and air-dried for MALDI-TOF analysis. The analysis was performed on an Autoflex III Smart Beam MALDI-TOF mass spectrometer (Bruker, Bremen, Germany) in the positive ion mode. For ^1H NMR spectral analysis, samples were dissolved in D_2O (30 mg/mL), and the spectra were carried out on a Bruker AV 500 MHz (Bruker, Karlsruhe, Germany).

2.4. Biofilm Formation

P. aeruginosa biofilms were cultured in 96-well polystyrene microtiter plates as previously described [16]. Briefly, *P. aeruginosa* was inoculated into LB medium at 28 °C overnight. Then, 100 mL of diluted cell culture (~2×10^7 colony-forming units, CFU) was inoculated into each well of a sterile flat-bottomed 96-well polystyrene micro-titer plate. The microtiter plate was incubated statically at 28 °C for 24 h to allow cell attachment and biofilm formation. *S. aureus* and *L. monocytogenes* biofilms were cultured at 37 °C with TSB medium and LB medium, respectively.

2.5. Biofilm Mass and Viability Analysis

In order to evaluate the anti-biofilm activity of COS-Strep conjugates, different treatments were conducted as indicated below. Blank LB broth, LB broth with COS, and LB broth with Strep were used as controls. Moreover, LB broth with the mixture of COS and Strep was also included as a control to determine the necessity of the conjugation. After biofilm formation, the 96-well plate was washed three times with phosphate buffer saline (PBS, pH 7.2) to remove the unattached cells. COS-conjugate and different controls were added into the washed biofilms separately, and the 96-well plates were then incubated at 28 °C for 24 h. Biofilms were washed three times with PBS prior to the analysis. The biofilm mass was determined by the crystal violet assay [17]. The sample was measured for absorbance at 590 nm with a TECAN Infinite M200 PRO multifunction microplate reader (TECAN, Grodig, Austria). To determine the cell viability of the biofilm, MTT [3-(4,5-dimethylthiazol-2-yl)-2,5-diphenyltetrazolium] assay was performed as previously described [18]. Briefly, 100 µL of 500 µg/mL MTT was added into each well and the plate was incubated for 3 h. MTT was then removed and the formed formazan was dissolved in 100 µL dimethyl sulfoxide (DMSO). Optical density (OD) of samples were measured at 490 nm using a TECAN Infinite M200 PRO multifunction microplate reader (TECAN, Grodig, Austria). The IC_{50} of anti-biofilm agents was analyzed using the standard broth microdilution method in accordance with the Clinical and Laboratory Standards Institute (CLSI) guidelines. All tests were performed in six replicates for each treatment. Each assay was performed with three biological repeats.

2.6. Fluorescence Microscopy Assay

One milliliter of *P. aeruginosa* (~2×10^7 CFU) in LB broth was transferred onto 10×10 mm glass coverslips (Citoglas, Guangzhou, China) placed on the bottom of the well of 24-well plates and cultivated at 28 °C for 24 h to allow biofilm formation. Unattached cells were removed and coverslips were washed three times with PBS. Formed biofilms were treated with COS-Strep conjugate and controls as indicated above for 24 h at 28 °C. After washing with PBS, 1 µg/mL 4,6-diamidino-2-phenylindole (DAPI, Abbkine, California, America) and 5 µg/mL WGA-FITC (Sigma-Aldrich, St. Louis, MO, USA) were added and incubated in dark for 30 min at 37 °C. Coverslips were then washed and fixed using a 4% paraformaldehyde solution for 30 min at 37 °C. The corresponding fluorescent images were taken by a fluorescent microscope LEICA CTR4000 (Leica, Barnack, Germany).

2.7. Cellular Toxicity Assay

Human umbilical vein endothelial cells (HUVECs) were obtained from the American Type Culture Collection (Manassas, VA, USA). The cells were grown in Dulbecco's modified eagle medium (DMEM) containing 10% fetal bovine serum (FBS) and 100 units/mL penicillin under a 5% CO_2 atmosphere at 37 °C. The toxicity assay was conducted as following: HUVEC cells were incubated in 96-well plates (3×10^3 cells/well) with Strep or COS-Strep at various concentrations ranging from 50 to 2000 µg/mL for 24 h. The cell toxicity was then evaluated by the MTT assay performed as above. Cell viability (%) was calculated as (absorbance of sample/absorbance of control) × 100.

2.8. qRT-PCR Analysis

2.8.1. Isolation of Total RNA

Two milliliters of bacterial cells (~2 × 10^7 CFU) in LB medium were cultured statically in a 35 × 10 mm style cell culture dish (Corning, New York, NY, USA) for biofilm formation. Drug treatment was conducted as described above. Total RNA was isolated as previously described with some modifications [18,19]. Biofilms were dislodged by 1 mL TRIzon reagent of Ultrapure RNA Kit (CWBio, Beijing, China) and the suspension was collected. The suspension was gently sonicated with a 0.5 cm probe with 10 KHz amplitude for 5 min in a noise isolating chamber JY92-IIN (Scientz, Ningbo, China) to release bacteria from biofilms without mechanical cell disruption. Total RNA was then extracted via acidic phenol–chloroform extraction. The yield and quality of RNA was determined with NanoDrop 2000C (Thermo, New York, NY, USA).

2.8.2. Synthesis of cDNA and RT-PCR

Purified RNA was reverse transcribed into cDNA with HiFiScript cDNA Synthesis Kit (CWBio, Beijing, China). Real-time PCR was performed using the Step One™ Real-Time PCR Instrument Thermal Cycling Block (Applied Biosystems Life Technologies, Foster City, California, USA) with the UltraSYBR Mixture Kit (CWBio, Beijing, China). The expression level of each target gene was normalized to that of the 16S rRNA. Each assay was performed in duplicates with three independent biological repeats. Fold change of mRNA level was calculated according to the $2^{-\Delta\Delta Ct}$ method. Primers used for real-time PCR were listed in Table 1.

Table 1. Primers used for the qRT-PCR.

Primer	Sequence (5′-3′)
algD-F	AGAAGTCCGAACGCCACA
algD-R	TCCAGCTCGCGGTAGAT
pelA-F	CCTTCAGCCATCCGTTCTTCT
pelA-R	TCGCGTACGAAGTCGACCTT
pslA-F	AAGATCAAGAAACGCGTGGAAT
pslA-R	TGTAGAGGTCGAACCACACCG
mexY-F	TTACCTCCTCCAGCGGC
mexY-R	GTGAGGCGGGCGTTGTG
mexZ-F	TTACCTCCTCCAGCGGC
mexZ-R	GTGAGGCGGGCGTTGTG
16S rRNA-F	AACCTGGGAACTGCATCCAA
16S rRNA-R	CTTCGCCACTGGTGTTCCTT

2.8.3. Statistical Analysis

Data are presented as means ± SD. A two-tailed Student's *t*-test was performed for the comparison between two groups and one-way analysis of variance (ANOVA) for multiple group analysis. The p-value < 0.05 or 0.01 was considered as statistically significantly different. All data were analyzed using Statistical Product and Service Solutions (SPSS) 13.0 software (SPSS Inc., Chicago, IL, USA).

3. Result

3.1. Synthesis and Characterization of COS-Strep Conjugates

The covalent conjugation between streptomycin and chitosan oligosaccharides was achieved by reduction of the resulting Schiff base formed by amino groups in chitosan oligosaccharide and aldehyde groups in streptomycin (Figure 1A), as described [20]. The product of conjugation was determined by MALDI-TOF-MS analysis (Figure 1B). Peaks had an m/z ratio of 905.6439, 1066.7164, 1227.8052, 1390.9264, 1550.0241, 1711.1075, that represented disaccharides (COS2), trisaccharides

(COS3), tetrasccharides (COS4), pentasaccharides (COS5), hexaoses (COS6), heptaoses (COS7) coupled with one streptomycin, respectively. The coupling between streptomycin and COS was evidenced by ^{1}H NMR analysis (Figure S2). The appearance of signals at 2.57 ppm in the spectrum of COS-Strep was likely attributed to methyl protons (Figure S2A). Weak signals at 9.66 ppm assigned to aldehyde protons in the spectrum of Strep disappeared in that of COS-Strep (Figure S2B). These results strongly suggested the formation of the COS-Strep conjugate.

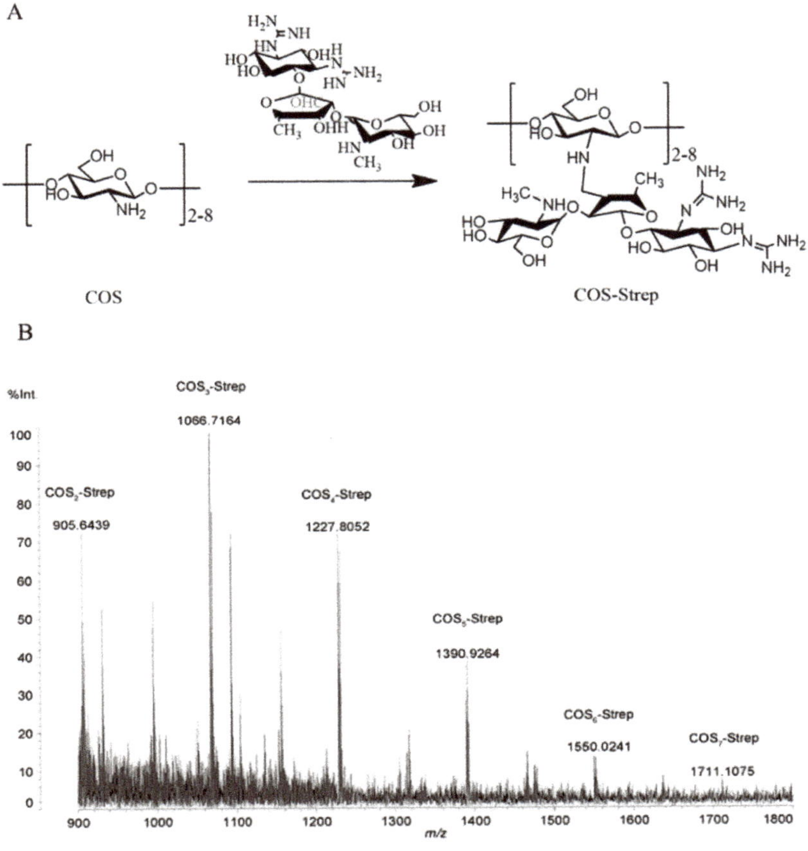

Figure 1. Reaction scheme of the chitosan oligosaccharides-streptomycin (COS-Strep) conjugate synthesis and characterization of synthesized products. Schematic diagram represented the reaction to synthesize of COS-Strep conjugates (**A**). The mass spectrum of COS-Strep conjugates by matrix-assisted laser desorption/ionization time of flight (MALDI-TOF) mass spectrometry (**B**).

3.2. *Inhibitory Effects of COS-Strep against* P. aeruginosa *biofilms*

Established *P. aeruginosa* biofilms were treated with COS-Strep to evaluate the anti-biofilm activity of the conjugate. COS-Strep had strongest capability in removing mature biofilms with a minimum effective concentration of 250 μg/mL; COS and Strep had no or weak anti-biofilm activity at 250 μg/mL (Figure 2A). Moreover, COS-Strep showed high efficacy on killing *P. aeruginosa* cells in the cell viability test. The IC_{50} value of COS-Strep is 88.35 μg/mL, which is 11-fold lower than that of streptomycin (>1000 μg/mL). For planktonic bacteria, the IC_{50} value of COS-Strep was slightly higher than that of streptomycin (Figure 2B). To be noted, a simple mixture with COS did not improve the anti-biofilm activity of streptomycin (Figure 2A). These results suggested that coupling with COS enhanced the antimicrobial efficiency of streptomycin against biofilm of *P. aeruginosa*.

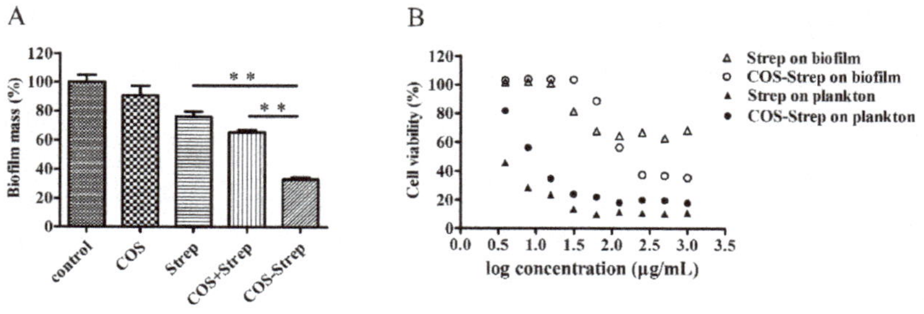

Figure 2. The anti-biofilm activity of COS-Strep conjugates on mature *Pseudomonas aeruginosa* biofilms. *P. aeruginosa* mature biofilms were treated with LB broth containing 250 μg/mL COS, streptomycin, COS-Strep and their mixture (COS + Strep, 250 + 250 μg/mL) for 24 h respectively. Blank medium was used as a control. The biofilm biomass was determined by crystal violet staining and normalized to the control (**A**). Established biofilms were exposed to COS-Strep with a series of concentrations for 24 h and the cell viability of *P. aeruginosa* was determined by MTT assay (**B**). Data are represented as means ± SD (n = 6). * $p < 0.05$ or ** $p < 0.01$.

3.3. The Degree of Polymerization of COS Influenced the Anti-Biofilm Efficacy of COS-Strep Conjugates

Studies showed that biological activities of COS were largely dependent on its degree of polymerization (DP) [2,21,22]. To investigate whether the DP of COS affects the anti-biofilm capacity of COS-Strep conjugates, two COS products with different DP, including COS (DP 2~8) and COS2 (DP 2~20) as well as Glucosamine and chitosan were conjugated with streptomycin to produce COS-Strep, COS2-Strep, GlcN-Strep and CS-Strep conjugates respectively. Four synthesized conjugates showed enhanced anti-biofilm activities against biofilms than streptomycin alone at 250 μg/mL (Figure 3). Moreover, two COS-streptomycin conjugates, COS-strep and COS2-Strep, removed more than 70% biofilms mass, while streptomycin was only capable of removing 22%.

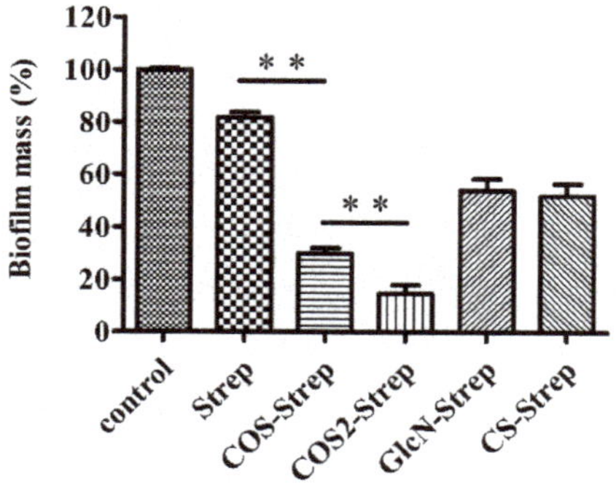

Figure 3. The anti-biofilm activity of COS-Strep with different polymerization degrees. Mature *P. aeruginosa* biofilms were exposed to 250 μg/mL COS-Strep, COS2-Strep, GlcN-Strep and chitosan-streptomycin conjugate (CS-Strep) for 24 h. The residual biofilm mass relative to the control was assessed by the crystal violet staining assay. Data are represented as means ± SD (n = 6). * $p < 0.05$; ** $p < 0.01$.

On the contrary, GlcN-Strep and CS-Strep conjugates only slightly enhanced the anti-biofilm activity compared to streptomycin (Figure 3). Among the two COS-Strep conjugates, COS2-Strep exhibited the highest anti-biofilm activity. These results indicated that the anti-biofilm activity of streptomycin can be enhanced by conjugating with COS rather than its structurally similar polymers or monosaccharide component. Furthermore, the anti-biofilm activity of COS-Strep conjugates was affected by the degree of polymerization of COS used in the conjugation process.

3.4. *Coupling with COS Did not Improve the Anti-Biofilm Activity of Streptomycin on* S. aureus *and* L. monocytogenes

To investigate the anti-biofilm activity of COS-Strep on other bacteria, we assessed the activity of COS-Strep on mature biofilms of *S. aureus* and *L. monocytogenes*, which are Gram-positive opportunistic human pathogens. COS-Strep or Strep alone did not show inhibition effects against biofilms of tested strains at 250 μg/mL (Figure 4).

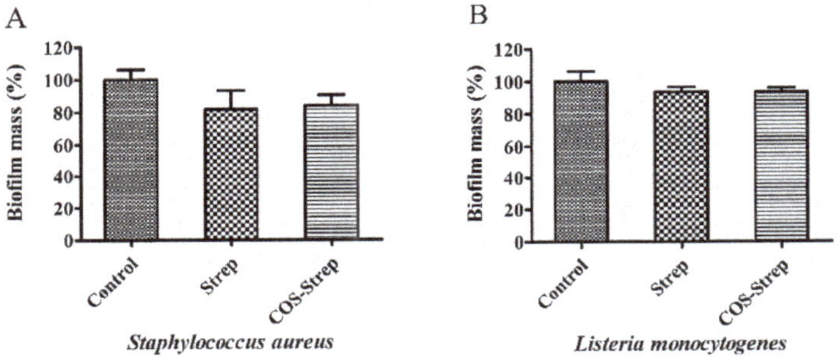

Figure 4. The anti-biofilm activity of COS-Strep conjugate on Gram-positive bacterial biofilms. *Staphylococcus aureus* (**A**) and *Listeria monocytogenes* (**B**) mature biofilms were exposed to COS-Strep for 24 h at 250 μg/mL. The biofilm mass was determined by crystal violet staining assay. Data are represented as means ± SD (n = 6).

3.5. *Cellular Toxicity*

HUVEC cells were used to determine potential side effects of the COS-Strep conjugate in cell viability analysis. Same as streptomycin (Figure 5A), COS-Strep had no obvious effects on the growth of the mammalian cell strain at 1 mg/mL (Figure 5B).

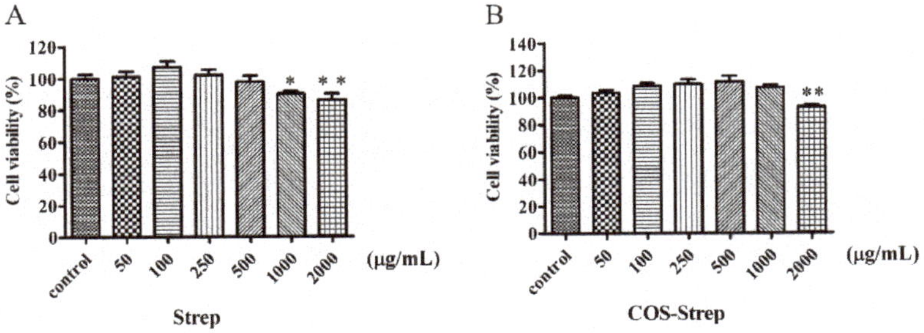

Figure 5. The cell toxicity of streptomycin (**A**) and COS-Strep (**B**) on HUVEC cells. Data are represented as means ± SD (n = 8). * $p < 0.05$ or ** $p < 0.01$, compared to the control group.

3.6. *Influence on* P. aeruginosa *Biofilm Related Gene Expressions under the COS-Strep Conjugate Treatment*

To explore the mechanism of the antibacterial activity of COS-Strep on *P. aeruginosa* biofilms, expression levels of several genes related to biofilm formation or drug-resistance were determined. Genes including *pslA*, *pelA*, and *algD*, which are related to biosynthesis of biofilm exopolysaccharides

Psl, Pel, and alignate [23,24]; *MexY*, and *mexZ* which encode proteins involved in MexX-MexY drug efflux pump system [25,26]; and *cdrA* which encode proteins to mediate bacterial aggregation and biofilm adherence [27], were selected as targets. Streptomycin treatment greatly upregulated the expression of *mexY* by 1.9 fold in biofilm cells, suggesting the activation of the MexX-MexY drug efflux pump system (Figure 6A). On the contrary, COS-Strep treatment slightly down-regulated the expression of *mexY* (Figure 6A), likely through upregulating the expression of its suppressor, *mexZ* (Figure 6B). Thus, COS-Strep treatment did not upregulate or even suppress the MexX-MexY system which was activated by streptomycin. Genes *pelA* and *algD* were also down-regulated by 0.68 and 0.75 fold, respectively with COS-Strep treatment compared to the control or streptomycin treated group (Figure 6C,D). On the other hand, the expression level of *pslA* and *cdrA* remained unaffected under COS-Strep treatment (Figure 6E,F). Therefore, the anti-biofilm activity of COS-Strep might be because of its ability to suppress the activation of the drug efflux pump system and the biosynthesis of specific exopolysaccharides.

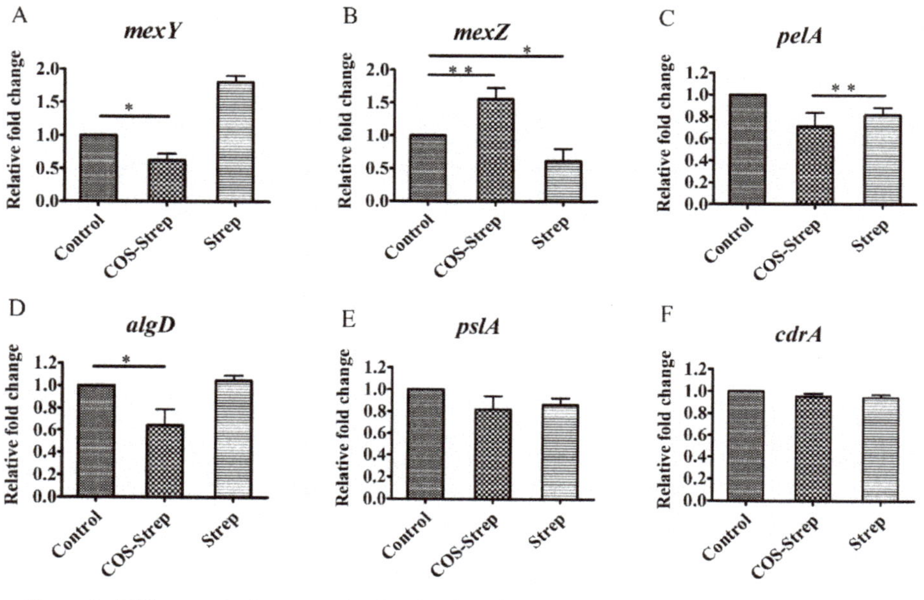

Figure 6. Differences in the expression levels of biofilm-related genes of *P. aeruginosa*. *mexY* (**A**), *mexZ* (**B**), *pelA* (**C**), *algD* (**D**), *pslA* (**E**), *and cdrA* (**F**) in *P. aeruginosa* following COS-Strep or streptomycin treatment. Data are represented as means ± SD (n = 3). * $p < 0.05$; ** $p < 0.01$.

3.7. *COS-Strep Treatment Reduced Biofilm Exopolysaccharides of* P. aeruginosa

In order to investigate the effect of COS-Strep on biofilm exopolysaccharides, we stained the biofilm with FITC labeled wheat germ agglutinin (WGA) lectin which bound to exopolysaccharide, and DAPI. We observed the reduction of signals with WGA-FITC and DAPI staining after COS-Strep treatment, suggesting its influence on both biofilm cell viability and exopolysaccharide (Figure 7).

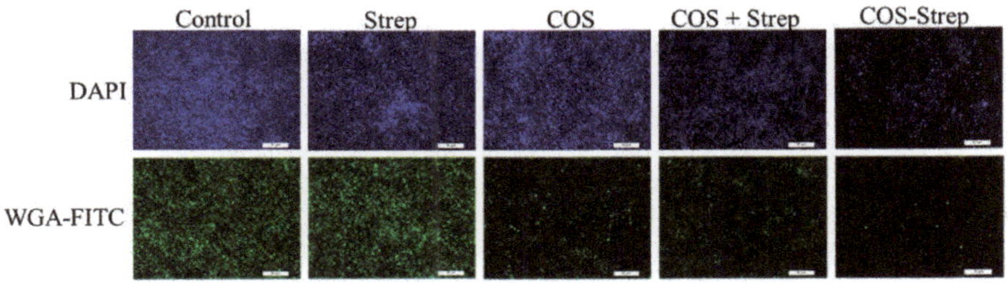

Figure 7. COS-Strep affected biofilm exopolysaccharides of *P. aeruginosa*. Drug treated biofilms were observed by fluorescence image assay. Shown are single-channel images of signal derived from staining with 4,6-diamidino-2-phenylindole (DAPI) (nucleus, blue, upper panel) and WGA-FITC (exopolysaccharide, green, lower panel). Scale bar, 50 μm.

4. Discussion

Streptomycin is a common aminoglycoside antibiotic which is used to treat a number of bacterial infections. However, pathogens in biofilms could greatly increase their drug resistance. It has been previously reported that chitosan coupling with streptomycin (CS-Strep) could eradicate biofilms of several Gram-positive organisms, but barely affect that of Gram-negative organisms such as *P. aeruginosa* [11]. However, the underlying molecular mechanism of the CS-Strep remained unclear. Moreover, poor water-solubility of CS-Strep might restrict its applications on anti-infection therapy. In this study, we prepared the chitosan oligosaccharide-streptomycin conjugate (COS-Strep), which has an improved water-solubility. Our data showed that the COS-Strep conjugate was much more effective in eradicating established biofilms of *P. aeruginosa* than streptomycin alone or their simple mixture (Figure 2). The efficacy of the anti-biofilm activity was affected by the DP of COS used for conjugation (Figure 3). The activity of COS-Strep on the *P. aeruginosa* biofilm was likely through inhibiting response of the MexX-MexY drug efflux pump system and synthesis of biofilm exopolysaccharides (Figure 6).

Surprisingly, unlike CS-Strep, the COS-Strep conjugate did not show an obvious anti-biofilm activity on Gram-positive organisms such as *S. aureus* and *L. monocytogenes* (Figure 4). However, COS-Strep effectively inhibited against *P. aeruginosa* biofilms (Figure 2), suggesting their opposite effects on tested organisms. Although COS and chitosan shared structural similarity, both showed anti-biofilm activity when conjugating with streptomycin, the mechanism behind the antimicrobial activity of the two conjugates might be different. Previous studies on the antibacterial activity of chitosan and COS indicated that chitosan had stronger bactericidal effects with gram-positive bacteria than gram-negative bacteria [28], while COS showed better activity against gram-negative bacteria [29]. These diverse activities might be relevant to the difference in the composition of cell walls and biofilm matrix of different organisms or the antibacterial action mode of COS and chitosan. The selective anti-biofilm activity of the COS-Strep conjugate on *P. aeruginosa* was likely determined by the glycan part of the conjugate, especially considering that streptomycin was not a suitable antibiotic for treatment of *P. aeruginosa* infection.

P. aeruginosa is a major clinical opportunistic pathogen. There is an increasing awareness of the important role of *P. aeruginosa* biofilm infections associated with specific tissue and implants such as the mucus plugs of the cystic fibrosis (CF) lungs, catheters, and contact lenses [30,31]. Antibiotic treatments for *P. aeruginosa* sometimes are inefficient due to its ability to form biofilms on various organic and inorganic surfaces. Studies have shown that the MexX-MexY drug efflux pump system plays a vital part in the intrinsic resistance of *P. aeruginosa* to aminoglycosides. The MexX-MexY system was regulated by *mexZ* which was a repressor of *mexY* expression [25,26]. To explore whether the antibacterial activity of COS-Strep on *P. aeruginosa* biofilms was through affecting MexX-MexY drug efflux pump system, the expression levels of several genes related to MexX-MexY drug efflux pump were determined under the treatment of COS-Strep. The results showed that COS-Strep did not induce the activation of the MexX-MexY system compared to streptomycin, (Figure 6). This result suggested that the COS-Strep conjugate suppressed the response of this drug-resistance machinery. The mechanism behind this activity requires further investigation.

We also found that expressions of exopolysaccharide biosynthesis genes were influenced under the COS-Strep treatment. In *P. aeruginosa* biofilms, Psl, Pel and alginate exopolysaccharides served as key structural components of the biofilm matrix [32]. Previous studies indicated that Psl and alginate were required for formation of biofilms, whereas Pel played an important role in controlling biofilm cell density and/or the compactness of biofilms [33]. Our studies showed that the expression of *pelA* and *algD* genes were suppressed under the treatment of COS-Strep (Figure 6C,D), but not *pslA* and *cdrA* (Figure 6E,F). CdrA, a biofilm matrix protein, is related to extracellular adhesion and promotes tight cellular interactions in biofilm aggregates [27]. The result indicated COS-Strep might impair the structural integrity of the biofilm by inhibiting the biosynthesis of Pel and alginate exopolysaccharides. Pel is a positively charged polysaccharide composed of partially acetylated 1-4 glycosidic linkages of *N*-acetylgalactosamine and *N*-acetylglucosamine [34]. WGA lectin usually recognizes *N*-acetylglucosamine-containing glycans. To further explore the possible influence of COS-Strep on biofilm exopolysaccharides, we determined the biofilm structure after drug treatment under a fluorescence microscope, using FITC (green fluorescent bioconjugates) labeled WGA lectin. Our results showed a significant reduction of green fluorescent signals after treatment with COS-Strep (Figure 7). It further supported that COS-Strep affected the structural integrity of biofilm exopolysaccharides.

5. Conclusions

In summary, our result highlighted that chitosan oligosaccharide coupling greatly increased the susceptibility of *P. aeruginosa* biofilms to streptomycin. COS-Strep treatments might suppress the response of the drug efflux pump system and inhibited the biosynthesis of Pel and alginate exopolysaccharides. Given chitosan oligosaccharide gain considerable attention as a biomaterial, due to its good water-solubility and low toxicity, this novel strategy might open up a new avenue to overcome the inherent resistance of biofilms to antibiotics, and come into wide use for combating biofilm-related problems in industrial and medical areas.

Supplementary Materials: The following are available online at http://www.mdpi.com/1660-3397/17/1/43/s1. Figure S1. The results of HPLC analysis of COS (DP2-8) and COS (DP 2-20) (A) and LC-MS results of COS and COS2; Figure S2. ^{1}H NMR spectra of COS, streptomycin, COS+Strep and COS-Strep conjugates. The Freeze-dried COS, Strep, the COS-Strep conjugate and a mixture of two molecules (mass ratio 1:1) were dissolved in deuterated water to a final concentration of 30mg/mL respectively. The spectra were recorded at 298 K in deuterium oxide on a Varian VNMRS-500 NMR spectrometer. Red arrow represented the methyl protons singal at 2.57 ppm in COS-Strep conjugates (A). Red arrow represented aldehyde proton singal at 9.66 ppm that was the functional group of streptomycin (B).

Author Contributions: Y.D. and Z.A.W. designed the study. R.L. and X.Y. were responsible for the acquisition of data. Z.A.W. and R.L. interpreted the experimental data. R.L. and Z.A.W. were the major contributors in drafting and revising the manuscript. Z.A.W. was final approval of the version to be submitted. All authors read and approved the final manuscript.

Funding: This research was funded by [National Natural Science Fund, China] grant number [NO. 31670809], [the Key Research Program of the Chinese Academy of Sciences] grant number [No. KFZD-SW-218] and [the Open Project Program of the Collaborative Innovation Center of Modern Bio-Manufacture, Anhui University] grant number [No. BM2016004].

Acknowledgments: Thanks to Yalu Yan for language polishing of this paper. Thanks to Jianjun Li for analyzing the NMR results.

Conflicts of Interest: The authors declare no conflict of interest.

References

1. Stoodley, P.; Sauer, K.; Davies, D.G.; Costerton, W.J. Biofilms as Complex Differentiated Communities. *Annu. Rev. Microbiol.* **2002**, *56*, 187–209. [CrossRef] [PubMed]

2. Carlson, R.P.; Taffs, R.; Davison, W.M.; Stewart, P.S. Anti-biofilm properties of chitosan-coated surfaces. *J. Biomater. Sci. Polym. Ed.* **2008**, *19*, 1035–1046. [CrossRef] [PubMed]
3. Lebeaux, D.; Ghigo, J.M.; Beloin, C. Biofilm-related infections: bridging the gap between clinical management and fundamental aspects of recalcitrance toward antibiotics. *Microbiol. Mol. Biol. Rev.* **2014**, *78*, 510–543. [CrossRef]
4. Nandakumar, V.; Chittaranjan, S.; Kurian, V.M.; Doble, M. Characteristics of bacterial biofilm associated with implant material in clinical practice. *Polym. J.* **2012**, *45*, 137–152. [CrossRef]
5. Miquel, S.; Lagrafeuille, R.; Souweine, B.; Forestier, C. Anti-biofilm Activity as a Health Issue. *Front. Microbiol.* **2016**, *7*, 592. [CrossRef] [PubMed]
6. Hengzhuang, W.; Wu, H.; Ciofu, O.; Song, Z.; Hoiby, N. Pharmacokinetics/pharmacodynamics of colistin and imipenem on mucoid and nonmucoid *Pseudomonas aeruginosa* biofilms. *Antimicrob. Agents Chemother.* **2011**, *55*, 4469–4474. [CrossRef] [PubMed]
7. Wang, H.; Wu, H.; Ciofu, O.; Song, Z.; Hoiby, N. In vivo pharmacokinetics/pharmacodynamics of colistin and imipenem in *Pseudomonas aeruginosa* biofilm infection. *Antimicrob. Agents Chemother.* **2012**, *56*, 2683–2690.
8. Wu, H.; Moser, C.; Wang, H.Z.; Hoiby, N.; Song, Z.J. Strategies for combating bacterial biofilm infections. *Int. J. Oral Sci.* **2015**, *7*, 1–7. [CrossRef] [PubMed]
9. Bechinger, B.; Gorr, S.U. Antimicrobial Peptides: Mechanisms of Action and Resistance. *J. Dent. Res.* **2017**, *96*, 254–260. [CrossRef] [PubMed]
10. Stewart, P.S.; Costerton, J.W. Antibiotic resistance of bacteria in biofilms. *Lancet (Lond. Engl.)* **2001**, *358*, 135–138. [CrossRef]
11. Zhang, A.; Mu, H.; Zhang, W.; Cui, G.; Zhu, J.; Duan, J. Chitosan coupling makes microbial biofilms susceptible to antibiotics. *Sci. Rep.* **2013**, *3*, 3364. [CrossRef]
12. Tre-Hardy, M.; Vanderbist, F.; Traore, H.; Devleeschouwer, M.J. In vitro activity of antibiotic combinations against *Pseudomonas aeruginosa* biofilm and planktonic cultures. *Int. J. Antimicrob. Agents* **2008**, *31*, 329–336. [CrossRef] [PubMed]
13. Thadathil, N.; Velappan, S.P. Recent developments in chitosanase research and its biotechnological applications: A review. *Food Chem.* **2014**, *150*, 392–399. [CrossRef] [PubMed]
14. Muanprasat, C.; Chatsudthipong, V. Chitosan oligosaccharide: Biological activities and potential therapeutic applications. *Pharmacol. Ther.* **2017**, *170*, 80–97. [CrossRef] [PubMed]
15. Zhang, G.; Liu, J.; Li, R.; Jiao, S.; Feng, C.; Wang, Z.A.; Du, Y. Conjugation of Inulin Improves Anti-Biofilm Activity of Chitosan. *Mar. Drugs* **2018**, *16*, 151. [CrossRef] [PubMed]
16. Pitts, B.; Hamilton, M.A.; Zelver, N.; Stewart, P.S. A microtiter-plate screening method for biofilm disinfection and removal. *J. Microbiol. Methods* **2003**, *54*, 269–276. [CrossRef]
17. Mosmann, T. Rapid colorimetric assay for cellular growth and survival: application to proliferation and cytotoxicity assays. *J. Immunol. Methods* **1983**, *65*, 55–63. [CrossRef]
18. Dumas, J.L.; van Delden, C.; Perron, K.; Kohler, T. Analysis of antibiotic resistance gene expression in *Pseudomonas aeruginosa* by quantitative real-time-PCR. *FEMS Microbiol. Lett.* **2006**, *254*, 217–225. [CrossRef]
19. Wu, D.Q.; Cheng, H.; Duan, Q.; Huang, W. Sodium houttuyfonate inhibits biofilm formation and alginate biosynthesis-associated gene expression in a clinical strain of *Pseudomonas aeruginosa* in vitro. *Exp. Ther. Med.* **2015**, *10*, 753–758. [CrossRef]
20. Djordjevic, D.; Wiedmann, M.; McLandsborough, L.A. Microtiter plate assay for assessment of Listeria monocytogenes biofilm formation. *Appl. Environ. Microbiol.* **2002**, *68*, 2950–2958. [CrossRef]
21. Pasquantonio, G.; Greco, C.; Prenna, M.; Ripa, C.; Vitali, L.A.; Petrelli, D.; Di Luca, M.C.; Ripa, S. Antibacterial activity and anti-biofilm effect of chitosan against strains of Streptococcus mutans isolated in dental plaque. *Int. J. Immunopathol. Pharmacol.* **2008**, *21*, 993–997. [CrossRef]
22. Costa, E.M.; Silva, S.; Tavaria, F.K.; Pintado, M.M. Study of the effects of chitosan upon Streptococcus mutans adherence and biofilm formation. *Anaerobe* **2013**, *20*, 27–31. [CrossRef] [PubMed]
23. Mann, E.E.; Wozniak, D.J. Pseudomonas biofilm matrix composition and niche biology. *FEMS Microbiol. Rev.* **2012**, *36*, 893–916. [CrossRef] [PubMed]
24. Franklin, M.J.; Nivens, D.E.; Weadge, J.T.; Howell, P.L. Biosynthesis of the *Pseudomonas aeruginosa* Extracellular Polysaccharides, Alginate, Pel, and Psl. *Front. Microbiol.* **2011**, *2*, 167. [CrossRef] [PubMed]
25. Aires, J.R.; Kohler, T.; Nikaido, H.; Plesiat, P. Involvement of an active efflux system in the natural resistance of *Pseudomonas aeruginosa* to aminoglycosides. *Antimicrob. Agents Chemother.* **1999**, *43*, 2624–2628. [CrossRef]

26. Westbrock-Wadman, S.; Sherman, D.R.; Hickey, M.J.; Coulter, S.N.; Zhu, Y.Q.; Warrener, P.; Nguyen, L.Y.; Shawar, R.M.; Folger, K.R.; Stover, C.K. Characterization of a *Pseudomonas aeruginosa* efflux pump contributing to aminoglycoside impermeability. *Antimicrob. Agents Chemother.* **1999**, *43*, 2975–2983. [CrossRef] [PubMed]
27. Reichhardt, C.; Wong, C.; Passos da Silva, D.; Wozniak, D.J.; Parsek, M.R. CdrA Interactions within the *Pseudomonas aeruginosa* Biofilm Matrix Safeguard It from Proteolysis and Promote Cellular Packing. *MBio* **2018**, *9*, e01376-18. [CrossRef] [PubMed]
28. No, H.K.; Park, N.Y.; Lee, S.H.; Meyers, S.P. Antibacterial activity of chitosans and chitosan oligomers with different molecular weights. *Int J. Food Microbiol* **2002**, *74*, 65–72. [CrossRef]
29. Lin, S.B.; Chen, S.H.; Peng, K.C. Preparation of antibacterial chito-oligosaccharide by altering the degree of deacetylation of beta-chitosan in a Trichoderma harzianum chitinase-hydrolysing process. *J. Sci. Food Agric.* **2009**, *89*, 238–244. [CrossRef]
30. Singh, P.K.; Schaefer, A.L.; Parsek, M.R.; Moninger, T.O.; Welsh, M.J.; Greenberg, E.P. Quorum-sensing signals indicate that cystic fibrosis lungs are infected with bacterial biofilms. *Nature* **2000**, *407*, 762–764. [CrossRef]
31. Delissalde, F.; Amabile-Cuevas, C.F. Comparison of antibiotic susceptibility and plasmid content, between biofilm producing and non-producing clinical isolates of *Pseudomonas aeruginosa*. *Int. J. Antimicrob. Agents* **2004**, *24*, 405–408. [CrossRef] [PubMed]
32. Colvin, K.M.; Irie, Y.; Tart, C.S.; Urbano, R.; Whitney, J.C.; Ryder, C.; Howell, P.L.; Wozniak, D.J.; Parsek, M.R. The Pel and Psl polysaccharides provide *Pseudomonas aeruginosa* structural redundancy within the biofilm matrix. *Environ. Microbiol* **2012**, *14*, 1913–1928. [CrossRef] [PubMed]
33. Ghafoor, A.; Hay, I.D.; Rehm, B.H. Role of exopolysaccharides in *Pseudomonas aeruginosa* biofilm formation and architecture. *Appl. Environ. Microbiol.* **2011**, *77*, 5238–5246. [CrossRef]
34. Jennings, L.K.; Storek, K.M.; Ledvina, H.E.; Coulon, C.; Marmont, L.S.; Sadovskaya, I.; Secor, P.R.; Tseng, B.S.; Scian, M.; Filloux, A.; et al. Pel is a cationic exopolysaccharide that cross-links extracellular DNA in the *Pseudomonas aeruginosa* biofilm matrix. *Proc. Natl. Acad. Sci. USA* **2015**, *112*, 11353–11358. [CrossRef] [PubMed]

marine drugs

MDPI

Article

Immunostimulatory Effects of Chitooligosaccharides on RAW 264.7 Mouse Macrophages via Regulation of the MAPK and PI3K/Akt Signaling Pathways

Yue Yang [1,2,3,4], Ronge Xing [1,2,4,*], Song Liu [1,2,4], Yukun Qin [1,2,4], Kecheng Li [1,2,4], Huahua Yu [1,2,4] and Pengcheng Li [1,2,4,*]

1 Key Laboratory of Experimental Marine Biology, Institute of Oceanology, Chinese Academy of Sciences, No. 7 Nanhai Road, Qingdao 266071, China; yy100462@163.com (Y.Y.); sliu@qdio.ac.cn (S.L.); ykqin@qdio.ac.cn (Y.Q.); lkc@qdio.ac.cn (K.L.); yuhuahua@qdio.ac.cn (H.Y.)

2 Laboratory for Marine Drugs and Bioproducts of Qingdao National Laboratory for Marine Science and Technology, No. 1 Wenhai Road, Qingdao 266237, China

3 College of Earth and Planetary Sciences, University of Chinese Academy of Sciences, Beijing 100049, China

4 Center for Ocean Mega-Science, Chinese Academy of Sciences, 7 Nanhai Road, Qingdao 266071, China

* Correspondence: xingronge@qdio.ac.cn (R.X.); pcli@qdio.ac.cn (P.L.); Tel.: +86-532-8289-8707 (P.L.); Fax: +86-532-8296-8780 (R.X.)

Received: 28 November 2018; Accepted: 7 January 2019; Published: 8 January 2019

Abstract: Chitooligosaccharides (COS), the hydrolyzed products of chitin and chitosan, can be obtained by various methods. In this study, water-soluble COS were prepared from α- and β-chitosan by microwave-assisted degradation and their immunostimulatory effects were investigated in RAW 264.7 macrophages. The results indicated that α-COS were more active than β-COS in promoting the production of nitric oxide (NO) and cytokines, such as tumor necrosis factor-α (TNF-α) and interleukin 6 (IL-6). Quantitative real-time reverse transcription polymerase chain reaction and Western blotting indicated that COS also enhanced the expression of inducible nitric oxide synthase (iNOS), cyclooxygenase-2 (COX-2), and TNF-α. Further analyses demonstrated that COS induced the phosphorylation of extracellular signal-regulated kinase (ERK), c-Jun N-terminal kinase (JNK), p38, p85 and Akt, and the nuclear translocation of p65, indicating that they are able to activate the mitogen-activated protein kinases (MAPKs) and phosphoinositide 3-kinases (PI3K)/Akt signaling pathways dependent on nuclear factor (NF)-κB activation. In conclusion, COS activate RAW 264.7 cells via the MAPK and PI3K/Akt signaling pathways and are potential novel immune potentiators.

Keywords: chitooligosaccharide; immunostimulatory activity; RAW 264.7 cells; mitogen-activated protein kinases (MAPK); phosphoinositide 3-kinases (PI3K)/Akt

1. Introduction

Immune responses are initiated by host defenses against invading pathogens via the innate and adaptive immune systems [1]. The immune responses of the elderly and patients with immunodeficiency diseases need to be enhanced. Therefore, immunoenhancing nutraceuticals and medicines have attracted a great deal of attention owing to their immunostimulatory activity. Macrophages and dendritic cells play pivotal roles in the immune system and activate immune responses via cytokine release, phagocytosis, and antigen presentation [2]. Macrophage activation is crucial for promoting immune activity [3]. Stimulated macrophages release various proinflammatory mediators and cytokines, including nitric oxide (NO), tumor necrosis factor-α (TNF-α), prostaglandin E_2 (PGE_2), interleukin-1β (IL-1β), and interleukin-6 (IL-6) [4,5]. These cytokines are secreted via activation of signaling pathways such as the mitogen-activated protein kinase (MAPK) and phosphoinositide 3-kinase (PI3K)/Akt, and via transcription factors like activator protein 1 (AP-1) and nuclear factor (NF)-κB.

Chitin is a naturally abundant substance exists in the fungal cell walls, exoskeletons of insects, and shells of crustaceans. An estimated 10^{11} tons of chitin are produced from living organisms annually [6]. Chitosan, a partially deacetylated product of chitin, has been widely studied and used in biomedical applications [7–9]. However, the pKa of chitosan is 6.5, and chitosan dissolves only under acidic conditions via the protonation of amino groups, which restricts its application. Nevertheless, chitosan is readily degraded into chitooligosaccharides (COS) by microwave irradiation, enzymes, or conventional heating. COS consist of 2–20 GlcN or GlcNAc units linked by β-1,4-*O*-glycoside bonds. The COS segments differ in the fraction of N-acetylated residues and the sequences of GlcN and GlcNAc residues [10].

COS possess many biological activities, including immunoregulatory, antiviral, anti-tumor, antibacterial, and antifungal activities [11]. Xing et al. [12] found that COS prepared by chemical hydrolysis, enzymatic hydrolysis, and microwave irradiation all improved innate and adaptive immunity, and COS degraded by microwave irradiation showed the finest activity. Through both in vitro and in vivo models, Zhang et al. [13] found that COS with a degree of polymerization (DP) of 3–8 promoted innate and adaptive immunity. Mei et al. [14], COS (DP 4–11) reported that COS (DP 4–11) exhibit strong immunostimulatory activity and protective effects in immunosuppressed mice. COS with chain lengths greater than six were more biologically active and had greater immunopotentiation activity than smaller COS [11].

Although some studies have reported on the immunoregulatory activity of COS, little is known of the molecular mechanisms involved. Therefore, it is not clear how COS exert their immunomodulatory activity. Feng et al. [15] demonstrated that COS promoted the release of IL-1β and TNF-α in macrophages. The promotion of cytokine gene transcription and protein expression by COS can affect immunity [16], but the detailed molecular mechanism of the immunomodulatory activity of COS is unclear, and the activity of β-COS has not been investigated. In this study, water-soluble α- and β-COS were obtained by microwave-assisted degradation. Then, the immunomodulatory activity of COS was investigated in RAW 264.7 cells, and the COS-induced signaling pathways were characterized to elucidate the molecular mechanisms.

2. Results

2.1. Characterization of COS

The IR spectra of α-chitosan (1856 kDa), β-chitosan (4574 kDa), α-COS (1874 Da), β-COS (2186 Da) were shown in Figure 1. The characteristic absorption peaks appeared at 1651 cm^{-1} (Amide I), 1591 cm^{-1} (N-H bending) and 1375 cm^{-1} (Amide III). The spectrum of α-COS and β-COS were similar to α- and β-chitosan with high molecular weight.

The ^{1}H NMR and ^{13}C NMR spectrum of α-chitosan (1856 kDa), β-chitosan (4574 kDa), α-COS (1874 Da) and β-COS (2186 Da) were shown in Figure 2. As shown in Figure 2C, the signal of α-COS (1874 Da) at 3.00 ppm was attributed to H2, the signals between 3.52 and 3.62 ppm were assigned to H5 and H6, the peaks at 3.75 ppm were attributed to H3 and H4. The peaks were similar to α-chitosan (1856 kDa) as shown in Figure 2A. The ^{13}C NMR spectrum of α-COS (1887 Da) was plotted in Figure 2G. The signals at 97.48, 55.67, 69.98, 76.18, 74.67, 59.80 were attributed to C1, C2, C3, C4, C5 and C6, respectively. These signals were also similar to those of the 1856-kDa chitosan (Figure 2E). As shown in Figure 2D,H, the ^{1}H NMR and ^{13}C NMR spectrum of β-COS (2186 Da) were plotted, and the signals were assigned. The signals of β-chitosan (4574 kDa) were identical with those of β-COS (2186 Da). Moreover, apart from a slight difference in signal intensity, the signals of β-chitosan and β-COS were also identical with those of α-chitosan and α-COS.

The difference of α- and β-COS originates from the antiparallel configuration of α-COS and the parallel structure of β-COS. The structure unit of COS was not destructed by microwave degradation demonstrated by the IR, ^{1}H NMR, and ^{13}C NMR spectra.

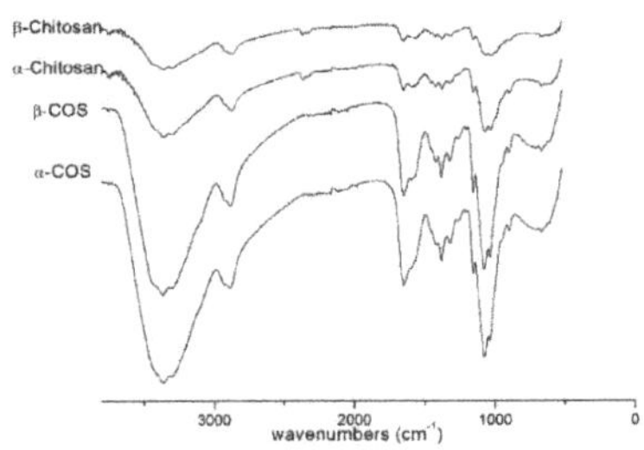

Figure 1. Fourier-transform infrared (FT-IR) spectra of chitosan and chitooligosaccharide (COS). The molecular weights were as follows: α-chitosan (1856 kDa), β-chitosan (4574 kDa), α-COS (1874 Da) and β-COS (2186 Da).

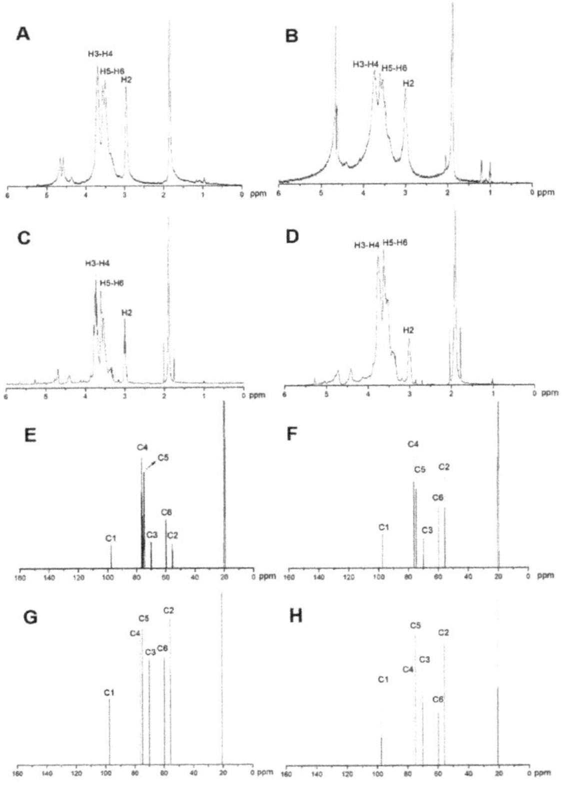

Figure 2. ^{1}H NMR and ^{13}C NMR spectra of chitosan and chitooligosaccharide (COS). (**A**) ^{1}H NMR spectrum of α-chitosan (1856 kDa). (**B**) ^{1}H NMR spectrum of β-chitosan (4574 kDa). (**C**) ^{1}H NMR spectrum of α-COS (1874 Da). (**D**) ^{1}H NMR spectrum of β-COS (2186 Da). (**E**) ^{13}C NMR spectrum of α-chitosan (1856 kDa). (**F**) ^{13}C NMR spectrum of β-chitosan (4574 kDa). (**G**) ^{13}C NMR spectrum of α-COS (1874 Da). (**H**) ^{13}C NMR spectrum of β-COS (2186 Da).

2.2. NO Production

To elucidate the immunological effect of COS, the cells were pretreated with various concentrations and configurations of COS, and NO production was measured using Griess reagent. As shown in Figure S1, the NO-promoting activity of α-COS was better than that of β-COS. The most effective COS had a molecular weight of 1874 Da (COS 1874 Da) and was chosen for further investigation. The results indicated that the production of NO by macrophages was enhanced by increasing the COS concentration from 12.5 to 200 μg/mL (Figure 3A). Furthermore, to eliminate lipopolysaccharide contamination, a ToxinSensor^{TM} Chromogenic LAL Endotoxin Assay Kit (GenScript, Piscatway, NJ, USA) was used to perform an endotoxin assay. The results showed that the samples were not contaminated by endotoxin.

2.3. Cell Viability

The cytocompatibility of different concentrations of COS in RAW 264.7 cells was evaluated by the MTT assay, and the blank control group was designated as 100% cell viability. The results showed that both α- and β-COS (100 μg/mL) had good biocompatibility after the pretreatment of RAW 264.7 cells for 24 h (Figure S2).

Figure 3B displays the effects of various concentrations of COS 1874 Da on macrophage viability. The cell viability with 12.5-200 μg/mL COS 1874 Da exceeded 80%, indicating that COS 1874 Da had no obvious toxicity in RAW 264.7 cells.

2.4. COS Induced the Production of Cytokines in Macrophages

To determine cytokine expression levels after COS treatment, cytometric bead array (CBA) experiments were conducted. Figure 4C,D shows that the production of TNF-α and IL-6 was obviously promoted by COS treatment (25, 50, 100 and 200 μg/mL) in a dose-dependent manner. The cytokine production was increased to nearly 20,000 ng/mL at a concentration of 200 μg/mL.

2.5. COS Enhanced Cytokine Gene and Protein Expression

To investigate whether COS can regulate the levels of cytokine transcription, RAW 264.7 cells were pretreated with 100 μg/mL COS 1874 Da for 0, 0.5, 1, 3 and 6 h. Then, the iNOS, COX-2, IL-6, and TNF-α gene levels were detected by real-time RT-PCR. Quantitative real-time PCR (Figure 4A) indicated that the expression of cytokine genes after a 360 min COS treatment was increased more than 20-fold compared with untreated cells, and the expression of COX-2 reached ca. 1000-fold. To validate these results, immunoblotting assays were performed. As shown in Figure 4B, the expression of TNF-α, IL-6, and COX-2 was obviously promoted after 180 min. These results confirmed the effect of COS on promoting inflammatory mediators in RAW 264.7 macrophages.

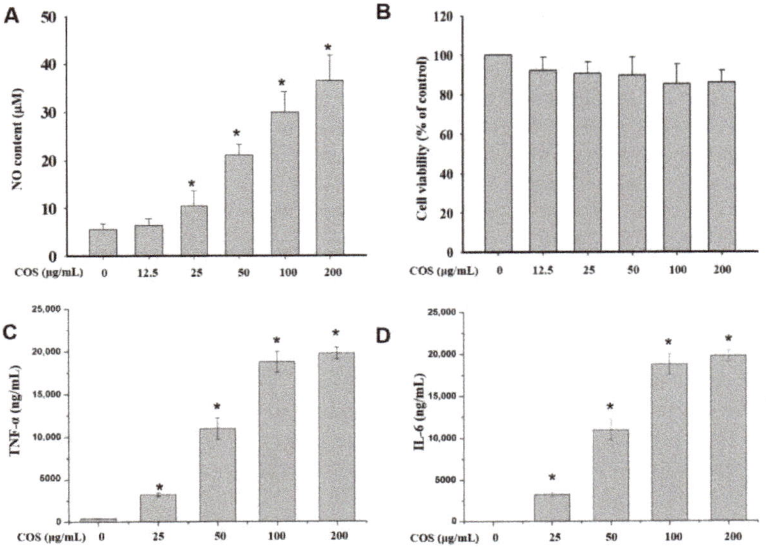

Figure 3. The effects of chitooligosaccharides (COS) on cell viability and cytokine production. RAW 264.7 cells were treated with COS (0–200 μg/mL) for 24 h. (**A**) The nitric oxide production on treatment with α-COS (1874 Da). (**B**) The cell viability on treatment with α-COS (1874 Da). (**C**) The production of tumor necrosis factor-α (TNF-α) on treatment with α-COS (1874 Da). (**D**) The production of interleukin-6 (IL-6) on treatment with α-COS (1874 Da). The values are presented as means ± SD (n = 3). (* $p < 0.05$ vs. control group).

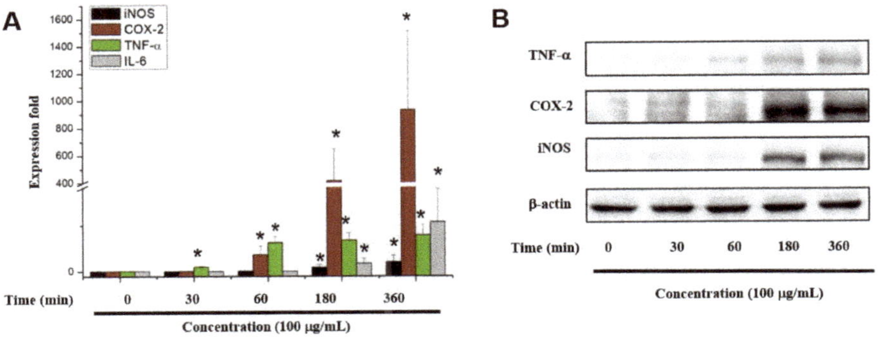

Figure 4. Effects of COS on the expression of cytokines in RAW 264.7 cells at the gene and protein levels. (**A**) Gene expression of inducible nitric oxide synthase (iNOS), TNF-α, IL-6, and cyclooxygenase (COX)-2 in RAW264.7 cells determined by real-time reverse transcription polymerase chain reaction after stimulation with 100 μg/mL COS (1874 Da). The expression data were normalized to glyceraldehyde 3-phosphate dehydrogenase and shown as fold-changes relative to the control (presented as means ± SD) (* $p < 0.05$ vs. control group). (**B**) The effects of 100 μg/mL COS (1874 Da) on the protein expression levels of TNF-α, iNOS, and COX-2.

2.6. COS Interferes with the NF-κB, MAPK and PI3K/Akt Signaling Pathways

Immunoblotting was used to examine the possible involvement of NF-κB in the induction of proinflammatory mediators by COS. As shown in Figure 5A, the expression of p65, a key subunit of NF-κB, increased in a time-dependent manner after COS treatment. Furthermore, 100 μg/mL

COS promoted the phosphorylation of IκBα and the upstream phosphorylation of IKKα/β complex (the upstream kinase of IκB) protein (Figure 5C). These results indicated that COS promotes IκBα degradation and activated the translocation of NF-κB.

To investigate the participation of the MAPK signaling pathway, cells were treated with COS for 0, 30, 60, 180 and 360 min, and then the phosphorylation of c-Jun N-terminal kinase (JNK), extracellular signal-regulated kinase (ERK), and p38 proteins was determined. The phosphorylation of ERK was obviously promoted at 30 min but decreased after 180 min (Figure 5B). The expression of p-JNK was promoted after treatment for 30 to 360 min. The phosphorylation of p38 was significantly promoted and reached a plateau after 180 min.

The phosphorylation of the members of the PI3K-Akt signaling pathway after COS treatment was also investigated. As shown in Figure 5D, the phosphorylated Akt levels peaked at 180 min. COS also promoted the phosphorylation of PDK1 in a time-dependent manner. Moreover, COS also stimulated p85 protein, the regulatory subunit of PI3K, which peaked at 60 min (Figure 5D).

To validate the involvement of MAPK, PI3K/Akt and NF-κB pathways in COS-induced NO production, the effects of specific inhibitors on NO production were determined in RAW 264.7 cells. As shown in Figure 5E, all the inhibitors suppressed the production of NO in COS-induced RAW 264.7 cells, further demonstrating that COS promote NO production by activating the MAPK, PI3K/Akt and NF-κB pathways.

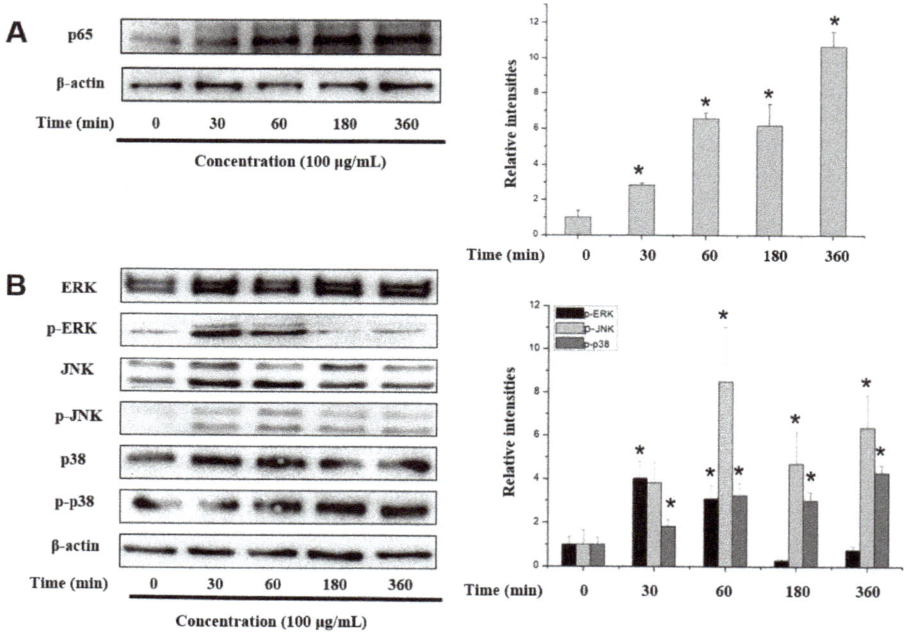

Figure 5. *Cont.*

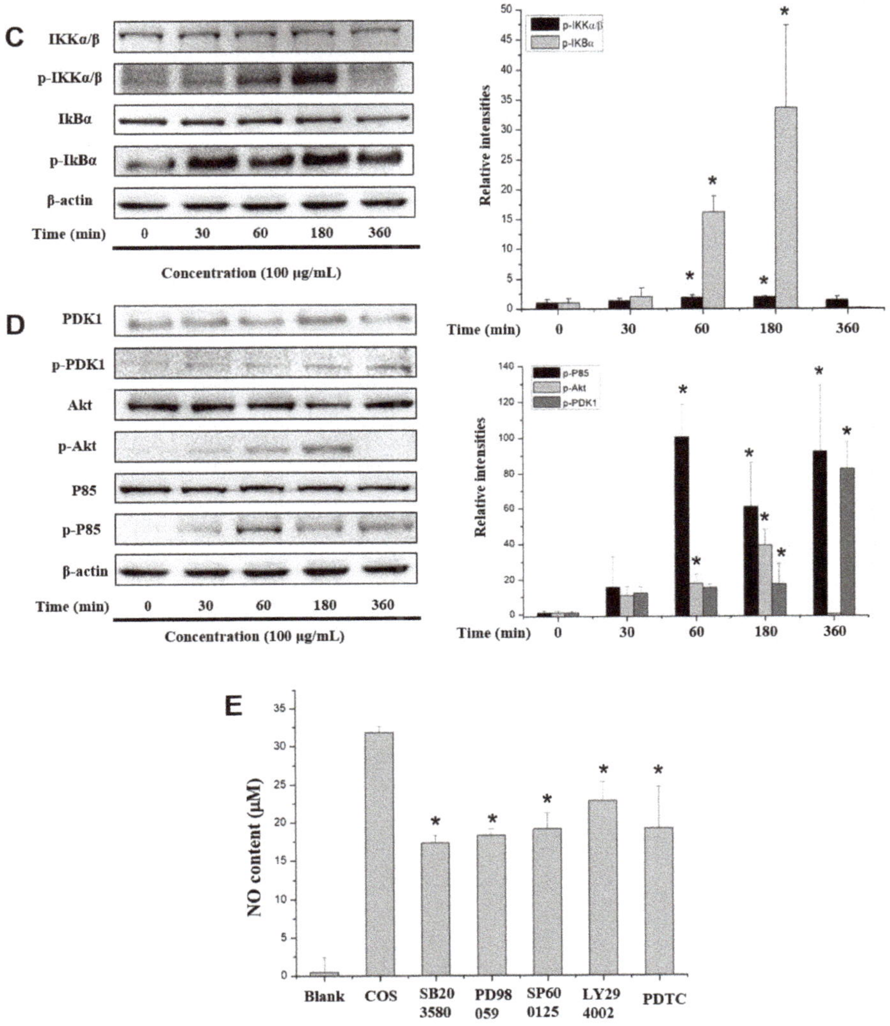

Figure 5. Determination of COS-induced signaling pathways. RAW 264.7 cells were stimulated with 100 μg/mL COS (1874 Da) for the indicated times (0–360 min). Then, cell proteins were extracted and subjected to Western blotting. The effects of COS (1874 Da) on the NF-κB p65 (**A**), MAPK (**B**), IKKα/β and IκBα (**C**), PI3K-Akt (**D**) signaling pathways were determined. The relative expression levels of protein were normalized by β-actin. (**E**) NO production in RAW 264.7 cells pretreated with or without inhibitors after stimulated with 100 μg/mL COS. Data are presented as mean ± SD. (* $p < 0.05$ vs. COS-treated group).

3. Discussion

NO, a small diffusible molecule, is a short-lived, endogenously produced gas synthesized mainly by iNOS [17]. As an effector molecule, NO may be responsible for eradicating invaded pathogens in macrophages [18]. Therefore, we determined the NO expression in RAW 264.7 cells treated with 100 μg/mL α- and β-COS. The results indicated that α-COS is more active at promoting NO production than β-COS. Then, we explored the molecular mechanisms of α-COS. After pretreatment with various concentrations of COS, the NO production in RAW 264.7 cells increased in a dose-dependent manner. Besides NO, pro-inflammatory cytokines are also pivotal in the destruction of pathogens. COS increased the production of two cytokines, TNF-α and IL-6, as determined by CBA and confirmed by RT-PCR and immunoblotting. Our results were consistent with the report by Wu et al. [19], who found that low-molecular-weight chitosan (3 and 50 kDa) considerably induced the expression of IL-6, TNF-α, NO, interferon-γ, and iNOS in a molecular weight- and concentration-dependent manner. Moreover, Wei et al. [16] also found that $(GLcN)_5$ and $(GLcN)_6$ promoted the gene expression and protein secretion of TNF-α, IL-1, and IFN-γ.

To explore the mechanisms of macrophage activation, we performed Western blot analysis of proteins involved in the NF-κB signaling pathway. The transcription factor NF-κB play vital roles in the innate and adaptive immune systems. NF-κB is related to the transcription of many mediators and proinflammatory cytokines genes, such as iNOS, IL-1β, TNF-α, and COX-2 [20–22]. As we demonstrated (Figure 5A), the subunit of NF-κB (p65) was phosphorylated on stimulation with COS. To explore the upstream pathway, the phosphorylation of IκB kinase enzyme complex (IKK α/β) and IκBα proteins were determined. The results showed that COS activated the IKK enzyme complex, which phosphorylated the downstream IκBα protein. Then, IκB proteins were ubiquitylated and degraded, which allowed NF-κB to translocate to the nucleus and promoted the production of its target genes. Our results were consistent with Zheng et al. [23], who found that low-molecular-weight chitosans exert immunostimulatory activity via activation of the AP-1 and NF-κB pathways and 3 kDa chitosan showed greater activity than 5 kDa chitosan in RAW264.7 macrophages. Li et al. [24] also found that five chitooligomers, ranging from dimers to hexamers, promoted the expression of NF-κB downstream genes. Our results demonstrated that besides COS of 3 kDa and COS below 1 kDa, COS of 2 kDa could also promote the translocation of NF-κB.

MAPK activates the transcription of several transcription factors, including NF-κB and AP-1 [25]. Based on the finding that COS promoted NF-κB activation, the phosphorylation levels of ERK, JNK, and p38 proteins were determined. This showed that COS activated the MAPK signaling pathway during macrophage activation. As shown in Figure 5C, COS promoted the phosphorylation of Akt and the p85 subunit. Furthermore, the upstream PDK1 was also increasingly phosphorylated by COS in RAW 264.7 cells. Therefore, the PI3K/Akt pathway, another important pathway in regulating immunity responses, also participated in the activation of RAW 264.7 macrophages induced by COS.

However, it has been reported that COS exerts an anti-inflammatory effect in macrophages by inhibiting the phosphorylation of MAPKs, NF-κB and AP-1 [26]. Kim et al. [27] reported that after oral intake of COS, the IL-12 and interferon-γ levels of elderly people were increased, while the production of IL-1β and TNF-α decreased; the results suggested that COS (3500 Da) has dual immunostimulatory and anti-inflammatory effects in the elderly. These findings are distinct from our results. The different biological activities of COS may result from the differences in molecular weight, degree of DP, N-acetylation, arrangement of acetyl groups, fraction of N-acetylated residues, and pattern of N-acetylation [28].

COS exert their immune-enhancing effect by the interaction with receptors on the macrophage membrane surface, such as Toll-like receptor 4 (TLR 4) [13], complement receptor 3 [29] and mannose receptor [30]. The COS we used in this study is a complex mixture, so it is not clear which component led to the immunostimulatory effect. Therefore, we need to further explore the receptors binding with COS. A remaining challenge is to identify the most active molecules using a component with a single DP.

4. Materials and Methods

4.1. Chemicals and Reagents

α-Chitosan with an average molecular weight of 1856 kDa and degree of deacetylation of 86.0% was provided by Qingdao Yunzhou Biochemical Corp. (Qingdao, China). *Loligo japonica* squid pens were obtained from Yongming Food Co., Ltd. (Liaoning, China). LPS (*Escherichia coli* 0111: B4), 1-(4,5-dimethylthiazol-2-yl)-3,5-diphenyltetrazolium bromide (MTT), sulfanilamide and naphthylethylenediamine dihydrochloride were obtained from Sigma (St. Louis, MO, USA). The Roswell Park Memorial Institute (RPMI) medium 1640 and Penicillin-Streptomycin were purchased from Gibco BRL (Life Technologies, Shanghai, China). The fetal bovine serum (FBS) was obtained from HyClone (Thermo Fisher Scientific, Logan, UT, USA). The kits for cDNA synthesis were purchased from Invitrogen (Carlsbad, CA, USA). The SYBR Premix Ex Taq kits were obtained from Takara Bio (Dalian, China). Primary antibodies to TNF-α, cyclooxygenase (COX)-2, p85, PDK1, Akt, IκBα, p65, c-Jun N-terminal kinase (JNK), extracellular signal-regulated kinase (ERK), p38, and phospho-specific antibodies to p85, PDK1, Akt, IκBα, p65, ERK, JNK, p38 and β-actin were purchased from Cell Signaling Technology (Beverly, MA, USA) except the primary antibody against inducible NO synthase (iNOS) from Abcam (Cambridge, MA, USA). Horseradish peroxidase (HRP)-conjugated goat anti-mouse, and goat anti-rabbit IgG antibodies were purchased from Abcam (Cambridge, MA, USA). The mouse inflammation cytometric bead array (CBA) kit was provided by BD Biosciences (San Diego, CA, USA). Inhibitors including SB203580 (a p38 inhibitor), PD98059 (an ERK inhibitor), SP600125 (a JNK inhibitor) and PDTC (a NF-κB inhibitor) were purchased from Selleck (Shanghai, China). LY294002 (a PI3K inhibitor) was provided by Calbiochem (San Diego, CA, USA).

4.2. Preparation of α- and β-Chitooligosaccharide

The preparation of β-chitosan from Loligo Japonica squid pens was followed by previously described [31]. The preparation of COS was performed by microwave irradiation method. Briefly, chitosan powder (5 g) was dissolved in 250 mL 2% acetic acid, then H_2O_2 (5 mL) was added before being heated in laboratory microwave reaction equipment with an infrared reaction thermometer under magnetic stirring. After the reaction, the average molecular weights of the resulting products were measured by gel permeation chromatography (GPC) analysis. The mixture was neutralized by NaOH and then dialyzed with 500 Da cut-off dialysis membrane.

4.3. Characterization of Chitosan and Chitooligosaccharide

The average molecular weight of COS was measured by GPC analysis performed on TSK 3000-PWXL column (Tosoh, Tokyo, Japan) eluted with the mobile phases (0.1 M CH3COONa and 0.2 M CH3COOH aqueous solution). Fourier transform infrared (FT-IR) spectra of chitosan and chitooligosaccharide were performed by a Thermo Scientific Nicolet iS10 FT-IR spectrometer. The NMR spectra (^{1}H and ^{13}C) were documented by a JEOL JNM-ECP600 spectrometer (JEOL, Tokyo, Japan).

4.4. Cell Culture

The RAW 264.7 cell line was provided by the American Type Culture Collection (Manassas, VA, USA). Cells were maintained in RPMI 1640 medium containing 10% FBS (inactivated by heating at 56 °C for 30 min), L-glutamine (2 mM) and 1% penicillin-streptomycin in a humidified atmosphere with 5% CO_2 at 37 °C.

4.5. Cell Proliferation Assay

RAW 264.7 macrophages were seeded onto 96-well flat-bottom culture plates (1×10^5 cells/well) and allowed to adhere overnight. Thereafter, fresh medium containing indicated contents of chitooligosaccharide (0–200 μg/mL) were introduced and incubated for 24 h. Then the supernatants were discarded, and cells were cultured with 100 μL MTT solution (0.5 mg/mL) for 4 h, and the formed formazan crystals were dissolved in 100 μL MTT stopping buffer. After overnight cultivation, the absorbance was determined at 550 nm using a microplate reader (Tecan, Männedorf, Switzerland).

4.6. NO and Cytokines Quantitation

Followed the treatment as described in Section 2.5, the culture supernatants were collected for determining NO and cytokines production. The NO levels were determined as nitrite NO_2^- by Griess reaction as previously reported [32]. The IL-6 and TNF-α levels were measured by C6 Plus flow cytometer (BD Biosciences, Sparks, MD, USA) using mouse inflammation cytometric bead array kits (San Diego, CA, USA).

4.7. The mRNA Expression Levels of Cytokines Determined by Reverse Transcription-Polymerase Chain Reaction

RAW 264.7 cells were treated by COS for different time periods (0, 30, 60, 180, 360 min). Then the total cellular RNA was extracted from various groups by Trizol® reagent (Invitrogen, Carlsbad, CA, USA). The concentrations of RNA were detected by Nanodrop spectrophotometer (NanoDrop Technologies, Wilmington, DE, USA) followed by cDNA synthesis. Then quantitative real-time polymerase chain reaction (PCR) was performed. The nucleotide sequences primers are shown in Table S1. QRT-PCR was carried out, and the fold increase of each gene was calculated using the $2^{-\Delta\Delta CT}$ method [33]. Housekeeping gene glyceraldehyde 3-phosphate dehydrogenase (GAPDH) was set as the internal reference.

4.8. Immunoblotting

For immunoblot analysis, RAW 264.7 macrophages were seeded in 6-well culture plates (5×10^5 cells/well) and cultured with COS for different time periods (0, 30, 60, 180, 360 min). Cells were scraped off, then the cytoplasmic and nuclear proteins were extracted. Briefly, cells were collected and lysed by 200 μL buffer (ComWin Biotech, Beijing, China). Then the total proteins were extracted by a Roche Complete protease inhibitor cocktail (Roche Diagnostics Ltd., Mannheim, Germany) and collected by centrifugation. Nuclear proteins were extracted using nuclear protein isolation kits (ComWin Biotech, Beijing, China) according to the manufacturer's instructions. The protein concentration was determined by BCA protein assay kits (Com Win Biotech). Then equal grams of proteins (40 μg) were loaded and separated by sodium dodecyl sulfate (SDS)-polyacrylamide gel electrophoresis (PAGE) and then transferred to a polyvinylidene fluoride (PVDF) membrane. After blocked by BSA and rinsed by TTBS, the membranes were incubated with primary and HRP-labeled antibodies. The blot was imaged by Tanon-5200 chemiluminescence detection system (Tanon Science, Shanghai, China). The band density was quantified by Quantity One software (Bio-Rad, Munich, Germany).

4.9. Statistical Analysis

Data were presented as mean ± SD, the significance among different groups was analyzed by one-way analysis of variance. p-values < 0.05 were regarded as statistically significant.

5. Conclusions

In conclusion, the NO production of macrophages pretreated with α- and β-COS was compared. The results suggested that α-COS is more active than β-COS. Therefore, α-COS was chosen for further study. The CBA, RT-PCR, and Western blotting results demonstrated that COS had immunostimulatory effects in RAW 264.7 cells. It promoted the secretion of NO and proinflammatory cytokines, including TNF-α, IL-6, and COX-2, via the PI3K-Akt and MAPK pathways and NF-κB activation. COS possesses great potential as a novel candidate for the treatment of immunosuppressive diseases and as a vaccine adjuvant.

Supplementary Materials: The following are available online at http://www.mdpi.com/1660-3397/17/1/36/s1, Figure S1: Nitric oxide production treated with α-chitooligosaccharide (α-COS) and β- chitooligosaccharide (β-COS) at the concentration of 100 μg/mL., Figure S2: The cell viability treated with α-COS and β-COS at the concentration of 100 μg/mL. Table S1: The primer sequences and conditions for RT-PCR.

Author Contributions: Data curation, S.L.; Methodology, K.L.; Software, H.Y.; Supervision, P.L.; Validation, Y.Q.; Writing—original draft, Y.Y.; Writing—review & editing, R.X.

Acknowledgments: We gratefully acknowledge Weicheng Hu for proving the cell culture room in Huaiyin Normal University (Jiangsu, China). This study was supported by the National Key R&D Program of China (2018YFC0311305), the Special projects of Foshan science and technology innovation team (2017IT100054), the Key Research Program of the Chinese Academy of Sciences (No. KFZD-SW-106) and the Key Research and Development Program of Shandong Province (2017YYSP018).

Conflicts of Interest: The authors declare no conflict of interest.

References

1. Wynn, T.A.; Chawla, A.; Pollard, J.W. Macrophage biology in development, homeostasis and disease. *Nature* **2013**, *496*, 445–455. [CrossRef] [PubMed]
2. Diskin, C.; Palsson-McDermott, E.M. Metabolic Modulation in Macrophage Effector Function. *Front. Immunol.* **2018**, *9*, 270. [CrossRef] [PubMed]
3. Schepetkin, I.A.; Quinn, M.T. Botanical polysaccharides: Macrophage immunomodulation and therapeutic potential. *Int. Immunopharmacol.* **2006**, *6*, 317–333. [CrossRef] [PubMed]
4. Laskin, D.L.; Sunil, V.R.; Gardner, C.R.; Laskin, J.D. Macrophages and tissue injury: Agents of defense or destruction? *Annu. Rev. Pharmacol. Toxicol.* **2011**, *51*, 267–288. [CrossRef] [PubMed]
5. Lee, J.; Choi, J.W.; Sohng, J.K.; Pandey, R.P.; Park, Y.I. The immunostimulating activity of quercetin 3-*O*-xyloside in murine macrophages via activation of the ASK1/MAPK/NF-kappaB signaling pathway. *Int. Immunopharmacol.* **2016**, *31*, 88–97. [CrossRef] [PubMed]
6. Elieh-Ali-Komi, D.; Hamblin, R. Michael Chitin and Chitosan: Production and Application of Versatile Biomedical Nanomaterials. *Int. J. Adv. Res.* **2016**, *4*, 411.
7. Yamamoto, H.; Kuno, Y.; Sugimoto, S.; Takeuchi, H.; Kawashima, Y. Surface-modified PLGA nanosphere with chitosan improved pulmonary delivery of calcitonin by mucoadhesion and opening of the intercellular tight junctions. *J. Control. Release* **2005**, *102*, 373–381. [CrossRef]
8. Wang, Y.-C.; Lin, M.-C.; Wang, D.-M.; Hsieh, H.-J. Fabrication of a novel porous PGA-chitosan hybrid matrix for tissue engineering. *Biomaterials* **2003**, *24*, 1047–1057. [CrossRef]
9. Fu, J.; Ji, J.; Yuan, W.; Shen, J. Construction of anti-adhesive and antibacterial multilayer films via layer-by-layer assembly of heparin and chitosan. *Biomaterials* **2005**, *26*, 6684–6692. [CrossRef]
10. Liaqat, F.; Eltem, R. Chitooligosaccharides and their biological activities: A comprehensive review. *Carbohydr. Polym.* **2018**, *184*, 243–259. [CrossRef]
11. Harish Prashanth, K.V.; Tharanathan, R.N. Chitin/chitosan: Modifications and their unlimited application potential—An overview. *Trends Food Sci. Technol.* **2007**, *18*, 117–131. [CrossRef]
12. Xing, R.; Liu, Y.; Li, K.; Yu, H.; Liu, S.; Yang, Y.; Chen, X.; Li, P. Monomer composition of chitooligosaccharides obtained by different degradation methods and their effects on immunomodulatory activities. *Carbohydr. Polym.* **2017**, *157*, 1288–1297. [CrossRef] [PubMed]
13. Zhang, P.; Liu, W.; Peng, Y.; Han, B.; Yang, Y. Toll like receptor 4 (TLR4) mediates the stimulating activities of chitosan oligosaccharide on macrophages. *Int. Immunopharmacol.* **2014**, *23*, 254–261. [CrossRef] [PubMed]
14. Mei, Y.X.; Chen, H.X.; Zhang, J.; Zhang, X.D.; Liang, Y.X. Protective effect of chitooligosaccharides against cyclophosphamide-induced immunosuppression in mice. *Int. J. Biol. Macromol.* **2013**, *62*, 330–335. [CrossRef] [PubMed]
15. Feng, J.; Zhao, L.; Yu, Q. Receptor-mediated stimulatory effect of oligochitosan in macrophages. *Biochem. Biophys. Res. Commun.* **2004**, *317*, 414–420. [CrossRef] [PubMed]
16. Wei, X.; Wang, Y.; Zhu, Q.; Xiao, J.; Xia, W. Effects of chitosan pentamer and chitosan hexamer in vivo and in vitroon gene expression and secretion of cytokines. *Food Agric. Immunol.* **2009**, *20*, 269–280. [CrossRef]
17. Xiong, Q.; Hao, H.; He, L.; Jing, Y.; Xu, T.; Chen, J.; Zhang, H.; Hu, T.; Zhang, Q.; Yang, X.; et al. Anti-inflammatory and anti-angiogenic activities of a purified polysaccharide from flesh of Cipangopaludina Chinensis. *Carbohydr. Polym.* **2017**, *176*, 152–159. [CrossRef] [PubMed]

18. Zhang, Y.; Liu, D.; Fang, L.; Zhao, X.; Zhou, A.; Xie, J. A galactomannoglucan derived from Agaricus brasiliensis: Purification, characterization and macrophage activation via MAPK and IkappaB/NFkappaB pathways. *Food Chem.* **2018**, *239*, 603–611. [CrossRef]
19. Wu, N.; Wen, Z.S.; Xiang, X.W.; Huang, Y.N.; Gao, Y.; Qu, Y.L. Immunostimulative Activity of Low Molecular Weight Chitosans in RAW264.7 Macrophages. *Mar. Drugs* **2015**, *13*, 6210–6225. [CrossRef] [PubMed]
20. Aikawa, N.; Shinozawa, Y.; Ishibiki, K.; Osahiko, A. Clinical analysis of multiple organ failure in burned patients. *Burns Incl. Therm. Injury* **1987**, *13*, 103–109. [CrossRef]
21. Von Asmuth, E.J.U.; Maessen, J.G.; Van Der Linden, C.J.; Buurma, W.A. Tumour necrosis factor alpha (TNF-alpha) and interleukin 6 in a zymosan-induced shock model. *Scand. J. Immunol.* **1990**, *32*, 313–319. [CrossRef] [PubMed]
22. Volman, J.H.T.; Hendriks, T.; Verhofstad, A.J.A.; Kullberg, B.-J.; Goris, R.J. Improved survival of TNF-deficient mice during the zymosan-induced multiple organ dysfunction syndrome. *Shock* **2002**, *17*, 468–472. [CrossRef] [PubMed]
23. Zheng, B.; Wen, Z.S.; Huang, Y.J.; Xia, M.S.; Xiang, X.W.; Qu, Y.L. Molecular Weight-Dependent Immunostimulative Activity of Low Molecular Weight Chitosan via Regulating NF-kappaB and AP-1 Signaling Pathways in RAW264.7 Macrophages. *Mar. Drugs* **2016**, *14*, 169. [CrossRef] [PubMed]
24. Li, X.; Zhou, C.; Chen, X.; Wang, J.; Tian, J. Effects of five chitosan oligosaccharides on nuclear factor-kappa B signaling pathway. *J. Wuhan Univ. Technol.-Mater. Sci. Ed.* **2012**, *27*, 276–279. [CrossRef]
25. Yang, Y.; Kim, S.C.; Yu, T.; Yi, Y.S.; Rhee, M.H.; Sung, G.H.; Yoo, B.C.; Cho, J.Y. Functional roles of p38 mitogen-activated protein kinase in macrophage-mediated inflammatory responses. *Mediat. Inflamm* **2014**, *2014*, 352–371. [CrossRef]
26. Ma, P.; Liu, H.-T.; Wei, P.; Xu, Q.-S.; Bai, X.-F.; Du, Y.-G.; Yu, C. Chitosan oligosaccharides inhibit LPS-induced over-expression of IL-6 and TNF-α in RAW264.7 macrophage cells through blockade of mitogen-activated protein kinase (MAPK) and PI3K/Akt signaling pathways. *Carbohydr. Polym.* **2011**, *84*, 1391–1398. [CrossRef]
27. Kim, H.M.; Hong, S.H.; Yoo, S.J.; Baek, K.S.; Jeon, Y.J.; Choung, S.Y. Differential effects of chitooligosaccharides on serum cytokine levels in aged subjects. *J. Med. Food* **2006**, *9*, 427–430. [CrossRef]
28. Aam, B.B.; Heggset, E.B.; Norberg, A.L.; Sorlie, M.; Varum, K.M.; Eijsink, V.G. Production of chitooligosaccharides and their potential applications in medicine. *Mar. Drugs* **2010**, *8*, 1482–1517. [CrossRef]
29. Wu, G.J.; Tsai, G.J. Chitooligosaccharides in combination with interferon-γ increase nitric oxide production via nuclear factor-κB activation in murine RAW264.7 macrophages. *Food Chem. Toxicol.* **2007**, *45*, 250–258. [CrossRef]
30. Han, Y.; Zhao, L.; Yu, Z.; Feng, J.; Yu, Q. Role of mannose receptor in oligochitosan-mediated stimulation of macrophage function. *Int. Immunopharmacol.* **2005**, *5*, 1533–1542. [CrossRef]
31. Yang, Y.; Xing, R.; Liu, S.; Qin, Y.; Li, K.; Yu, H.; Li, P. Immunostimulatory effects of sulfated chitosans on RAW 264.7 mouse macrophages via the activation of PI3K/Akt signaling pathway. *Int. J. Biol. Macromol.* **2018**, *108*, 1310–1321. [CrossRef] [PubMed]
32. Baek, K.-S.; Hong, Y.D.; Kim, Y.; Sung, N.Y.; Yang, S.; Lee, K.M.; Park, J.Y.; Park, J.S.; Rho, H.S.; Shin, S.S.; et al. Anti-inflammatory activity of AP-SF, a ginsenoside-enriched fraction, from Korean ginseng. *J. Ginseng Res.* **2015**, *39*, 155–161. [CrossRef] [PubMed]
33. Livak, K.J.; Schmittgen, T.D. Analysis of Relative Gene Expression Data Using Real-Time Quantitative PCR and the $2-\Delta\Delta$CT Method. *Methods* **2001**, *25*, 402–408. [CrossRef] [PubMed]

marine drugs

MDPI

Article

Chitosan Oleate Salt as an Amphiphilic Polymer for the Surface Modification of Poly-Lactic-Glycolic Acid (PLGA) Nanoparticles. Preliminary Studies of Mucoadhesion and Cell Interaction Properties

Dalila Miele [1], Silvia Rossi [1], Giuseppina Sandri [1], Barbara Vigani [1], Milena Sorrenti [1], Paolo Giunchedi [2,*], Franca Ferrari [1] and Maria Cristina Bonferoni [1,*]

1 Department of Drug Sciences, University of Pavia, 27100 Pavia, Italy; dalila.miele01@universitadipavia.it (D.M.); silvia.rossi@unipv.it (S.R.); giuseppina.sandri@unipv.it (G.S.); barbara.vigani@unipv.it (B.V.); milena.sorrenti@unipv.it (M.S.); franca.ferrari@unipv.it (F.F.)

2 Department of Chemistry and Pharmacy, University of Sassari, 07100 Sassari, Italy

* Correspondence: pgiunc@uniss.it (P.G.); cbonferoni@unipv.it (M.C.B.); Tel.: +39-079-228-754 (P.G.); +39-0382-987-357 (M.C.B.)

Received: 30 September 2018; Accepted: 12 November 2018; Published: 15 November 2018

Abstract: Most of the methods of poly-lactic-glycolic acid (PLGA) preparation involve the passage through the emulsification of a PLGA organic solution in water followed by solvent evaporation or extraction. The choice of the droplet stabilizer during the emulsion step is critical for the dimensions and the surface characteristics of the nanoparticles (NPs). In the present work, a recently described ionic amphiphilic chitosan derivative, chitosan oleate salt (CS-OA), was proposed for the first time to prepare PLGA NPs. A full factorial design was used to understand the effect of some formulation and preparation parameters on the NP dimensions and on encapsulation efficiency (EE%) of Nile red, used as a tracer. On the basis of the DoE study, curcumin loaded NPs were prepared, having 329 ± 42 nm dimensions and 68.75% EE%. The presence of a chitosan coating at the surface was confirmed by positive zeta potential and resulted in mucoadhesion behavior. The expected improvement of the interaction of the chitosan surface modified nanoparticles with cell membrane surface was confirmed in Caco-2 cell culture by the internalization of the loaded curcumin.

Keywords: chitosan oleate salt; amphiphilic polymer; PLGA; nanoparticles; mucoadhesion; Caco-2 cell culture; nile red; curcumin

1. Introduction

Poly-lactic-glycolic acid (PLGA) is one of the most widely used biodegradable polymers in nanoparticle (NP) formulations, thanks to possible modulation of biodegradation rate by means of the choice of suitable PLGA grades and thanks to good regulatory position, as they are well accepted by FDA and EMA [1,2].

Most of the methods of PLGA NPs preparation involve the passage through the emulsification of a PLGA organic solution in water followed by solvent evaporation or extraction. The choice of the droplet stabilizer during the emulsion step is critical for the dimensions and the surface characteristics of the NPs. The most used stabilizer in the literature is PVA [3]. Few other polymers were demonstrated to be useful to stabilize nanoemulsions, such as carbomer and poloxamer, while other macromolecules, such as cellulose derivatives and gelatin, resulted in NPs with acceptable dimensions only when used in association with PVA [4]. In most cases the zeta potential resulted negative, with the only exception of the association between PVA and the cationic gelatin A [4].

A growing interest can be seen in recent years in the literature for PLGA NPs coating to modify the surface to cationic charge. Positively charged NPs can in fact more efficiently interact with negatively charged cellular membranes triggering cell uptake [5–8]. From this perspective, the coating with chitosan is in many cases a first choice for its low cost, good biocompatibility, and interesting biological properties such as mucoadhesion [9], that in turn can support the efficiency of nanosystems for mucosal vaccination [10,11]. Moreover, chitosan coated PLGA NPs are described as useful tools to improve transfection in nucleic acids delivery [12,13]. An early systematic study was performed to assess the possible employment of chitosan as stabilizing agent in the preparation of NPs, with and without PVA. While chitosan alone resulted not suitable to stabilize the particles, PVA-chitosan blends led to NPs of low dimensions and positive surface charge [14]. A further approach involves the preparation of PVA-stabilized NPs coated in a second step by chitosan electrostatic adsorption [6,15,16].

Polymeric surfactants present peculiar efficiency in the stabilization of nanoemulsions, due to the multiple contact points of the hydrophobic moieties with the o/w interface and steric effect of hydrated hydrophilic chains [17]. If a derivative of a bioactive polymer is used, some of the polymer properties can be maintained by the nanoemulsion. Recently, some evidence was given of the ability of a new amphiphilic chitosan salt, chitosan oleate CS-OA [18], obtained by ionic interaction between chitosan and oleic acid, to stabilize an essential oil nanoemulsion [19]. It was observed that a low energy method could be combined with the self-assembling behavior of chitosan after electrostatic interaction with the hydrophobic moieties of oleic acid. Nanoemulsions of dimensions in the nanometric range were obtained, depending on chitosan concentration and resulted physically stable for at least three months. The zeta potential of the nanoemulsion confirmed that the chitosan derivative was adsorbed at the droplet interface thanks to affinity of oleic chains for hydrophobic phase, while chitosan backbone resulted arranged towards the aqueous medium [19]. Chitosan oleate maintained in this case an antimicrobial effect, in accordance with literature findings [20,21]. Nanoemulsions based on alpha tocopherol and stabilized by means of chitosan oleate salt were studied on fibroblast and keratinocyte cell lines, on ex vivo human biopsies, and in vivo on a rat burn model, showing the biological effects of both chitosan and oleic acid on the wound healing promotion [22,23].

In the present work, the physical stabilization of nanoemulsions by chitosan oleate was for the first time exploited in the preparation of chitosan coated PLGA NPs. The peculiar arrangement of the hydrophobically modified polymer at the oil to water interface around the droplets should in fact result in the exposure of polysaccharide chains towards the aqueous environment so that solvent removal would lead to the occurrence of PLGA NPs coated with a chitosan shell. In the perspective of a Quality by Design-based pharmaceutical development, the DoE approach is more and more encouraged. In this frame, screening factorial designs are a useful instrument to study the relevance of formulation, preparation and assessment variables on product properties [24,25]. A screening full factorial design was here used to understand the effect of the ratio between chitosan and oleic acid, of chitosan concentration and of stirring rate on the NP dimensions and on encapsulation efficiency of Nile red used as a tracer. To confirm the interaction with the biological substrates, curcumin loaded NPs were prepared and tested for mucoadhesion properties and internalization in Caco-2 substrates. Curcumin was chosen as a hydrophobic model molecule for its largely studied behavior, and the possibility to compare the results obtained with the proposed new CS-OA based systems with those obtained with NPs previously described in the literature [26–28].

2. Results and Discussion

Figure 1 shows the results of the preliminary study performed to assess the relationship between the amount of CS-OA used during the preparation of the nanoparticles and their final dimensions. The CS-OA was obtained in situ by electrostatic interaction between the polysaccharide and the oleic acid, at a 1:1 stoichiometric ratio. Increasing polymer dispersion volumes were added during the emulsification step to stabilize the dispersion of PLGA ethyl acetate solution in water. Final CS concentrations resulted in a range between 725 and 840 μg/mL, while the amount of ethyl acetate

PLGA solution and polymer concentration were maintained constant. The three samples prepared with the lowest volumes of CS-OA dispersion corresponded to the highest mean particle size values, of 7.99 (±1.87) μm, 3.11 (±0.82) μm, and 1.54 (±0.23) μm. These samples were characterized by laser diffraction apparatus and showed a clear decrease of the percentage of dispersion exceeding the nanometer dimensions with the increase in chitosan derivative volume. By further increasing the CS-OA amount, the resulting particulate dimensions decreased below 1000 nm. The comparison between the two series of data can of course be considered just indicative, as the measurements of the dimensions are obtained with two different apparatus, but nevertheless suggested the use of CS-OA concentrations in a higher range. To better assess the relevance of CS-OA amount, CS to OA ratio, and of a preparative parameter such as ULTRA-TURRAX speed, a DoE-based evaluation was performed on Nile red loaded NPs.

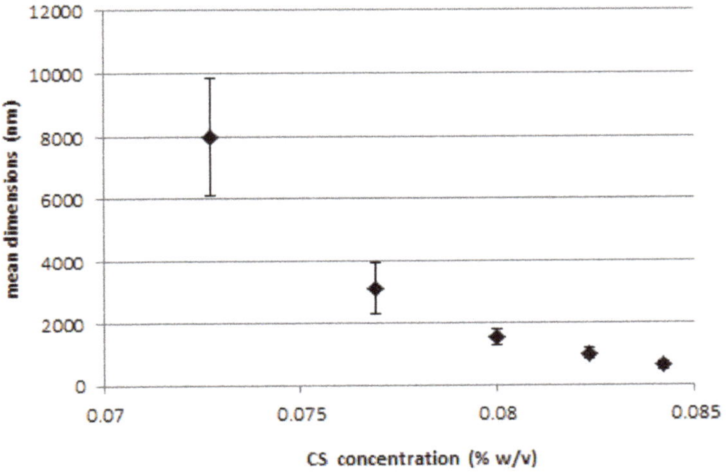

Figure 1. Dimensions of the dispersion (mean ± SD; n = 3) for different chitosan (CS) final concentrations.

2.1. Relevance of Formulation and Preparation Parameters on Nile Red Loaded NPs through DoE Study

In this phase of the development study, the volume of CS-OA dispersion was maintained constant (at 10 mL) and Nile red-loaded NPs were prepared by checking the possible further reduction of the dimensions by increasing the stirring rate and the initial chitosan concentration. The relevance of hydrophobic modification level was evaluated by comparing CS-OA at 1:0.2 and at 1:1 chitosan:oleic acid molar ratio, in a range between a low substitution and the maximum stoichiometric ratio.

Stirring rate range was from 13,500 rpm, slightly higher than the stirring rate used in Phase 1, to 20,500 rpm, the highest rate for the used apparatus.

Chitosan concentration was studied in the range 0.1% (*w*/*v*) slightly higher than the maximum one considered in Phase 1, and 0.2% (*w*/*v*), that in a previous work allowed the authors to obtain nanoemulsions of a few hundred nanometers in size [19].

Nile red was encapsulated in the NPs as a fluorescent tracer, for its hydrophobic character, compatible with loading in PLGA core of the NPs. A full factorial was designed and both the dimensions of the PLGA NPs and the encapsulation efficiency of Nile red were evaluated as a response.

Table 1 reports the data obtained for the eight samples and for the three central points of the Full Factorial 2^3 experimental design.

All the data come from analysis replicates (whose variability is described by the standard deviation values) while the replicates necessary for the variability evaluation of the model were performed on the central point. Each set of data was evaluated for standardized skewness and standardized kurtosis and the values resulted within the range expected for data from a normal distribution.

Apart from the two samples with the lowest concentration of chitosan and the lowest ratio between chitosan and oleic acid, whose dimensions were as high as 1830 nm and 1186 nm for 13,500 and 20,500 rpm stirring rate, respectively, in all other cases the average size is maintained in the range of NP systems. All the samples analyzed have an encapsulation efficiency higher than 65%, and as high as 89.58% in the case of the sample prepared with chitosan concentration 0.2% (*w*/*v*), CS-OA ratio 1:1 and stirring rate 13,500 rpm.

Table 1. Dimensions and encapsulation efficiency (EE%) (mean ± SD; n = 4) of the samples prepared according to the 2^3 full factorial experimental design taking into account, as factors, the chitosan (CS) concentration 0.1–0.2% (*w*/*v*), the stoichiometric ratio chitosan: oleic acid (CS-OA) (1:0.2–1:1), and the ULTRA-TURRAX stirring speed (13,500–24,000 rpm).

Independent Variables (Factors)			Dependent Variables (Responses)	
CS Conc (% *w*/*v*)	CS-OA Ratio	Stirring Rate (rpm)	Dimensions nm (±SD)	EE% (±SD)
−1	−1	−1	1829 (±303)	70.83 (±1.31)
1	−1	−1	610 (±47)	80.92 (±0.06)
−1	1	−1	627 (±16)	85.42 (±1.72)
1	1	−1	591 (±26)	89.58 (±0.09)
−1	−1	1	1186 (±197)	68.35 (±7.37)
1	−1	1	832 (±93)	79.39 (±2.54)
−1	1	1	634 (±19)	72.19 (±5.60)
1	1	1	620 (±24)	86.51 (±1.33)
0	0	0	760 (±23)	71.28 (±0.80)
0	0	0	759 (±17)	72.68 (±2.04)
0	0	0	733 (±32)	76.62 (±1.36)

The model used to fit the data of NP dimensions is as follows.

$$\text{dimensions} = 834{,}636 - 202{,}875{*}A - 248{,}125{*}B - 48{,}125{*}C + 190{,}375{*}A{*}B + 110{,}875{*}A{*}C + 57{,}125{*}B{*}C$$

The Pareto chart for NP dimensions (Figure 2) and the ANOVA table (Table 2), show that both chitosan concentration and stoichiometric ratio between chitosan (CS) and hydrophobic agent (OA) significantly influence the response. Both these effects have a negative sign, so that the higher concentration (0.2% *w*/*v*) and the higher CS:OA ratio (1:1) contribute to decrease the average size of the particles. The effect of concentration factor confirms the trend observed in the preliminary part of the study (Figure 1). The effect of hydrophobic modification seems to confirm its importance for the anchoring of CS-OA at oil to water interface. This is in line with literature data that found poor stabilization of the emulsion with chitosan alone [14]. It is conceivable however that the theoretical stoichiometry between chitosan and oleic acid does not correspond to the final composition of the modified polymer, as it is likely that not all the amino groups of the polymer are involved in the interaction with the fatty acid.

The graph of interaction between concentration and polymer ratio and hydrophobic agent shows a very clear interdependence, confirmed by the statistics that see this significant interaction (Figure 3). However, each of the factors assumes a marked importance in decreasing the particle size when the other factor is at the lowest level, and the stability of the dispersion is probably more critical.

The Pareto chart shows that the mechanical agitation during preparation is not significant, contrary to what could be expected.

Table 2. ANOVA table obtained from the statistical analysis of the 2^3 full factorial design for the effects of the three factors considered and of their binary interactions on NP dimensions.

Source	Sum of Squares	d.f.	Mean Square	F-Ratio	*p*-Value
A: CS concentration	329,266	1	329,266	11.13	0.0290
B: CS:OA ratio	492,528	1	492,528	16.64	0.0151
C: rpm	18,528.1	1	185,28.1	0.63	0.4731
AB	289,941	1	289,941	9.80	0.0352
AC	98,346.1	1	98,346.1	3.32	0.1424
BC	26,106.1	1	26,106.1	0.88	0.4008
Total error	118,385	4	29,596.2		
Total (corr.)	1.3731×10^6	10			

R^2 = 91.3752 percent; R^2 (adjusted for d.f.) = 78.4381 percent.

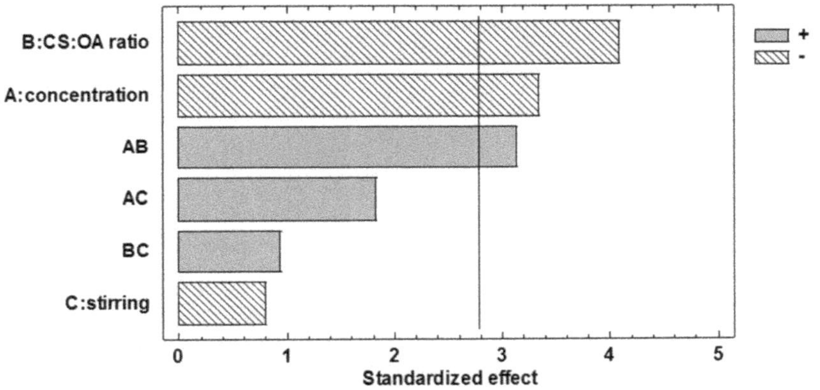

Figure 2. Pareto chart obtained from the statistical analysis of the 2^3 full factorial design and illustrating the effects of the three factors considered and of their interactions on poly-lactic-glycolic acid (PLGA) nanoparticle (NP) dimensions.

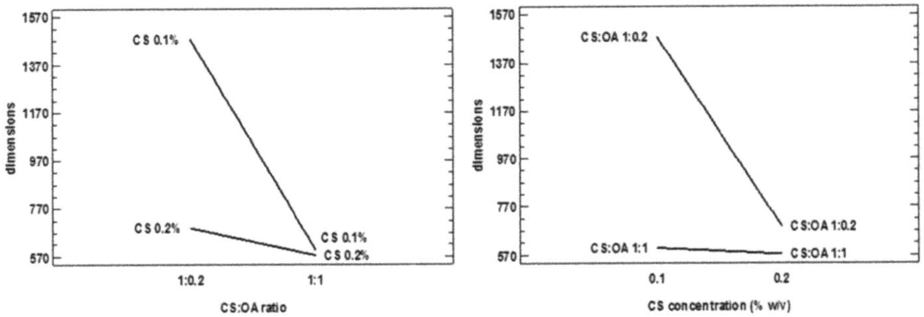

Figure 3. Interaction plots obtained from the statistical analysis of the 2^3 full factorial design and illustrating the interactions between the factors concentration (CS % *w*/*v*) and chitosan:oleic acid (CS:OA) ratio.

The model used in the case of EE% as response is as follows.

$$EE\% = 77.6151 + 4.94963*A + 4.27651*B - 2.54119*C - 0.332076*A*B + 1.38938*A*C - 1.53579*B*C$$

In this case a reduced model obtained by exclusion of the not significant interaction with the lowest coefficient was chosen.

Regarding the effect of the factors on the efficiency of encapsulation, the Pareto graph (Figure 4) and the corresponding ANOVA (Table 3), suggest that also in the case of EE% response, the chitosan concentration and the molar ratio between the polymer and the hydrophobic agent have a significant and positive effect. This is in line with their relevance on nanoemulsion stabilization during nanoparticle preparation as it seemed conceivable that quick and efficient coating of the droplets should help the retention of the marker inside the NPs.

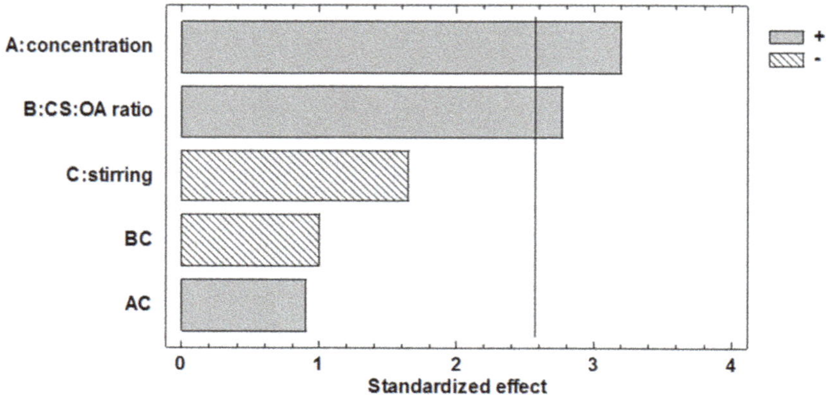

Figure 4. Pareto chart obtained from the statistical analysis of the 23 full factorial design illustrating the effects of the three factors considered and their interactions on Nile red encapsulation efficiency (EE%) in PLGA NP.

Table 3. ANOVA table obtained from the statistical analysis of the 23 full factorial design for the effects of the three factors considered and their binary interactions on encapsulation efficiency (EE%).

Source	Sum of Squares	d.f.	Mean Square	F-Ratio	p-Value
A: CSconcentration	195.991	1	195.991	10.24	0.0240
B: CS-OA ratio	146.308	1	146.308	7.64	0.0396
C: stirring	51.6612	1	51.6612	2.70	0.1614
AC	15.4429	1	15.4429	0.81	0.4103
BC	18.8691	1	18.8691	0.99	0.3664
Total error	95.7231	5	19.1446		
Total (corr.)	523.996	10			

R^2 = 81.7321 percent; R^2 (adjusted for d.f.) = 63.4641 percent.

2.2. Curcumin Loaded NPs

Considering the results of the DoE study on critical parameters, the following conditions were chosen to prepare chitosan coated PLGA NPs: chitosan concentration 0.2% (w/v), chitosan:oleic acid ratio 1:1, and 24,000 rpm ULTRA-TURRAX stirring rate. As reported in Table 1, however, the dimensions of the NPs were even in this case higher than 500 nm. To further reduce the dimensions, acetone 5% v/v was added together with the hydrophobic phase. It is reported in the literature that acetone, as water miscible solvent, during addition to aqueous environment is subject to quick diffusion. This effect lowers the interfacial tension and makes the dispersion of the droplets finer, resulting in turn in small NP dimensions [29].

According to this mechanism, the dimensions of the CS-OA stabilized NPs were reduced, making possible a direct comparison of CS-OA-stabilized NPs with samples obtained by using PVA to stabilize the nanoemulsion, according to the procedure described in the literature [3]. The comparison of the two nanosystems, prepared with CS-OA and with PVA, both unloaded and loaded with curcumin, was performed by considering dimensions, polydispersion index, and zeta potential (Table 4). EE% values are also given in Table 4 in the case of curcumin loaded systems.

Considering the dimensions, the NPs obtained by using CS-OA as stabilizer, both unloaded (CS-OA PLGA) and curcumin loaded (Cur-CS-OA PLGA), were in a range of few hundred nanometers, comparable to the results obtained by using PVA. As the dimensions, at the same process conditions, are influenced mainly by surfactant effect of the polymers during emulsification, these results confirm the efficiency of CS-OA as amphiphilic polymer in emulsion stabilization. EE% was slightly higher for PVA NPs (~82%) with respect to CS-OA NPs (~70%). EE% differences can be here explained by a different arrangement of curcumin at the NP surface. This could represent also a possible explanation for the different zeta potential values observed for unloaded and curcumin loaded NPs. Zeta potential is clearly positive for both the unloaded and curcumin loaded CS-OA NPs, confirming the presence of a chitosan shell at the NP surface.

In both the systems the NPs showed EE% values quite high, in line with the hydrophobic nature of curcumin and its good affinity for the PLGA core. On the basis of EE% values, the curcumin colloidal concentration was calculated, ranging between approximately 82 μg/mL in the case of Cur-CS-OA PLGA and almost 100 μg/mL in the case of Cur-PVA PLGA. In both cases a clear improvement of concentration was observed with respect to curcumin solubility, that literature reports as low as 11 ng/mL [30].

Table 4. Characterization of CS-OA-stabilized NPs prepared with acetone and comparison with PVA stabilized NPs, unloaded and loaded with curcumin (mean ± SD, $n = 3$).

	Dimensions (nm)	Poly Dispersion Index	Zeta Potential (mV)	EE (%)	Curcumin Concentration (μg/mL)
CS-OA PLGA	346 ± 88	0.32 ± 0.10	59.0 ± 2.34	-	-
PVA PLGA	310 ± 74	0.68 ± 0.15	−26.33 ± 1.52	-	-
Cur-CS-OA PLGA	329 ± 42	0.501 ± 0.016	35.45 ± 3.35	68.75 ± 0.83	82.5 ± 0.99
Cur-PVA PLGA	274 ± 9	0.648 ± 0.083	−0.09 ± 2.4	81.99 ± 1.58	98.1 ± 1.47

Figure 5 reports some representative TEM images of CS-OA PLGA NPs. The NPs observed in TEM analysis, like those reported in Figure 5, showed dimensions of few hundred nanometers, in accordance with the results of PCS analysis shown in Table 4, although the two methods differ by physical principle, sampling, and information obtained. From the morphological point of view, TEM images show nonaggregated, spherical NPs. In particular, for those CS-OA PLGA NPs in which the chitosan coating was partially interrupted, like in the images selected for Figure 5, it was possible to appreciate a less dense homogeneous core corresponding to the PLGA inner matrix, and the presence of a more dense surface outer layer conceivably represented by the chitosan coating.

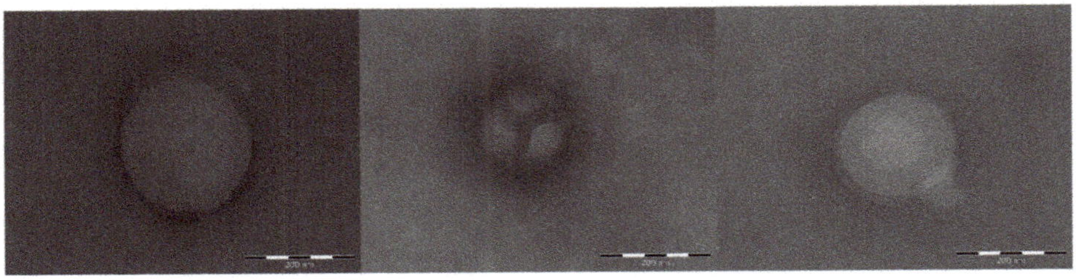

Figure 5. Representative TEM images of CS-OA PLGA nanoparticles. Bars: 200 nm.

2.2.1. Curcumin Loaded NPs Mucoadhesion Behavior

The mucoadhesion behavior of the NPs is illustrated in Figure 6. In particular, Figure 6 shows the results of the test performed in vitro based on the interaction between the NPs and a commercial mucin dispersion. The difference in absorption (ΔA) between the measured absorbance A and the theoretical one (Atheor), indicated as interaction parameter, was proposed in the literature [31] and gives a measure of the interaction between the mucin and the NPs. When no interaction takes place, ΔA = 0 while values of ΔA > 0 indicate a strong interaction between the mucin and the micelles. This approach was previously validated for NP systems [32] by correlation of the positive values of interaction parameter with positive interaction between NP surface and mucin assessed with different other in vitro and ex vivo tests. A positive mucoadhesive interaction clearly occurs here with Cur-CS-OA PLGA chitosan-coated NPs while it is not visible for uncoated ones, as it could be expected for the chitosan presence on the NP surface thanks to its well-known mucoadhesive behavior.

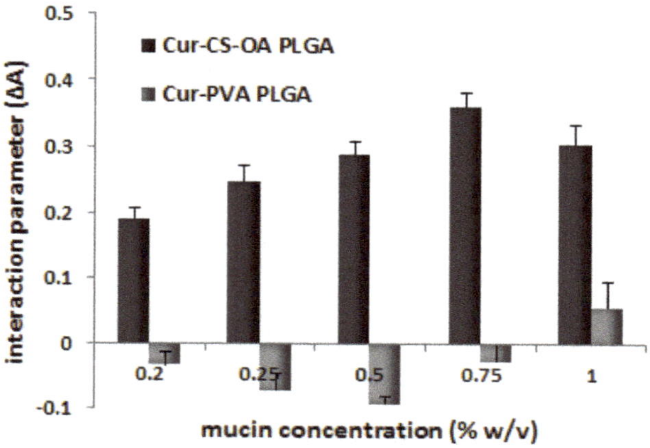

Figure 6. Interaction parameter (mean ± SD, $n = 4$) as a function of mucin concentration for Cur-CS-OA and Cur-PVA NPs. The differences between the two samples were statistically significant at all the mucin concentrations (Mann–Whitney, $p < 0.05$).

2.2.2. Curcumin Loaded NPs. Interaction with Caco-2 Cell Lines

Figure 7 confirms the good biocompatibility of the curcumin loaded samples in a range of curcumin concentrations up to 25 μg/mL. In all cases cell viability was around 80% of the controls, without differences between the free curcumin in DMSO and the two NP samples. This result is in line with what was observed by Beloqui et al. [27] that on the basis of cytotoxicity studies, treated Caco-2 cells with NPs combining poly(lactide-co-glycolide) acid (PLGA) and a polymethacrylate polymer with curcumin concentration of 75 μg/mL. Therefore, Caco-2 cells seem less sensitive to curcumin effect than other cell lines such as A2780 CP or MDA-MB-231 studied by Yallapu et al. [33] or some tumoral cells studied by other authors [26,34] that found 25 μM curcumin both free and loaded in NPs strongly cytotoxic, close in many cases to DL_{50} values.

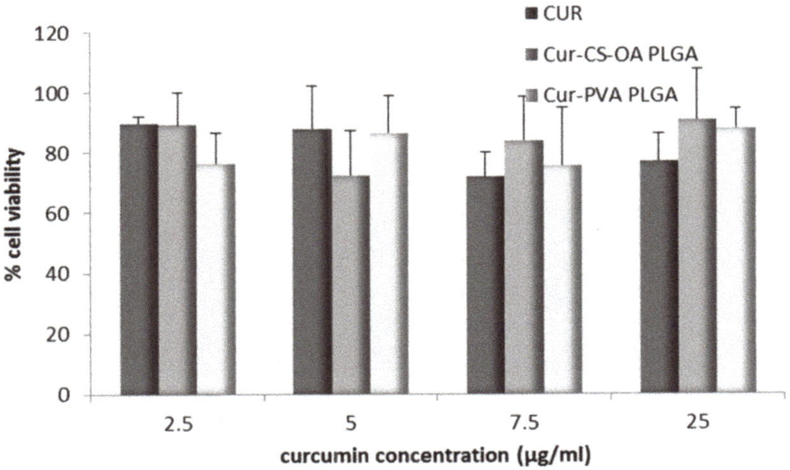

Figure 7. Biocompatibility with Caco-2 cell lines for the samples Cur-CS-OA PLGA, Cur-PVA PLGA, and free curcumin at different curcumin concentrations, as % of cell vitality with respect to the controls after 24 h (mean ± SD, $n = 8$).

The association of curcumin with Caco-2 cells grown 48 h on microscope slides is illustrated in Figure 8a,b. The pictures in Figure 8a are representative images of clusters of cells whose nuclei are stained in red by propidium iodide, while the blue staining indicates the curcumin presence in cytoplasm. In Figure 8b, the curcumin quantified in the cells by image analysis elaboration of the Confocal Laser Scanning Microscopy (CLSM) fluorescence signal, is illustrated for each sample. Cur-CS-OA PLGA sample shows strong positive association to the cells. The good internalization of free curcumin inside the cells is probably determined by its hydrophobic character, that allows easy passage of the cell membranes of the molecule once it is in solution.

Figure 9a,b refers to cells grown on transwell membranes. In this experimental set the Caco-2 cells reach full polarization and are able to express tight junctions. Also in this case, curcumin can be seen inside the cells, as indicated by the blue staining around the nuclei and along the Z axis. Figure 9b shows the results of fluorescence quantification. CS-OA coated NPs seem to be responsible of good internalization in cells, slightly lower than that of free curcumin, but higher than that of PVA NPs.

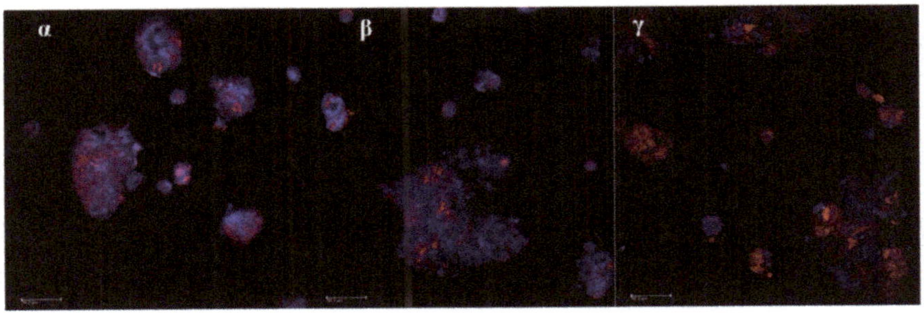

(a)

Figure 8. *Cont.*

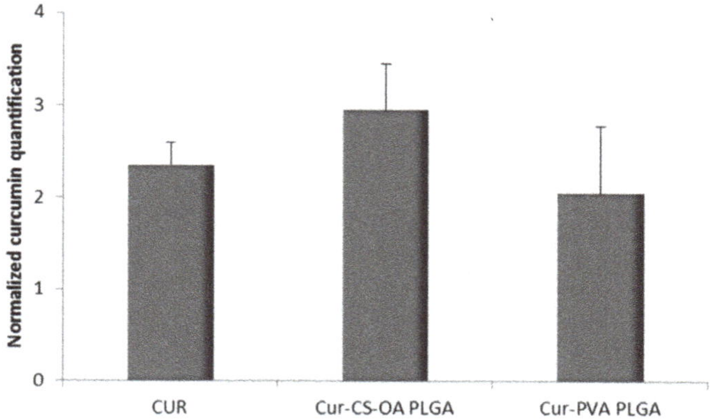

(b)

Figure 8. (**a**) Representative CLSM photomicrographs of Caco-2 cell substrates grown after 48 h on microscope slides and treated 24 h with the samples. (α) Free curcumin; (β) Cur-CS-OA PLGA; (γ) Cur-PVA-PLGA. Bar: 50 μm; (**b**) CLSM fluorescence quantification, obtained by image analysis, of the amount of curcumin associated to the cells grown on microscope slides (mean ± SD; $n = 3$).

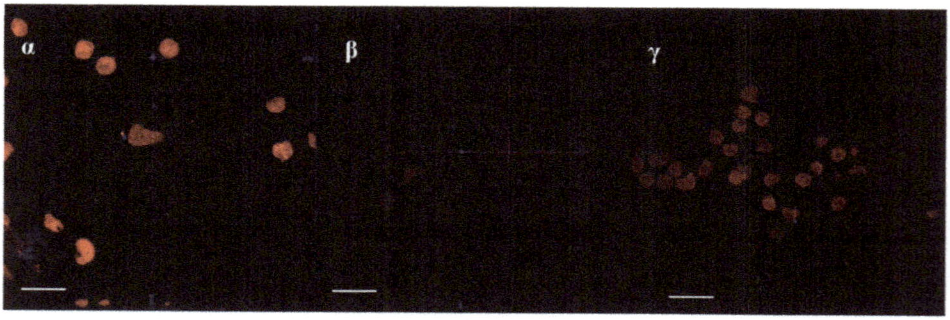

(a)

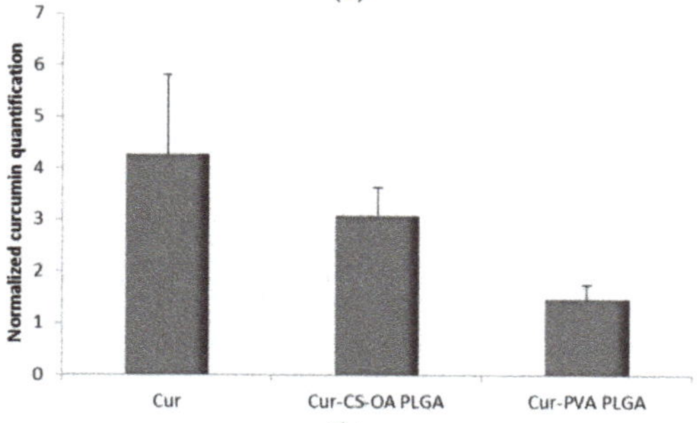

(b)

Figure 9. (**a**) Representative CLSM photomicrographs with z planes of Caco-2 cell substrates grown on transwell membranes, and treated for 3 h with the samples. (α) Free curcumin; (β) Cur-CS-OA PLGA; (γ) Cur-PVA PLGA. Bar: 20 μm; (**b**) CLSM fluorescence quantification, obtained by image analysis, of the amount of curcumin associated to the Caco-2 cells grown on transwell membrane (mean ± SD; $n = 3$).

In no case curcumin could be quantified in the acceptor compartment, in line also in this case with other author results, that did not find quantifiable Papp values for curcumin through Caco-2 cells [27]. However, it was possible to measure the curcumin concentration by fluorescence analysis in the apical compartment at the end of the 3 h test. On the basis of these results the amount of curcumin associated with Caco-2 substrate treated with the samples was calculated by difference. The results are illustrated in Figure 10 and support what previously observed by CLSM pictures. In the case of Cur-CS-OA PLGA sample about 40% of the curcumin put in contact with the cell substrates seems associated with the cell layers. Statistically significant differences can be seen between Cur-CS-OA PLGA and both curcumin and Cur-PVA PLGA (one-way ANOVA, post-hoc Fisher's test).

The transepithelial electrical resistance (TEER) profiles during the three hours of contact of the samples with the substrates (Figure 11) show that no decrease occurred, even with the CS-OA-coated sample, indicating that the presence of the chitosan layer around the NPs does not influence in this case the tight junction structure. This result was not expected, as there are many example in the literature reporting that chitosan-based NPs open tight junctions. The result obtained in this case could be due to a concentration effect, as previously observed with chitosan coated PLGA nanoparticles on Calu3 [35], or to tight association of chitosan with the NPs in line with previous studies on chitosan palmitate polymeric micelles in which it was put in evidence that among different substitution grades, only the less substituted and more hydrophilic derivative was able to maintain the capability to decrease TEER values [36].

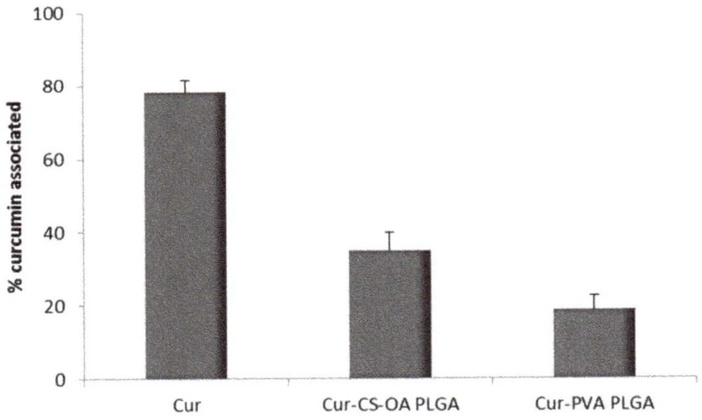

Figure 10. Percentage of curcumin associated to the Caco-2 cell substrates (mean ± SD; $n = 8$) detected by fluorescence analysis. Statistically significant differences (one-way ANOVA, post-hoc Fisher's test, $p < 0.05$): Cur vs. Cur-CS-OA PLGA, Cur vs. Cur-PVA PLGA, Cur-CS-OA PLGA, and vs. Cur-PVA PLGA.

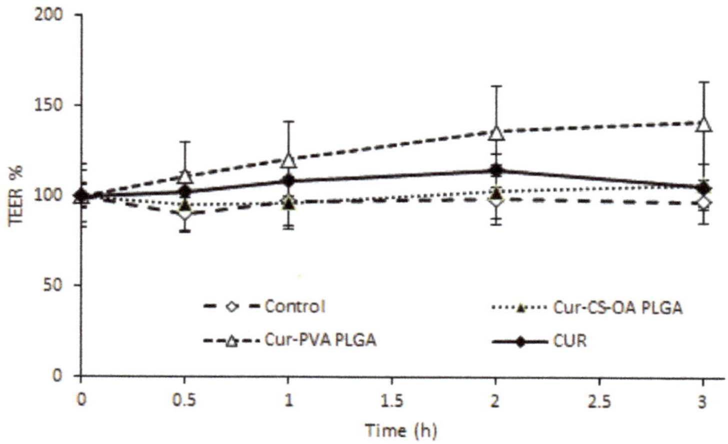

Figure 11. Transepithelial/endothelial electrical resistance (TEER) % profiles of Caco-2 substrates on transwell membranes after contact with Cur-CS-OA PLGA, with Cur-PVA PLGA, and with free curcumin (mean ± SD; $n = 4$).

3. Materials and Methods

3.1. Materials

The following materials were used, chitosan (CS) was obtained as HCl salt from low molecular weight (LMW, chitosan base, deacetylation degree 80% (Sigma-Aldrich, Milan, Italy), by addition of HCl 0.5 N to chitosan until complete dissolution, dialysis in bidistilled water for 24 h and freeze-drying (HetoDrywinner, Analitica de Mori, Milan, Italy). Oleic acid was from Fluka (Milan, Italy). PLGA Resomer RG 503H, Low MW grade poly-vinyl-alcohol (PVA), Nile red and curcumin were all from Sigma-Aldrich. Acetone, acetic acid, sodium acetate, and sodium chloride were acquired from Carlo Erba (Milan, Italy).

3.2. Preparation of the Chitosan Coated NPs

Chitosan oleate (CS-OA) was obtained in situ, as previously described [19,22], by self-assembling during the preparation of the samples. Briefly, oleic acid dissolved in acetone was added to chitosan HCl solution at either 0.1 or 0.2% *w*/*v* and acetone was removed under stirring for about 20 min. The ratio between chitosan and oleic acid was calculated as molar ratio taking into account the molecular weight of glucosamine unit and the theoretical free amino groups of chitosan. Considering the 80% deacetylation degree in accordance with the used chitosan grade, a 1:1 ratio corresponded to 1.4 mg of oleic acid per each mg of chitosan.

In a first step a 0.1% (*w*/*v*) of chitosan concentration and 1:1 stoichiometric ratio with oleic acid were used. 2.5 mL of ethyl acetate solution containing 12 mg PLGA were added to 3 mL distilled water. Emulsification started at 9500 rpm by means of ULTRA-TURRAX T25 (Janke & Kunkel, IKA® Labortechnik, Germany) equipped with 10 mm probe (S25 N-10 G) and after 5 min different volumes of CS-OA dispersion, between 8 and 16 mL, were added. After 10 min, ethyl acetate was removed under stirring at 40 °C for about 45 min. The weight lost during evaporation was assessed and the initial volume reconstituted with distilled water.

3.3. Dimensional and Zeta Potential Characterization of Dispersed Phase

The particle size of the dispersed phase was measured by laser diffraction, Microtrac (Microtrac® SRA 150 ASVR, Honeywell, Phoenix, AZ, USA) for samples exceeding the nanometer range. For the samples in the nanometric range the dimensions and the Polydispersity Index (PI) were measured by Photon Correlation Spectroscopy (PCS) (N5 Submicron Particle Size Analyzer Beckman Coulter, Milan, Italy). PCS analysis were performed at 90° detection angle after dilution in 0.22 µm filtered bidistilled water. PI indicates the width of the size distribution ranging between 0 (monodispersity) and 1. At least three replicates were performed. Zeta potential measurements were performed by means of a Zetasizer® Nanoseries (Malvern Instruments Ltd., Worcestershire, UK). Three measurements were performed for each sample.

For TEM analysis the samples have been layered on 300 mesh cupper grids. The images have been obtained with a JEOL JEM1200EX II apparatus (JEOL Ltd., Tokyo, Japan).

3.4. Nile Red Loaded NPs

For Nile red-loaded NPs, a full factorial 2^3 design was used to study the following formulation and preparation factors (independent variables) each of them set at two levels as hereafter indicated, chitosan concentration 0.1% w/v (−1) and 0.2% w/v (+1), chitosan to oleic acid ratio 1:0.2 (−1) and 1:1 (+1), and ULTRA-TURRAX speed at 13,500 rpm (−1) and 20,500 rpm (+1). In this study, 100 µL of 1 mg/mL Nile red in ethyl acetate were added together with 2.5 mL of 4.8 mg/mL ethyl acetate PLGA solution to 10 mL of chitosan oleate aqueous dispersion prepared as previously described. Two response (dependent) variables, that is nanoparticle dimensions and Nile red encapsulation efficiency, were considered. According with the 2^3 full factorial design, eight experiments were performed. Moreover, one central point was added and replicated three times. All the experiments were performed in a randomized sequence.

Nile Red Encapsulation Efficiency (EE%) Evaluation

Nile red was quantified by UV–Vis detection (Perkin Elmer Instrument Lambda 25 UV–Vis Spectrometer, Monza, Italy) in CH_3CN and acetate buffer 0.1 M pH 4.0, 80:20 mixture, where it was previously verified that all the NP components could be solubilized. Absorbance was read at 552 nm, where the maximum of absorbance was found in the solvent used. The encapsulation efficiency (EE%) was calculated as the percentage ratio between the amount of the tracer quantified in the NPs and the amount added to the formulation. To determine the EE% the samples, after centrifugation 10 min at 6000 rpm to remove by precipitation the amount not encapsulated, the supernatant was diluted in CH_3CN and acetate buffer mixture and spectrophotometrically read.

3.5. Preparation of Curcumin Loaded NPs

Curcumin loaded NPs were obtained with the same solvent evaporation procedure (Figure 12) described above for Nile red loaded NPs. 1.2 mg of curcumin dissolved in 500 µL of acetone were added together with 2.5 mL of 4.8 mg/mL ethyl acetate PLGA solution to 10 mL of chitosan oleate aqueous dispersion prepared as previously described, to obtain a final concentration of 120 µg/mL. In this case, to stabilize the nanoemulsion, the CS-OA dispersion obtained as previously described from 0.2% w/v chitosan and 1:1 chitosan and oleic acid ratio was used. For comparison purposes, NPs stabilized with 2% w/v PVA solution according to the literature [37] were prepared. In both cases, ULTRA-TURRAX homogenization was performed at 20,500 rpm.

Curcumin Quantification and EE% Evaluation

Curcumin was quantified by UV–Vis detection in CH_3CN and acetate buffer 0.1 M pH 4.0, 80:20 mixture. Absorbance was read at 431 nm wavelength. To determine the EE% of the samples (after centrifugation at 10 min at 6000 rpm to remove by precipitation the amount not encapsulated) the supernatant was diluted in CH_3CN and acetate buffer mixture and spectrophotometrically read.

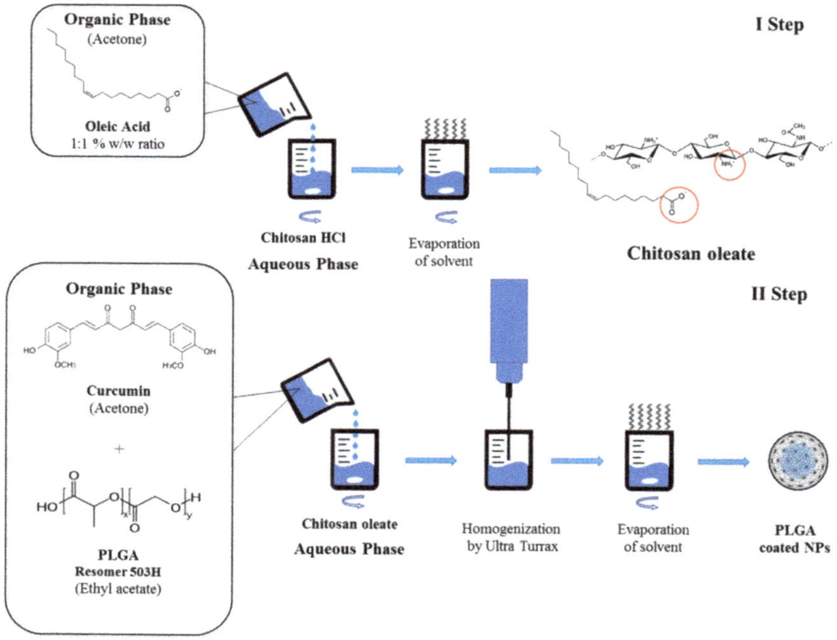

Figure 12. Schematic representation of the preparation method of chitosan-coated NPs.

3.6. Mucoadhesion Evaluation

For the in vitro test, different concentrations, ranging between 0.1% and 1.0% *w*/*v* of mucin type I (Sigma-Aldrich, Milan, Italy), were prepared and put in contact with 200 µL of NP sample for 2 min. Turbidimetric measurements were carried out using a spectrophotometer (UV–Vis Lamba 25, Perkin Elmer, Milan, Italy) at $\lambda = 500$ nm. The mixtures of samples and mucin at increasing concentrations, were compared with the dispersions containing the same concentration of mucin as in the mixture [32]. The turbidimetry values were also elaborated according to the method described in the literature [31]: the effective absorbance (A) was that of the mixture of mucin and NPs. The theoretical absorbance (Atheor) was calculated by adding the absorbance of NPs and that of mucin dispersion at the same concentration. The interaction parameter was the difference in absorption (ΔA) between the measured absorbance and the theoretical one.

3.7. Caco-2 Biocompatibility Test

Caco-2 cell culture was grown in a polystyrene flask in complete culture medium consisting of DMEM added with 1% *v*/*v* of a penicillin–streptomycin–amphotericin 100× solution (pen/strep/amph; Euroclone, Milan, Italy), 10% *v*/*v* of inactivated fetal FBS bovine serum (Fetal Bovine Serum; Euroclone, Milan, Italy) and 1% *v*/*v* of nonessential amino acids 100× (Mem Nonessential Amino Acid Solution 100×; Sigma-Aldrich, Milan, Italy). The cells were grown in an incubator (CO_2 Incubator, PBI International, Milan, Italy) at 37 °C, in a humidified atmosphere, containing 5% of CO_2.

For the cytotoxicity test, Caco-2 cells were seeded (0.35×10^5 cells per well) in 96-well plates (Cellstar 96 Well Culture Plate, Greiner Bio-One, Frickenhausen, Germany) with an area of 0.36 cm^2. After seeding, the plates were placed in the incubator for 24 h, then the cells were washed with 100 µL of PBS, and the samples were added.

NPs loaded with curcumin were tested on cell lines to assess biocompatibility at final curcumin concentration ranging from 2.5 to 25 µg/mL concentration. After 24 h of contact with the samples, a MTT test was performed. The MTT test is based on conversion of tetrazolium salt (3-(4,5-dimetiltiazol-2-)-2,5-diphenyltetrazolium bromide) to formazan by mitochondrial dehydrogenases of vital cells [38]. Briefly, 50 μL of 2.5 mg/mL MTT solution (Sigma-Aldrich, Milan, Italy) in HBSS (Hank's Buffered Salt Solution) pH 7.4 was put in contact with each cell substrate for 3 h. After removing the reagent, the substrates were washed with 200 μL of PBS. Then 100 μL of DMSO was put in each well. The absorbance was read at 570 nm by means of an ELISA plate reader (Imark Absorbance Reader, Biorad, Milan, Italy). Cell viability was calculated as percentage ratio between the absorbance of each sample and the absorbance of controls (cell substrates in growth medium).

3.8. Cell Uptake Studies

Cell uptake was evaluated by means of confocal laser scanning microscopy (CLSM). This was performed both on cells grown 48 h on slides and on cells grown on transwell membranes. In the first case the cells were seeded in 24-well plates. At the bottom of each well was a 13 mm diameter slide (Coverglass Borosilicate, VWR International, Milan, Italy) on which the cells were made to adhere and grow for 24 h. The samples were added and left in contact with the cells another 24 h, after which the cell substrates were washed with 500 μL of PBS and fixed with a 3% *v*/*v* glutaraldehyde solution in PBS for one hour at 4 °C. The glutaraldehyde was removed and the wells were washed twice with 500 μL of PBS.

Cells were also seeded on transwell membranes (0.4 μm pores, 1.13 cm^2 surface, Cellstar® permeable support tissue culture plate, Greiner bio one®, Milano, Italy) and grown 20 ± 1 days until complete confluence. Monolayer integrity was verified by checking TEER values. The basolateral compartment was filled with 1.5 mL of DMEM without Phenol red to avoid fluorescence interferences. Five-hundred microliters of each sample was diluted in DMEM at a final curcumin concentration of 24 μg/mL and placed in donor chamber. After 3 h curcumin was quantified by fluorescence analysis in the apical and basolateral compartment by means of a microplate reader (Plate reader, Synergy HT, 14041014) at 485 nm excitation and 528 nm emission. The cell substrates were washed with PBS, treated 10 min with paraformaldehyde and washed twice with PBS.

Nuclei were stained just before the microscope analysis with 150 μL of propidium iodide (PI) 20 μg/mL in PBS for 5 min in the dark. The PI was then removed and the cells washed with 200 μL of PBS. The slides were examined using a laser scanning confocal microscope (CLSM, Leica TCS SP5II, Leica Microsystems CMS GmbH, Milan, Italy), which allows visualization of fluorescence of propidium iodide (λex = 520 nm and λem = 630 nm) and of curcumin (λex = 440 nm and λem = 520 nm). The fluorescence was quantified on all the microphotographs collected (at least 3 for each sample) by means of an Image analysis program (ImageJ 1.46r, NIH, Bethesda, MD, USA). The blue intensity of curcumin was normalized per each image by the red fluorescence of nuclei.

3.9. Statistical Analysis

Statistical evaluations were performed by means of Statgraphics 5.0, Statistical Graphics Corporation, MD, USA. Differences were determined according to one-way ANOVA and were considered significant at $p < 0.05$. The same statistical package was used to analyze the results of the full factorial design.

4. Conclusions

The results obtained in this study appear promising for the application of an ionic chitosan derivative, such as the chitosan oleate salt, in the easy preparation of nanoparticles with hydrophobic cores that are surface modified with a hydrophilic polysaccharide corona. The high zeta potential values confirm the presence of chitosan at the nanoparticle surface. Chitosan coating can be advantageous for its well-known biological properties and for increased possibilities of further derivatization. Efficiency of the chitosan derivative in PLGA NP preparation resulted comparable to that of PVA. Clear improvement of mucoadhesion behavior has been obtained for CS-OA-based NPs. Further work will be necessary to better understand the mechanism of association between chitosan and oleic acid and its final stoichiometry. Also, the interaction of the nanoparticles with biological substrates and the possible improvement of absorption enhancement properties would deserve better investigation, although the preliminary results here obtained confirm a positive cell internalization of the surface modified nanoparticles, likely due to the interaction of cationic chitosan with the anionic cell membrane. Considering the good potentiality of the PLGA core in the loading of hydrophobic drugs and the mucoadhesion and penetration enhancement properties of the chitosan shell, applications in the delivery of poorly soluble and poorly absorbable drugs can be envisaged.

In a more general perspective, the use of amphiphilic derivatives of bioactive polymers, like chitosan, as nanoemulsion stabilizers in solvent evaporation methods can be proposed as a useful approach for surface modification of nanoparticles with bioactive polymeric shells.

Author Contributions: Conceptualization, M.C.B.; Methodology, M.C.B., S.R., G.S., F.F.; Formal Analysis, M.S.; Investigation, D.M., B.V.; Data Curation, D.M., S.R., G.S., B.V.; Writing—Original Draft Preparation, M.C.B., P.G.; Writing—Review & Editing, M.C.B., P.G.; Supervision, M.C.B., P.G.

Funding: This research received no external funding.

Conflicts of Interest: The authors declare no conflict of interest.

References

1. Danhier, F.; Ansorena, E.; Silva, J.M.; Coco, R.; Le Breton, A.; Preat, V. PLGA-based nanoparticles: An overview of biomedical applications. *J. Control. Release* **2012**, *161*, 505–522. [CrossRef] [PubMed]
2. Mir, M.; Ahmed, N.; Rehman, A.U. Recent applications of PLGA based nanostructures in drug delivery. *Colloids Surf. B Biointerfaces* **2017**, *159*, 217–231. [CrossRef] [PubMed]
3. Astete, C.E.; Sabliov, C.M. Synthesis and characterization of PLGA nanoparticles. *J. Biomater. Sci. Polym. Ed.* **2006**, *17*, 247–289. [CrossRef] [PubMed]
4. Vandervoort, J.; Ludwig, A. Biocompatible stabilizers in the preparation of PLGA nanoparticles: A factorial design study. *Int. J. Pharm.* **2002**, *238*, 77–92. [CrossRef]
5. Tahara, K.; Sakai, T.; Yamamoto, H.; Takeuchi, H.; Hirashima, N.; Kawashima, Y. Improved cellular uptake of chitosan-modified PLGA nanospheres by A549 cells. *Int. J. Pharm.* **2009**, *382*, 198–204. [CrossRef] [PubMed]
6. Alqahtani, S.; Simon, L.; Astete, C.E.; Alayoubi, A.; Sylvester, P.W.; Nazzal, S.; Shen, Y.; Xu, Z.; Kaddoumi, A.; Sabliov, C.M. Cellular uptake, antioxidant and antiproliferative activity of entrapped a-tocopherol and c-tocotrienol in poly(lactic-co-glycolic) acid (PLGA) and chitosan covered PLGA nanoparticles (PLGA-Chi). *J. Colloid Interface Sci.* **2015**, *445*, 243–251. [CrossRef] [PubMed]
7. He, C.; Hua, Y.; Yin, L.; Tang, C.; Yin, C. Effects of particle size and surface charge on cellular uptake and biodistribution of polymeric nanoparticles. *Biomaterials* **2010**, *31*, 3657–3666. [CrossRef] [PubMed]
8. Yameen, B.; Choi, W.I.; Vilos, C.; Swami, A.; Shi, J.; Farokhzad, O.C. Insight into nanoparticle cellular uptake and intracellular targeting. *J. Control. Release* **2014**, *190*, 485–499. [CrossRef] [PubMed]
9. Martínez-Pérez, B.; Quintanar-Guerrero, D.; Tapia-Tapia, M.; Cisneros-Tamayo, R.; Zambrano-Zaragoza, M.L.; Alcalá-Alcalá, S.; Mendoza-Muñoz, N.; Piñón-Segundo, E. Controlled-release biodegradable nanoparticles: From preparation to vaginal applications. *Eur. J. Pharm. Sci.* **2018**, *115*, 185–195. [CrossRef] [PubMed]
10. Pawar, D.; Mangal, S.; Goswami, R.; Jaganathan, K.S. Development and characterization of surface modified PLGA nanoparticles for nasal vaccine delivery: Effect of mucoadhesive coating on antigen uptake and immune adjuvant activity. *Eur. J. Pharm. Biopharm.* **2013**, *85*, 550–559. [CrossRef] [PubMed]
11. Rose, F.; Wern, J.E.; Gavins, F.; Andersen, P.; Follmann, F.; Foged, C. A strong adjuvant based on glycol-chitosan-coated lipid-polymer hybrid nanoparticles potentiates mucosal immune responses against the recombinant Chlamydia trachomatis fusion antigen CTH522. *J. Control. Release* **2018**, *271*, 88–97. [CrossRef] [PubMed]
12. Nafee, N.; Taetz, S.; Schneider, M.; Schaefer, U.F.; Lehr, C. Chitosan-coated PLGA nanoparticles for DNA/RNA delivery: effect of the formulation parameters on complexation and transfection of antisense oligonucleotides. *Nanomedicine* **2007**, *3*, 173–183. [CrossRef] [PubMed]

13. Jagani, H.V.; Josyula, V.R.; Palanimuthu, V.R.; Hariharapura, R.C.; Gang, S.S. Improvement of therapeutic efficacy of PLGA nanoformulation of siRNA targeting anti-apoptotic Bcl-2 through chitosan coating. *Eur. J. Pharm. Sci.* **2013**, *48*, 611–618. [CrossRef] [PubMed]
14. Kumar, R.M.N.V.; Bakowsky, U.; Lehr, C.M. Preparation and characterization of cationic PLGA as DNA carriers. *Biomaterials* **2004**, *25*, 1771–1777. [CrossRef]
15. Badran, M.M.; Mady, M.M.; Ghannam, M.M.; Shakeel, F. Preparation and characterization of polymeric nanoparticles surface modified with chitosan for target treatment of colorectal cancer. *Int. J. Biol. Macromol.* **2017**, *95*, 643–649. [CrossRef] [PubMed]
16. Kang, B.S.; Choi, J.S.; Lee, S.E.; Lee, J.K.; Kim, T.H.; Jang, W.S.; Tunsirikongkon, A.; Kim, J.K.; Park, J.S. Enhancing the in vitro anticancer activity of albendazole incorporated into chitosan-coated PLGA nanoparticles. *Carbohydr. Polym.* **2017**, *159*, 39–47. [CrossRef] [PubMed]
17. Tadros, T. Polymeric surfactants in disperse systems. *Adv. Colloid Interface Sci.* **2009**, *147–148*, 281–299. [CrossRef] [PubMed]
18. Bonferoni, M.C.; Sandri, G.; Dellera, E.; Rossi, S.; Ferrari, F.; Mori, M.; Caramella, C. Ionic polymeric micelles based on chitosan and fatty acids and intended for wound healing. Comparison of linoleic and oleic acid. *Eur. J. Pharm. Biopharm.* **2014**, *87*, 101–106. [CrossRef] [PubMed]
19. Bonferoni, M.C.; Sandri, G.; Rossi, S.; Usai, D.; Liakos, I.; Garzoni, A.; Fiamma, M.; Zanetti, S.; Athanassiou, A.; Caramella, C.; et al. A novel ionic amphiphilic chitosan derivative as a stabilizer of nanoemulsions: Improvement of antimicrobial activity of *Cymbopogon citratus* essential oil. *Colloids Surf. B Biointerfaces* **2017**, *152*, 385–392. [CrossRef] [PubMed]
20. Liu, X.F.; Guan, Y.L.; Yang, D.Z.; Li, Z.; Yao, K.D. Antibacterial action of chitosan and carboxymethylated chitosan. *J. Appl. Polym. Sci.* **2001**, *79*, 1324–1335.
21. Zheng, C.J.; Yoo, J.S.; Lee, T.G.; Cho, H.Y.; Kim, Y.H.; Kim, W.G. Fatty acid synthesis a target for antibacterial activity of unsaturated fatty acids. *FEBS Lett.* **2005**, *579*, 5157–5162. [CrossRef] [PubMed]
22. Bonferoni, M.C.; Riva, F.; Invernizzi, A.; Dellera, E.; Sandri, G.; Rossi, S.; Marrubini, G.; Bruni, G.; Vigani, B.; Caramella, C.; et al. Alpha tocopherol loaded chitosan oleate nanoemulsions for wound healing. Evaluation on cell lines and ex vivo human biopsies, and stabilization in spray dried Trojan microparticles. *Eur. J. Pharm. Biopharm.* **2018**, *123*, 31–41. [CrossRef] [PubMed]
23. Bonferoni, M.C.; Sandri, G.; Rossi, S.; Dellera, E.; Invernizzi, A.; Boselli, C.; Icaro Cornaglia, A.; Del Fante, C.; Perotti, C.; Vigani, B.; et al. Association of Alpha Tocopherol and Ag Sulfadiazine Chitosan Oleate Nanocarriers in Bioactive Dressings Supporting Platelet Lysate Application to Skin Wounds. *Mar. Drugs* **2018**, *16*, 56. [CrossRef] [PubMed]
24. Pramod, K.; Tahir, M.A.; Charoo, N.A.; Ansari, S.H.; Ali, J. Pharmaceutical product development: A quality by design approach. *Int. J. Pharm. Investig.* **2016**, *6*, 129–138. [CrossRef] [PubMed]
25. Bonferoni, M.C.; Rossi, S.; Ferrari, F.; Stavik, E.; Pena-Romero, A.; Caramella, C. Factorial analysis of the influence of dissolution medium on drug release from carrageenan-diltiazem complexes. *AAPS PharmSciTech* **2000**, *1*, e15. [PubMed]
26. Anand, P.; Nair, H.B.; Sung, B.; Kunnumakkara, A.B.; Yadav, V.R.; Tekmal, R.R.; Aggarwal, B.B. Design of curcumin-loaded PLGA nanoparticles formulation with enhanced cellular uptake, and increased bioactivity in vitro and superior bioavailability in vivo. *Biochem. Pharmacol.* **2010**, *79*, 330–338. [CrossRef] [PubMed]
27. Beloqui, A.; Coco, R.; Memvanga, P.B.; Ucakar, B.; des Rieux, A.; Preat, V. pH-sensitive nanoparticles for colonic delivery of curcumin in inflammatory bowel disease. *Int. J. Pharm.* **2014**, *473*, 203–212. [CrossRef] [PubMed]
28. Chuah, L.H.; Roberts, C.J.; Billa, N.; Abdullah, S.; Rosli, R. Cellular uptake and anticancer effects of mucoadhesive curcumin-containing chitosan nanoparticles. *Colloids Surf. B Biointerfaces* **2014**, *116*, 228–236. [CrossRef] [PubMed]
29. Bouchemal, K.; Briancon, S.; Perrier, E.; Fessi, H. Nanoemulsion formulation using spontaneous emulsification: Solvent, oil and surfactant optimization. *Int. J. Pharm.* **2004**, *280*, 241–251. [CrossRef] [PubMed]
30. Kaminaga, Y.; Nagatsu, A.; Akiyama, T.; Sugimoto, N.; Yamazaki, T.; Maitani, T.; Mizukami, H. Production of unnatural glucosides of curcumin with drastically enhanced water solubility by cell suspension cultures of Catharanthus roseus. *FEBS Lett.* **2003**, *555*, 311–316. [CrossRef]

31. He, P.; Davis, S.S.; Illum, L. In vitro evaluation of the mucoadhesive properties of chitosan microspheres. *Int. J. Pharm.* **1998**, *166*, 75–88. [CrossRef]
32. Bonferoni, M.C.; Sandri, G.; Ferrari, F.; Rossi, S.; Larghi, V.; Zambito, Y.; Caramella, C. Comparison of different in vitro and ex vivo methods to evaluate mucoadhesion of glycol-palmitoyl chitosan micelles. *J. Drug Deliery Sci. Technol.* **2010**, *20*, 419–424. [CrossRef]
33. Yallapu, M.M.; Gupta, B.K.; Jaggi, M.; Chauhan, S.C. Fabrication of curcumin encapsulated PLGA nanoparticles for improved therapeutic effects in metastatic cancer cells. *J. Colloid Interface Sci.* **2010**, *351*, 19–29. [CrossRef] [PubMed]
34. Mohanty, C.; Sahoo, S.K. The in vitro stability and in vivo pharmacokinetics of curcumin prepared as an aqueous nanoparticulate formulation. *Biomaterials* **2010**, *31*, 6597–6611. [CrossRef] [PubMed]
35. Nafee, N.; Schneider, M.; Schaefer, U.F.; Lehr, C.M. Relevance of the colloidal stability of chitosan/PLGA nanoparticles on their cytotoxicity profile. *Int. J. Pharm.* **2009**, *381*, 130–139. [CrossRef] [PubMed]
36. Bonferoni, M.C.; Sandri, G.; Dellera, E.; Rossi, S.; Ferrari, F.; Zambito, Y.; Caramella, C. Palmitoyl Glycol Chitosan Micelles for Corneal Delivery of Cyclosporine. *J. Biomed. Nanotechnol.* **2016**, *12*, 231–240. [CrossRef] [PubMed]
37. Mukerjee, A.; Vishwanatha, J.K. Formulation, characterization and evaluation of curcumin-loaded PLGA nanospheres for cancer therapy. *Anticancer Res.* **2009**, *29*, 3867–3875. [PubMed]
38. Stockert, J.C.; Horobin, R.W.; Colombo, L.L.; Blazquez-Castro, A. Tetrazolium salts and formazan products in Cell Biology: Viability assessment, fluorescence imaging, and labeling perspectives. *Acta Histochem.* **2018**, *120*, 159–167. [CrossRef] [PubMed]

marine drugs

MDPI

Article

Influence of Preparation Methods of Chitooligosaccharides on Their Physicochemical Properties and Their Anti-Inflammatory Effects in Mice and in RAW264.7 Macrophages

Ángela Sánchez [1,2], María Mengíbar [1], Margarita Fernández [2], Susana Alemany [2], Angeles Heras [1,*] and Niuris Acosta [1,*]

1 Instituto de Estudios Biofuncionales, Departamento de Química en Ciencias Farmacéuticas, Facultad de Farmacia, Universidad Complutense de Madrid, 28040 Madrid, Spain; assanchez@iib.uam.es (Á.S.); marianmengibar@hotmail.es (M.M.)

2 Instituto de Investigaciones Biomédicas "Alberto Sols", Consejo Superior de Investigaciones Científicas & Universidad Autónoma de Madrid, (CSIC-UAM), 28029 Madrid, Spain; marfermar47@gmail.com (M.F.); salemany@iib.uam.es (S.A.)

* Correspondence: aheras@ucm.es (A.H.); facosta@ucm.es (N.A.); Tel.: +34-913943284 (A.H. & N.A.)

Received: 25 September 2018; Accepted: 24 October 2018; Published: 2 November 2018

Abstract: The methods to obtain chitooligosaccharides are tightly related to the physicochemical properties of the end products. Knowledge of these physicochemical characteristics is crucial to describing the biological functions of chitooligosaccharides. Chitooligosaccharides were prepared either in a single-step enzymatic hydrolysis using chitosanase, or in a two-step chemical-enzymatic hydrolysis. The hydrolyzed products obtained in the single-step preparation were composed mainly of 42% fully deacetylated oligomers plus 54% monoacetylated oligomers, and they attenuated the inflammation in lipopolysaccharide-induced mice and in RAW264.7 macrophages. However, chitooligosaccharides from the two-step preparation were composed of 50% fully deacetylated oligomers plus 27% monoacetylated oligomers and, conversely, they promoted the inflammatory response in both in vivo and in vitro models. Similar proportions of monoacetylated and deacetylated oligomers is necessary for the mixtures of chitooligosaccharides to achieve anti-inflammatory effects, and it directly depends on the preparation method to which chitosan was submitted.

Keywords: chitooligosaccharides; anti-inflammatory action; RAW264.7 macrophage

1. Introduction

Inflammation is a response of the organism to injury, and a prolonged or intense inflammatory event can lead to the development of several diseases. Different cell types and inflammatory mediators such as cytokines act in coordination to resolve the inflammatory event successfully [1]. Lipopolysaccharide (LPS) is a common pathogen-associated molecular-pattern contained in large amounts in the cell walls of Gram-negative bacteria, and stimulates cells of the innate immune system by its ligation to Toll-like receptor 4 (TLR4) [2]. Different cell types, such as neutrophils and macrophages, respond to LPS by releasing potent inflammatory mediators [3,4]. Neutrophils are typically the first leukocytes to be recruited to the inflammatory site and are capable of eliminating pathogens by multiple mechanisms [5,6]. Macrophages are also inflammatory cells with the capacity to acquire a variety of different functional phenotypes in response to the extracellular signals [7,8].

Mitogen-activated protein kinases (MAPKs) are highly conserved families of serine/threonine protein kinases involved in a variety of fundamental cellular processes which play a key role in signal transduction [9,10]. These MAPK signaling pathways induce a secondary response by increasing the expression of inflammatory cytokines and chemokines. The binding of LPS to TLR4 engages multiple signal transduction pathways, including three groups of MAPK: extracellular-signal-regulated kinases (ERKs); the cJun NH_2-terminal kinases (JNKs); and the p38 MAP kinases [11]. The importance of the different MAPKs in controlling cellular responses to the environment by regulating gene expression has made them a priority for research related to many human diseases [9]. Indeed, the ERK, JNK, and p38 pathways are all molecular targets for drug development [12].

Chitosan, the main derivative of chitin, is the essential polymer to produce chitooligosaccharides (COSs), which are linear co-oligomers of *N*-acetyl glucosamine (GlcNAc) and glucosamine (GlcN) units in varying proportions. COSs have been reported to exhibit numerous biological functions, such as antibacterial, anti-inflammatory, antioxidant, immunity-enhancing, antitumor, etc. [13–16]. The biological effects of COSs depend on their degree of polymerization (DP) or average molecular weight (Mw), the degree of *N*-acetylation (DA), and/or the pattern of *N*-acetylation (PA), which in turn depends on the source of chitosan and, most importantly, on the hydrolysis strategy [17]. The relation between the biological function and the structure of COSs is still not well understood [18], making it difficult to establish a hypothesis about their structure–function relationship. The bioactivities of COSs are often tested using relatively poorly characterized chitooligomers, so it is essential to use well-defined and highly purified COS preparations with defined physicochemical characteristics to understand their bioactivity [13].

Currently, COSs are produced by different physical and chemical methods [19–22], but enzymatic procedures present significant advantages, especially when COSs will be used for biomedical applications [23–25]. Partial enzymatic hydrolysis of chitosan with specific enzymes such as chitosanases has been proposed as an alternative to the other hydrolysis methods [26] because the resulting COS can be defined [27].

The focus of this study was to clarify the relationship between the preparation methods of COSs, their physicochemical structure, and their effects related to (anti)-inflammatory properties. Our group optimized the reproducibility of COS preparation methods, and we prepared several COSs by enzymatic depolymerization, with and without previous chemical degradation of chitosan. The structure and composition of chitooligosaccharides were studied in detail and the roles of the anti-inflammatory properties of these COSs using in vitro and in vivo models were evaluated.

2. Results

2.1. Structural and Physicochemical Characterization of COSs

The chitosanolytic activity was checked by HP-SEC, and COSs with lower Mw than initial chitosan were successfully obtained by both methods (Table 1). Low molecular weight chitosan (LMWC) with 32 kDa was obtained in the first step of the two-step process (P2), which led to P2COS (Mw 5 kDa), with lower Mw than P1COS (Mw 8 kDa). In the ^{1}H-NMR spectra, the proton signals (H1–H6) showed the preservation of chitosan structure in both P1COS and P2COS (Figure 1). A slight signal assigned to 5-hydroxymethyl-2-furfural (HMF) was observed in P2COS (Figure 1C). Using ^{13}C-NMR, it was checked that the internal structures of P1COS and P2COS were not altered in their preparation processes (Figure 2). The pattern of *N*-acetylation was 0.8 and 0.9 respectively for P1COS and P2COS, corresponding to a random pattern of acetylated monomers distribution [28].

Table 1. Average molecular weight (Mw), degree of *N*-acetylation (DA), zeta potential (ζ), pattern of *N*-acetylation (PA), and percentage of acetylated oligomers. P1COS: chitooligosaccharide (COS) prepared using the one-step method; P2COS; COS prepared using the two-step method.

Sample	Mw (kDa)	DA (%)	ζ (mV)	PA	A_0 (%)	A_1 (%)	A_2 (%)	A_3 (%)	A_4–A_{24} (%)
P1COS	8	13	56.4 ± 4.9	0.8	42	54	3	1	0
P2COS	5	11	33.1 ± 1.9	0.9	50	27	14	9	0

(A_0), mono- (A_1), di- (A_2), and triacetylated (A_3) oligomers.

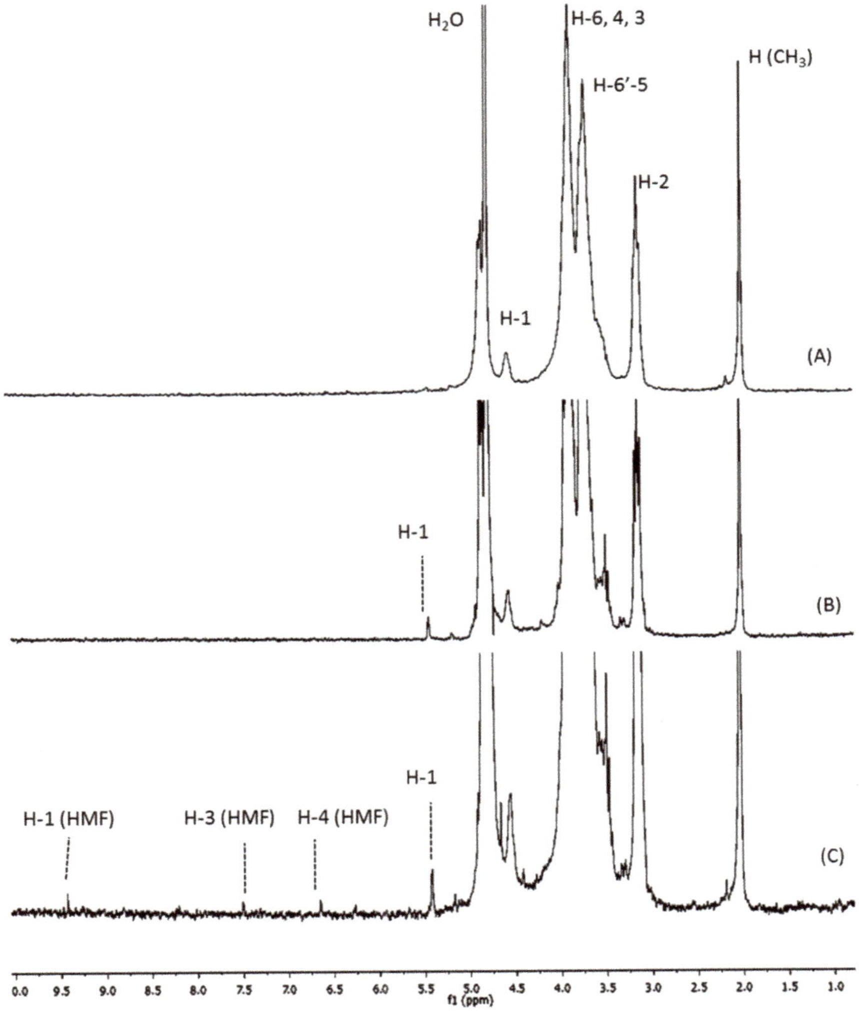

Figure 1. ^{1}H-NMR spectra. (**A**) Native chitosan; (**B**) P1COS; (**C**) P2COS. (**B**,**C**) show the signal of H1 corresponding to deacetylated reducing ends. (**C**): The assignments of 5-hydroxymethyl-2-furfural (HMF) were H-1 (9.43 ppm), H-3 (7.51 ppm), and H-4 (6.66 ppm) [29].

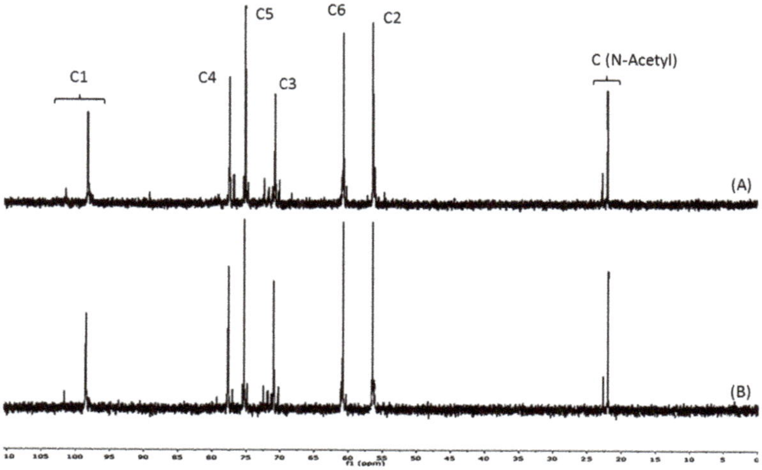

Figure 2. ^{13}C-NMR spectra. (**A**) P1COS obtained in the one-step enzymatic method; (**B**) P2COS obtained in the two-step chemical-enzymatic method.

Both P1COS and P2COS were analyzed by MALDI-TOF-MS to determinate their composition and abundance of the degree of polymerization (Table 1 and Figure 3). COSs showed the typical profile of molecular composition for chitooligosaccharides, and their DP ranged from 3 to 24 in P1COS and from 3 to 17 in P2COS. This result is in concordance with the lower Mw determined previously for this fraction by HP-SEC. Both COSs were composed of fully deacetylated oligomers (A_0) and mono-(A_1), di-(A_2), and tri-acetylated (A_3) oligomers. Larger acetylated oligomers were not detected (Table 1).

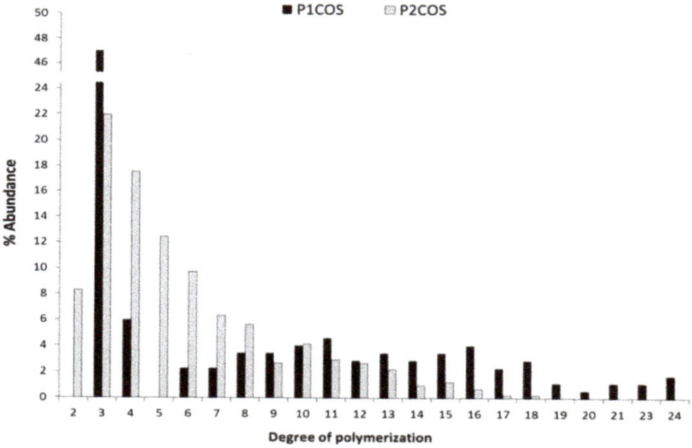

Figure 3. The abundance of the percentage of the degree of polymerization present in both mixtures of P1COS and P2COS.

2.2. Role of P1COS and P2COS in the Peritoneal Migration of Neutrophils

Intraperitoneal injection of LPS in mice induces the accumulation of neutrophils in the peritoneum [30]. To test the implication of P1COS and P2COS in anti-inflammatory response in vivo, we injected mice with LPS, P1COS, and P2COS, as well as LPS together with P1COS or P2COS. Twenty-four hours later, the neutrophil population recruitment to the peritoneum was determined by flow cytometry (Figure 4). P1COS promoted a decrease in the neutrophil population in LPS-induced mice, meaning that P1COS was able to attenuate the acute inflammatory response. Conversely, P2COS generated the most elevated neutrophil recruitment to the peritoneum, even higher than LPS, indicating a pro-inflammatory behavior for this COS. To further analyze the role of P1COS and P2COS in inflammation, we next decided to study how they modulate the LPS response in vitro using RAW264.7 macrophage.

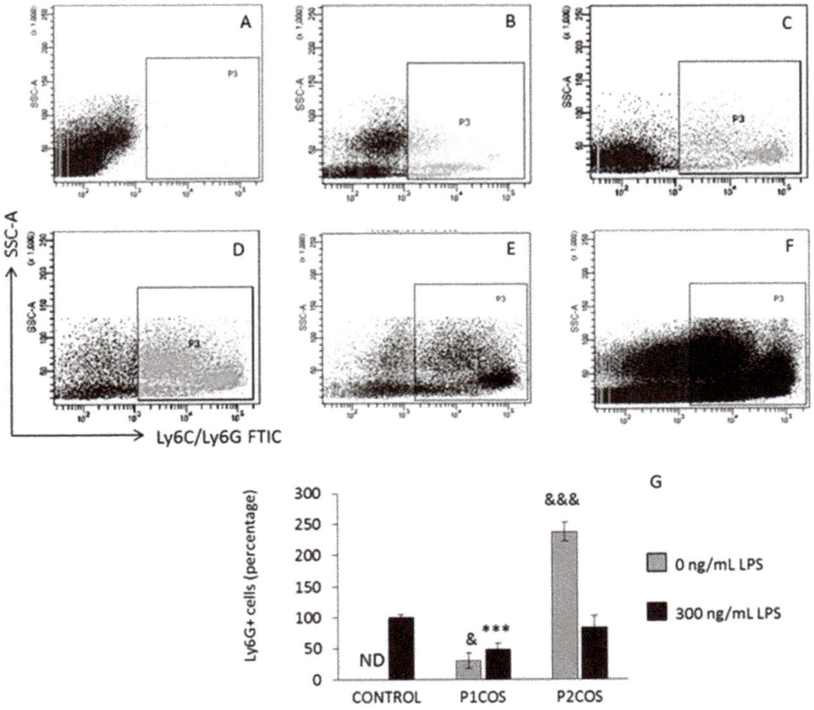

Figure 4. Neutrophils population from mice treated with lipopolysaccharide (LPS), P1COS, P2COS, LPS plus P1COS, and LPS plus P2COS. Mice received an intraperitoneal injection of LPS (1 mg/kg) or of either P1COS or P2COS (10 mg/kg) alone or together with LPS, and 24 h later the levels of circulating neutrophils Ly6G+ cells were analyzed by flow cytometry. (**A–F**) Representative flow cytometry graphs showing the percentage of circulating Ly6G+ cells. (**A**) Control group; (**B**) P1COS; (**C**) P2COS; (**D**) LPS; (**E**) LPS and P1COS; (**F**) LPS and P2COS. (**G**) The means ± SD (n = 6) of the frequency of cells relative to the total number of circulating cells. Asterisks represent the significance with respect to the control LPS-induced mice and "&" with respect to the control without LPS. The 100% inflammation corresponds to $2.1 \times 10^5 \pm 2.5 \times 10^4$ Ly6G+ cells. ND: not detectable.

2.3. *Role of P1COS and P2COS on LPS-Activated RAW264.7 Macrophage Cells*

First, we analyzed the cytotoxicity of P1COS and P2COS on RAW264.7 cells by assaying the viability of the cells incubated with different concentrations of both compounds. P1COS did not affect the viability of the cells at any of the concentrations tested (Figure 5). On the contrary, P2COS affected the viability of macrophage at 5 mg/mL, decreasing the cell survival about 60%. Therefore, 2 mg/mL of P2COS was used for in vitro experiments.

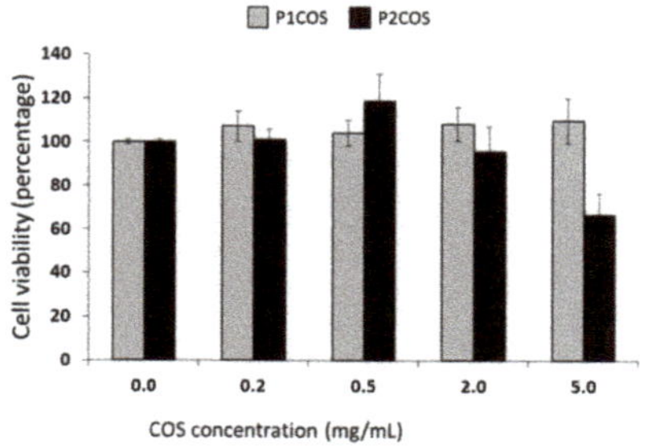

Figure 5. Effects of P1COS and P2COS on the viability of RAW264.7 cells. Cells were treated for 4 h with P1COS or P2COS (0–5 mg/mL), and relative cell viability was measured. The panel shows the mean ± SD from three independent experiments relative to the total cell viability in non-treated cells. Asterisk represents the significance with respect to the non-treated control.

Subsequently, RAW264.7 macrophage cells were treated with P1COS or P2COS, with or without LPS, to assess the effect on the activation state of ERK, JNK, and p38α by Western blotting. The activation levels of these kinases were evaluated by determining their phosphorylation state [9]. Both P1COS and P2COS significantly attenuated the activation of ERK and JNK in LPS-induced macrophage (Figure 6B,D). On the other hand, p38α was attenuated by P1COS but not by P2COS, which promoted a strong increase in its activation levels (Figure 6C). Interestingly, stimulation of cells with P2COS increased the phosphorylation of both p38α and ERK. Indeed p38α phosphorylation was even higher when it was stimulated with P2COS rather than with LPS. However, P1COS did not activate any of the MAP kinases in this cell system.

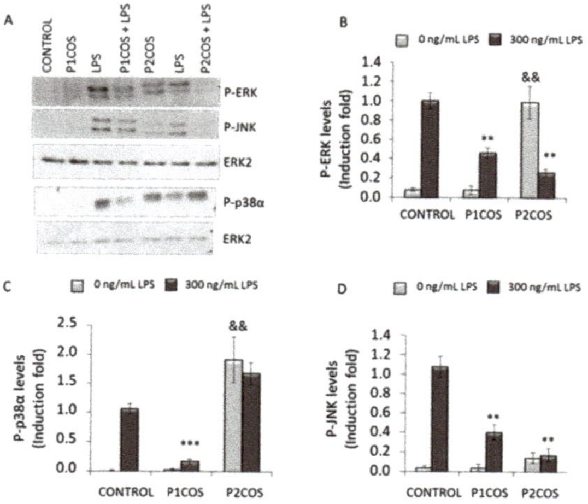

Figure 6. Extracellular-signal-regulated kinase (ERK), cJun NH_2-terminal kinase (JNK), and p38α phosphorylation levels in RAW264.7 cells treated with P1COS or P2COS with or without LPS. Cells were stimulated with LPS (300 ng/mL) or either P1COS or P2COS (2 mg/mL) with or without LPS for 30 min. P-ERK, P-JNK, and P-p38α were analyzed by Western blots, and the total protein ERK2 was analyzed as loading controls. (**A**) Representative Western blots of all experimental conditions. (**B–D**) The graphs show the means ± SD (n = 3) of protein levels fold induction relative to the total of phosphorylated protein in LPS-induced cells, after normalizing values. Asterisk represents the significance with respect to the control LPS-induced cells and "&&" with respect to the control without LPS.

To investigate whether P2COS activates RAW264.7 in the same way as LPS, cells were pre-incubated with two different compounds: polymyxin-B, known to inhibit TLR4 activation [31], and cytochalasin-B, as an actin cytoskeleton disruptor [32], and then stimulated with P2COS. The presence of polymyxin-B did not affect the activation of p38α and ERK promoted by P2COS in RAW264.7 cells (Figure 7A,B). However, the presence of cytochalasin-B was able to partially inhibit the effect of P2COS, drastically decreasing activation levels of ERK and p38α (Figure 7C,D).

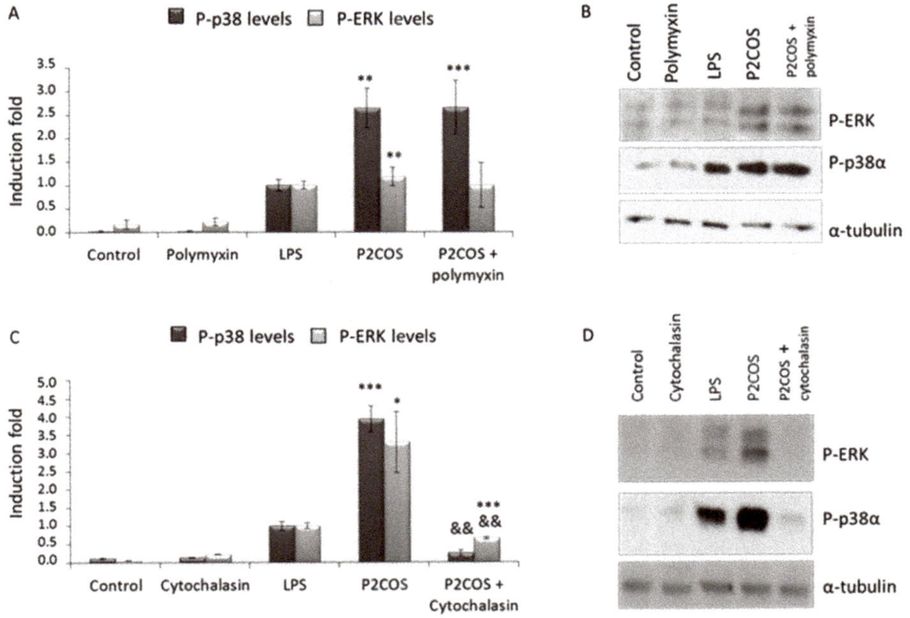

Figure 7. Protein levels of P-ERK and P-p38α in RAW264.7 after P2COS treated (2 mg/mL) for 30 min. Cells were pre-incubated or not with polymyxin-B (1 μg/mL) or cytochalasin-B (10 μg/mL) for 30 min before stimulation with COS, after which the levels of P-ERK and P-p38 were determined by Western blot analysis. As a loading control, membranes were blotted with anti-α-tubulin. (**B**,**D**) Representative Western blots of all experimental conditions. (**A**,**C**) The graphs show the means ± SD (n = 3) of protein levels fold induction relative to the total phosphorylated protein in LPS-induced cells, after normalizing values. Asterisk represents the significance with respect to the non-treated cells and "&&" with respect to the P2COS plus polymyxin-B or cytochalasin-B respectively.

3. Discussion

3.1. The Relation between P1COS and P2COS Preparation Methods and Their Composition

Due to the action of the chitosanase, which specifically breaks glycosidic bonds GlcN–GlcN or GlcN–GlcNAc, higher-intensity signals corresponding to the new deacetylated reducing ends generated (5.4 ppm, assigned to H-1 of GlcN) were detected in P1COS and P2COS [26,33], and a slight increase of this signal was seen in P2COS. In the acidic hydrolysis step of P2, major unstable 2,5-anhydro-D-mannose reducing ends would be produced, leading to the generation of Schiff bases that in turn contribute to HMF formation [29]. The intermediate products of Maillard reactions are advanced glycation end products (AGEs) that emit fluorescence [34], but we found a negligible signal in P2COS. The random pattern of acetylation determined for P1COS and P2COS suggests that the preparation methods did not affect the internal structure of COSs.

As in the chitosanolytic hydrolysis, the GlcN–GlcN or GlcN–GlcNAc glycosidic bonds are attacked by the nitrous acid [29], decreasing the substrate viscosity. Therefore, the double hydrolysis of P2 facilitates the production of COS with lower Mw. The molecular composition was described as $D_{n\text{-}m}A_m$, where m has values between 0 and 3 and n has values between the minimum and the maximum DP [23,35]. P2COS had a slightly higher percentage of fully deacetylated sequences (A0 = 50%) than P1COS (A0 = 42%), in concordance with results obtained by ^{1}H-NMR. Conversely, monoacetylated oligomers (A1 = 54%) were dominant in P1COS and more abundant than in P2COS (A1 = 27%). Therefore, COSs with a higher percentage of A0 oligomers and lower Mws were generated in P2 as we previously described for chitosan from another source [36].

3.2. Role of P1COS and P2COS in LPS-Induced Mice and LPS-Activated RAW264.7 Macrophage Cells

It has been reported that the Mw and DP distribution of COSs influence their anti-inflammatory capacity [37,38] and that this is dose-dependent [39], showing a better anti-inflammatory activity for COS with Mw lower than 10 kDa. It has been proposed that the anti-inflammatory effects of COS in LPS-induced mice could be due to the formation of a stable water-soluble COS–LPS complex through electrostatic interactions [40], making the interaction between LPS and its receptor TLR4 [41] difficult and promoting a partial inhibition of its effect. The interaction of COS–LPS significantly depends on the LPS structure, concentration, COS Mw, and the parameters of the medium where the complexing occurs [42]. Hydroxyl groups of COS would be donors of a proton to form hydrogen bonds, and their *N*-acetyl groups would be collaborating in the hydrophobic interaction that together would stabilize the complex [43,44].

The protein ERK is involved in the regulation of main functions in differentiated cells (e.g., mitosis or apoptosis), and many different stimuli activate the ERK pathway [9,45–47]. JNK and p38α MAPK, also called stress-activated protein kinases, have been implicated in a variety of cellular processes, including cell proliferation, differentiation, and death [48]. The natural peptide polymyxin-B is a potent antibiotic that binds to LPS and neutralizes it [31]. P2COS was able to activate inflammation in a TLR4-independent way since ERK and p38α were activated in the presence of polymyxin-B (Figure 7A,B). However, the inflammation promoted by P2COS was significantly attenuated in the presence of cytochalasin-B since the activation levels of P-ERK1 and P-p38α decreased drastically (Figure 7C,D), meaning that this P2COS needs to be internalized by the macrophage to promote inflammation. The attenuation of p38α was stronger than ERK, which remained active. Therefore, it seems that the activation promoted by P2COS is not exclusively by phagocytosis, since significant levels of P-ERK were detected.

Both P1COS and P2COS showed similar DA (Table 1), but P1COS contained a higher proportion of fully deacetylated (A0) and monoacetylated (A1) oligomers (42% and 54%, respectively) than P2COS, which was composed of 50% of A0 and 27% of A1 oligomers. The higher proportion of A0 and A1 oligomers of P1COS could be crucial to establishing a stable complex with the LPS. This composition would contribute to stabilizing the LPS–COS complex. P1COS prepared by the enzymatic single-step method seems to be an optimal option to produce COSs with anti-inflammatory activity, and the different composition of P2COS would not promote the LPS–COS complex formation, making it difficult to attenuate the inflammatory response.

The composition of P2COS probably allows it to complex with LPS as described above, promoting the attenuation of MAPK in LPS-induced RAW264.7 cells (Figure 6). However, preparation method P2 would influence its pro-inflammatory behavior, promoting the activation of ERK and p38 MAPK, and resulting in P2COS being recognized by cells as an alarm signal. Compared to P1COS, the higher presence of deacetylated reducing ends would also contribute to pro-inflammatory effects. The HMF detected, a common product of Maillard reactions and generated by heat in some food [49], showed no evidence of toxicity [50]. However, the participation of this compound in more advanced stages of Maillard reactions cannot be discarded [51,52]. This fact could contribute to the pro-inflammatory effects shown for P2COS in mice and in the RAW264.7 macrophage. The AGEs are produced in the cell as a consequence of carbohydrate and protein degradation promoted by cellular aging. The negligible presence of AGEs that are closely related to cardiovascular diseases [34] could contribute to the pro-inflammatory response of P2COS. Many intracellular receptors recognize different exogenous molecules [53]. Macrophages have receptors for AGEs (RAGEs) [54] through which they activate the ERK pathways between others [55]. These RAGEs could recognize part of P2COS, but more experiments would be needed to investigate this interaction. Based upon this observation, it seems that the preparation of COSs by a single-step process based on an enzymatic hydrolysis of chitosan is a better option for the generation of COSs with anti-inflammatory properties.

4. Materials and Methods

4.1. Preparation of COSs

Two kinds of COS were prepared from chitosan (89 kDa; DA 17%) obtained from fresh North Atlantic shrimp shells *Pandalus borealis* (Novamatrix, Sandvika, Norway). This chitosan (0.5%, *w*/*w* in 0.5 M acetic acid) was filtered through a series of glass Buchner funnels (250 to 16 μm), precipitated with 10% (*w*/*v*) NaOH aqueous solution, and washed to neutrality with distilled water before its use. One Mw range fraction of COS (Mw 5–10 kDa) was enzymatically prepared using chitosanase EC 3.2.1.132 from *Streptomyces griseus* (Sigma-Aldrich, St. Louis, MO, USA) in the single-step process (P1). The COS was named P1COS, was dialyzed against distilled water until complete salt elimination, and freeze-dried. The other method to prepare COS was performed in two steps (P2). In the first stage, chitosan was depolymerized with nitrous acid [56] to obtain a low molecular weight chitosan (LMWC), which was enzymatically degraded in the second stage with chitosanase EC 3.2.1.132. One Mw range fraction of COS (Mw 5–10 kDa) was isolated, dialyzed, and freeze-dried, and it was named P2COS. All details of preparation methods were previously reported [36]. Prior to stimulation of the anti-inflammatory effect, an exhaustive physicochemical characterization of COS was performed. Both processes were monitored by HP-SEC, and a standard chitosan curve was used to determine the Mw of LMWC, P1COS, and P2COS [57].

4.2. Structural and Physicochemical Characterization of COS

^{1}H-NMR spectra were obtained on a 300 MHz Bruker Advance Spectrometer (Bruker Ettinglen, Bremen, Germany). Chitooligosaccharides were dissolved (0.5%, *w*/*v*) in 1% DCl/D_2O (Sigma-Aldrich), measurements were recorded at 25 °C, the acquisition time was 1 s with 32 scans, and DA was determined according to [58]. ^{13}C-NMR spectra were obtained on an Agilent DD2 600 Spectrometer (Agilent Technologies, Santa Clara, CA, USA). Samples were prepared as described above. The acquisition time was 1.5 s with 5788 scans and 600 MHz. The PA was determined as described in [28]. MALDI-TOF-MS was performed in a Bruker Ultraflex MALDI-TOF mass spectrometer (Bruker-Daltonik, Bremen, Germany) in positive ion mode as detailed by Madhuprakash, El Gueddari, Moerschbacher, and Podile [59].

4.3. Animal Model

Wild type C57BL/6 mice between the ages of 10–12 weeks were used for in vivo experiments. The animals were handled in accordance with Institutional Guidelines for the Care and Use of Laboratory Animals in research, the relevant European Council Directive (2010/63/EU), and Spanish law (R.D.1201/2005), with the approval of the Ethics Committee of the Consejo Superior de Investigaciones Científicas. Mice were intraperitoneally injected with LPS (*Salmonella enterica* serotype Typhimurium, Sigma-Aldrich, 1 mg/kg) alone or together with P1COS or P2COS (10 mg/kg), which were previously dissolved in PBS and sterilized by filtration through a 0.2 μm filter. After 24 h, peritoneal cells were isolated and stained with Anti-Gr1 (Ly6C/Ly6G) FITC (Bioscience, Madrid, Spain). The neutrophil population was determined by flow cytometry (FC 500 MPL, Beckman-Coulter, Indianapolis, IN, USA).

4.4. Cell Culture, Stimuli, and Western Blotting Analysis

Murine RAW264.7 macrophage was cultured in Dulbecco's modified Eagle's medium (DMEM) supplemented with 10% heat-inactivated fetal bovine serum (FBS), 25 mM HEPES, 100 U/mL penicillin, 0,5 μg/mL streptomycin, and 2 mM glutamine. Cells were cultured at 37 °C in a humidified atmosphere (5% CO_2). For in vitro studies, COSs were prepared in culture medium and sterilized by filtration. Prior to stimulation with P1COS or P2COS, non-toxic concentrations of COSs were selected after evaluating their cytotoxicity in the range 0.2 to 5 mg/mL for 4 h [60] by 3-(4,5-dimethylthiazol-2-yl)-2,5-diphenyltetrazolium bromide (MTT) test. For experiments, raw cells were cultured overnight in DMEM with 0.1% FBS. Subsequently, cells were treated with 2 mg/mL of P1COS or P2COS with or without LPS (300 ng/mL) for 30 min. After that, cells were collected and protein extracts were generated and subjected to Western blot analysis [61] using anti-phospho-Erk1/2 (P-ERK, P-p44/42MAPK, Cell-Signaling, Leiden, The Netherlands), anti-phospho-p38α (P-p38, P-T180/Y182, Cell Signaling, Leiden, The Netherlands), and anti-phospho-Jnk1/2 (P-JNK, P-T183/Y185 JNK1/2, Promega-Biotech, Madrid, Spain) antibodies. In some experiments, cells were pre-treated with 1 μg/mL of polymyxin-B (Sigma-Aldrich, St. Louis, MO, USA) or 10 μg/mL of cytochalasin-B (*Drechslera dematioidea*, Sigma-Aldrich, St. Louis, MO, USA) for 30 min before COS treatment.

4.5. Statistical Analysis

Statistical significance was determined by applying student's *t*-test using GraphPad-Prism software. Results shown are mean ± standard error. *p*-values are represented in the figures with asterisks: * $p < 0.05$, ** $p < 0.01$, and *** $p < 0.001$.

5. Conclusions

P1COS prepared by the single-step enzymatic method was able to attenuate the inflammatory response in LPS-induced mice and in LPS-activated murine RAW264.7 macrophage cells. Preparation of COS by this method generates oligomers with a lower proportion of fully deacetylated oligomers compared to our proposed two-step methods. Moreover, its balance with acetylated oligomers seems to be a crucial requirement for using P1COSs as anti-inflammatory agents. On the contrary, the high proportion of fully deacetylated reducing ends and the lower percentage of acetylated oligomers of P2COS could contribute to destabilizing the LPS–COS complex, decreasing its anti-inflammatory effect. In addition, the intermediate products of the Maillard reactions of P2COS could contribute to its pro-inflammatory action in vivo and in vitro. The development of detailed methods to prepare COSs and to study their physicochemical structure is essential to establishing a relationship with their biological function. The use of COSs as anti-inflammatory agents in biotechnological applications will depend on a good knowledge of the structure–function relation.

Author Contributions: A.S. performed the experiments and wrote original manuscript; M.M. designed the experiments and analyzed the data; M.F. and S.A. designed experiments, methodology, and analyzed the data of cell culture and COS anti-inflammatory response; N.A. and A.H. conceived the experiments, formally analyzed the data, wrote-reviewed and edited the paper.

Funding: This research was funded by MAT2010-21016-C02-01 (A.H.) and SAF2014-52009-R (S.A.) grants from the Spanish Ministry of the Economy and Competitiveness.

Conflicts of Interest: The authors declare no conflict of interest.

References

1. Medzhitov, R. Origin and physiological roles of inflammation. *Nature* **2008**, *454*, 428–435. [CrossRef] [PubMed]
2. Kawai, T.; Akira, S. The role of pattern-recognition receptors in innate immunity: Update on Toll-like receptors. *Nat. Immunol.* **2010**, *11*, 373–384. [CrossRef] [PubMed]
3. Abreu, M.T.; Thomas, L.S.; Arnold, E.T.; CLukasek, K.; Michelsen, K.S.; Arditi, M. TLR signaling at the intestinal epithelial interface. *J. Endotoxin Res.* **2003**, *9*, 322–330. [CrossRef] [PubMed]

4. Arndt, P.G.; Suzuki, N.; Avdi, N.J.; Malcolm, K.C.; Worthen, G.S. Lipopolysaccharide-induced c-Jun NH2-terminal kinase activation in human neutrophils: Role of phosphatidylinositol 3-Kinase and Syk-mediated pathways. *J. Boil. Chem.* **2004**, *279*, 10883–10891. [CrossRef] [PubMed]
5. Kolaczkowska, E.; Kubes, P. Neutrophil recruitment and function in health and inflammation. *Nat. Rev. Immunol.* **2013**, *13*, 159–175. [CrossRef] [PubMed]
6. Perobelli, S.M.; Galvani, R.G.; Gonçalves-Silva, T.; Xavier, C.R.; Nóbrega, A.; Bonomo, A. Plasticity of neutrophils reveals modulatory capacity. *Braz. J. Med Boil. Res.* **2015**, *48*, 665–675. [CrossRef] [PubMed]
7. Sica, A.; Mantovani, A. Macrophage plasticity and polarization: In vivo veritas. *J. Clin. Investig.* **2012**, *122*, 787–795. [CrossRef] [PubMed]
8. Stout, R.D.; Suttles, J. Functional plasticity of macrophages: Reversible adaptation to changing microenvironments. *J. Leukocite Boil.* **2004**, *76*, 509–513. [CrossRef] [PubMed]
9. Johnson, G.L.; Lapadat, R. Mitogen-activated protein kinase pathways mediated by ERK, JNK, and p38 protein kinases. *Science* **2002**, *298*, 1911–1912. [CrossRef] [PubMed]
10. Manning, G.; Whyte, D.B.; Martinez, R.; Hunter, T. Sudarsanam, S. The protein kinase complement of the human genome. *Science* **2002**, *298*, 1912–1934. [CrossRef] [PubMed]
11. Sabio, G.; Davis, R.J. TNF and MAP kinase signalling pathways. *Semin. Immunol.* **2014**, *26*, 237–245. [CrossRef] [PubMed]
12. English, J.M.; Cobb, M.H. Pharmacological inhibitors of MAPK pathways. *Trends Pharmacol. Sci.* **2002**, *23*, 40–45. [CrossRef]
13. Li, K.; Xing, R.; Liu, S.; Li, P. Advances in preparation, analysis and biological activities of single chitooligosaccharides. *Carbohydr. Polym.* **2016**, *139*, 178–190. [CrossRef] [PubMed]
14. Ngo, D.H.; Vo, T.S.; Ngo, D.N.; Kang, K.H.; Je, J.Y.; Pham, N.D.; Byun, H.G.; Kim, S.K. Biological effects of chitosan and its derivatives. *Food Hydrocoll.* **2015**, *51*, 200–216. [CrossRef]
15. Xu, Q.; Liu, M.; Liu, Q.; Wang, W.; Du, Y.; Yin, H. The inhibition of LPS-induced inflammation in RAW264.7 macrophages via the PI3K/Akt pathway by highly N-acetylated chitooligosaccharide. *Carbohydr. Polym.* **2017**, *174*, 1138–1143. [CrossRef] [PubMed]
16. Zou, P.; Yang, X.; Wang, J.; Li, Y.; Yu, H.; Zhang, Y.; Liu, G. Advances in characterization and biological activities of chitosan and chitosan oligosaccharides. *Food Chem.* **2016**, *190*, 1174–1181. [CrossRef] [PubMed]
17. Santos-Moriano, P.; Woodley, J.M.; Plou, F.J. Continuous production of chitooligosaccharides by an immobilized enzyme in a dual-reactor system. *J. Mol. Catal. B Enzym.* **2016**, *133*, 211–217. [CrossRef]
18. Chen, M.; Zhu, X.; Li, Z.; Guo, X.; Ling, P. Application of matrix-assisted laser desorption/ionization time-of-flight mass spectrometry (MALDI-TOF-MS) in preparation of chitosan oligosaccharides (COS) with degree of polymerization (DP) 5–12 containing well-distributed acetyl groups. *Int. J. Mass Spectrom.* **2010**, *290*, 94–99. [CrossRef]
19. Tsao, C.T.; Chang, C.H.; Lin, Y.Y.; Wu, M.F.; Han, J.L.; Hsieh, K.H. Kinetic study of acid depolymerization of chitosan and effects of low molecular weight chitosan on erythrocyte rouleaux formation. *Carbohydr. Res.* **2011**, *346*, 94–102. [CrossRef] [PubMed]
20. Wu, S. Preparation of water soluble chitosan by hydrolysis with commercial a-amylase containing chitosanase activity. *Food Chem.* **2011**, *128*, 769–772. [CrossRef]
21. Xia, Z.; Wu, S.; Chen, J. Preparation of water soluble chitosan by hydrolysis using hydrogen peroxide. *Int. J. Boil. Macromol.* **2013**, *59*, 242–245. [CrossRef] [PubMed]
22. Xing, R.; Liu, Y.; Li, K.; Yu, H.; Liu, S.; Yang, Y.; Chen, X.; Li, P. Monomer composition of chitooligosaccharides obtained by different degradation methods and their effects on immunomodulatory activities. *Carbohydr. Polym.* **2017**, *157*, 1288–1297. [CrossRef] [PubMed]
23. Cabrera, J.C.P.; Cutsem, P. Preparation of chitooligosaccharides with degree of polymerization higher than 6 by acid or enzymatic degradation of chitosan. *Biochem. Eng. J.* **2005**, *25*, 165–172. [CrossRef]
24. Hamer, S.N.; Cord-Landwehr, S.; Biarnés, X.; Planas, A.; Waegeman, H.; Moerschbacher, B.M.; Kolkenbrock, S. Enzymatic production of defined chitosan oligomers with a specific pattern of acetylation using a combination of chitin oligosaccharide deacetylases. *Sci. Rep.* **2015**, *5*, 8716. [CrossRef] [PubMed]
25. Jung, W.J.; Park, R.D. Bioproduction of Chitooligosaccharides: Present and Perspectives. *Mar. Drugs* **2014**, *12*, 5328–5356. [CrossRef] [PubMed]
26. Vårum, K.M.; Holme, H.K.; Izume, M.; Torger-Stokke, B.; Smidsrød, O. Determination of enzymatic hydrolysis specificity of partially N-acetylated chitosans. *Biochim. Biophys. Acta* **1996**, *1291*, 5–15. [CrossRef]

27. Aam, B.B.; Heggset, E.B.; Norberg, A.L.; Sørlie, M.; Vårum, K.M.; Eijsink, V.G.H. Production of Chitooligosaccharides and Their Potential Applications in Medicine. *Mar. Drugs* **2010**, *8*, 1482–1517. [CrossRef] [PubMed]
28. Weinhold, M.X.; Sauvageau, J.C.M.; Kumirska, J.; Thöming, J. Studies on acetylation patterns of different chitosan preparations. *Carbohydr. Polym.* **2009**, *78*, 678–684. [CrossRef]
29. Tømmeraas, K.; Vårum, K.M.; Christensen, B.E.; Smidsrød, O. Preparation and characterization of oligosaccharides produced by nitrous acid depolymerisation of chitosans. *Carbohydr. Res.* **2001**, *333*, 137–144. [CrossRef]
30. Soria-Castro, I.; Krzyzanowska, A.; Pelaez, M.L.; Regadera, J.; Ferrer, G.; Montoliu, L.; Rodriguez-Ramos, R.; Fernandez, M.; Alemany, S. Cot/tpl2 (MAP3K8) mediates myeloperoxidase activity and hypernociception following peripheral inflammation. *J. Boil. Chem.* **2010**, *285*, 33805–33815. [CrossRef] [PubMed]
31. Cardoso, L.S.; Araujo, M.I.; Góes, A.M.; Pacífico, L.G.; Oliveira, R.R.; Oliveira, S.C. Polymyxin B as inhibitor of LPS contamination of Schistosoma mansoni recombinant proteins in human cytokine analysis. *Microb. Cell Fact.* **2007**, *6*, 1. [CrossRef] [PubMed]
32. MacLean-Fletcher, S.; Pollard, T.D. Mechanism of action of cytochalasin B on actin. *Cell* **1980**, *20*, 329–341. [CrossRef]
33. Ishiguro, K.; Yoshie, N.; Sakurai, M.; Inoue, Y. A 1H-NMR study of a fragment of partially N-deacetylated chitin produced by lysozyme degradation. *Carbohydr. Res.* **1992**, *237*, 333–338. [CrossRef]
34. Jung, W.K.; Park, P.J.; Ahn, C.B.; Je, J.Y. Preparation and antioxidant potential of maillard reaction products from (MRPs) chitooligomer. *Food Chem.* **2014**, *145*, 173–178. [CrossRef] [PubMed]
35. Mengíbar, M.; Ganan, M.; Miralles, B.; Carrascosa, A.V.; Martínez-Rodriguez, A.J.; Peter, M.G.; Heras, A. Antibacterial activity of products of depolymerization of chitosans with lysozyme and chitosanase against Campylobacter jejuni. *Carbohydr. Polym.* **2011**, *84*, 844–848. [CrossRef]
36. Sánchez, Á.; Mengíbar, M.; Rivera-Rodríguez, G.; Moerchbacher, B.; Acosta, N.; Heras, A. The effect of preparation processes on the physicochemical characteristics and antibacterial activity of chitooligosaccharides. *Carbohydr. Polym.* **2017**, *157*, 251–257. [CrossRef] [PubMed]
37. Fernandes, J.C.; Spindola, H.; de Sousa, V.; Santos-Silva, A.; Pintado, M.E.; Malcata, F.X.; Carvalho, J.E. Anti-Inflammatory Activity of Chitooligosaccharides in vivo. *Mar. Drugs* **2010**, *8*, 1763–1768. [CrossRef] [PubMed]
38. Qiao, Y.; Bai, X.; Du, Y. Chitosan oligosaccharides protect mice from LPS challenge by attenuation of inflammation and oxidative stress. *Int. Immunopharmacol.* **2011**, *11*, 121–127. [CrossRef] [PubMed]
39. Yoon, H.J.; Moon, M.E.; Park, H.S.; Im, S.Y.; Kim, Y.H. Chitosan oligosaccharide (COS) inhibits LPS-induced inflammatory effects in RAW 264.7 macrophage cells. *Biochem. Biophys. Res. Commun.* **2007**, *358*, 954–959. [CrossRef] [PubMed]
40. Davydova, V.N.; Yermak, I.M.; Gorbach, V.I.; Krasikova, I.N.; Solov'eva, T.F. Interaction of Bacterial Endotoxins with Chitosan. Effect of Endotoxin Structure, Chitosan Molecular Mass, and Ionic Strength of the Solution on the Formation of the Complex. *Biochemistry* **2000**, *65*, 1082–1090. [PubMed]
41. Yermak, I.M.; Davidova, V.N.; Gorbach, V.I.; Luk'yanov, P.A.; Solov'eva, T.F.; Ulmer, A.J.; Buwitt-Beckmann, U.; Rietschel, E.T.; Ovodov, Y.S. Forming and immunological properties of some lipopolysaccharide–chitosan complexes. *Biochimie* **2006**, *88*, 23–30. [CrossRef] [PubMed]
42. Davydova, V.N.; Naberezhnykh, G.A.; Yermak, I.M.; Gorbach, I.N.; Solov'eva, T.F. Determination of Binding Constants of Lipopolysaccharides of Different Structure with Chitosan. *Biochemistry* **2006**, *71*, 332–339. [CrossRef]
43. Naberezhnykh, G.A.; Gorbach, V.I.; Likhatskaya, G.N.; Davidova, V.N.; Solov'eva, T.F. Interaction of Chitosans and Their N-Acylated Derivatives with Lipopolysaccharide of Gram-Negative Bacteria. *Biochemistry* **2008**, *73*, 432–441. [CrossRef] [PubMed]
44. Naberezhnykh, G.A.; Gorbach, V.I.; Kalmykova, E.N.; Solov'eva, T.F. Determination of the parameters of binding between lipopolysaccharide and chitosan and its N-acetylated derivative using a gravimetric piezoquartz biosensor. *Biophys. Chem.* **2015**, *198*, 9–13. [CrossRef] [PubMed]
45. Cagnol, S.; Chambard, J.C. ERK and cell death: Mechanisms of ERK-induced cell death–apoptosis, autophagy and senescence. *FEBS J.* **2010**, *277*, 2–21. [CrossRef] [PubMed]
46. Khavari, T.A.; Rinn, J. Ras/Erk MAPK signaling in epidermal homeostasis and neoplasia. *Cell Cycle* **2007**, *6*, 2928–2931. [CrossRef] [PubMed]

47. Mebratu, Y.; Tesfaigzi, Y. How ERK1/2 activation controls cell proliferation and cell death: Is subcellular localization the answer? *Cell Cycle* **2009**, *8*, 1168–1175. [CrossRef] [PubMed]
48. Minakami, M.; Kitagawa, N.; Iida, H.; Anan, H.; Inai, T. p38 mitogen-activated protein kinase and c-jun NH2-terminal protein kinase regulate the accumulation of a tight junction protein, ZO-1, in cell–cell contacts in HaCaT cells. *Tissue Cell* **2015**, *47*, 1–9. [CrossRef] [PubMed]
49. Capuano, E.; Fogliano, V. Acrylamide and 5-hydroxymethylfurfural (HMF): A review on metabolism, toxicity, occurrence in food and mitigation strategies. *LWT–Food Sci. Technol.* **2011**, *44*, 793–810. [CrossRef]
50. NTP. NTP toxicology and carcinogenesis studies of 5-(Hydroxymethyl)-2-furfural (CAS No. 67-47-0) in F344/N rats and B6C3F1 mice (gavage studies). *Natl. Toxicol. Program Tech. Rep. Ser.* **2010**, *554*, 7–13, 15–19, 21–31.
51. Tomas, D.; Karin, K.; Stephanie, D.; Imre, B. Analysis of Amadori compounds by high-performance cation exchange chromatography coupled to tandem mass spectrometry. *Anal. Chem.* **2005**, *77*, 140–147.
52. Zeng, L.; Qin, C.; Chi, W.; Wang, L.; Ku, Z.; Li, W. Browning of chitooligomers and their optimum preservation. *Carbohydr. Polym.* **2007**, *67*, 551–558. [CrossRef]
53. Basta, G. Receptor for advanced glycation end products and atherosclerosis: From basic mechanisms to clinical implications. *Atherosclerosis* **2008**, *196*, 9–21. [CrossRef] [PubMed]
54. Akira, S.; Uematsu, S.; Takeuchi, O. Pathogen recognition and innate immunity. *Cell* **2006**, *124*, 783–801. [CrossRef] [PubMed]
55. Ott, C.; Jacobs, K.; Haucke, E.; Navarrete Santos, A.; Grune, T.; Simm, A. Role of advanced glycation end products in cellular signaling. *Redox Boil.* **2014**, *2*, 411–429. [CrossRef] [PubMed]
56. Allan, G.G.; Peyron, M. Molecular weight manipulation of chitosan I: Kinetics of depolymerization by nitrous acid. *Carbohydr. Res.* **1995**, *277*, 257–272. [CrossRef]
57. Mengíbar, M.; Mateos-Aparicio, I.; Miralles, B.; Heras, A. Influence of the physico-chemical characteristics of chito-oligosaccharides (COS) on antioxidant activity. *Carbohydr. Polym.* **2013**, *97*, 776–782. [CrossRef] [PubMed]
58. Hirai, A.; Odani, H.; Nakajima, A. Determination of degree of deacetylation of chitosan by 1H- NMR spectroscopy. *Polym. Bullettin* **1991**, *26*, 87–94. [CrossRef]
59. Madhuprakash, J.; El Gueddari, N.E.; Moerchbacher, B.M.; Podile, A.R. Production of bioactive chitosan oligosaccharides using the hypertransglycosylating chitinase-D from serratia proteamaculans. *Bioresour. Technol.* **2015**, *198*, 503–509. [CrossRef] [PubMed]
60. Hansen, M.B.; Nielsen, S.E.; Berg, K. Re-examination and further development of a precise and rapid dye method for measuring cell growth/cell kill. *J. Immunol. Methods* **1989**, *119*, 203–210. [CrossRef]
61. Rodríguez, C.; López, P.; Pozo, M.; Duce, A.M.; López-Pelaéz, M.; Fernández, M.; Alemany, S. COX2 expression and Erk1/Erk2 activity mediate Cot-induced cell migration. *Cell. Signal* **2008**, *20*, 1625–1631. [CrossRef] [PubMed]

marine drugs

MDPI

Article

Reclamation of Marine Chitinous Materials for Chitosanase Production via Microbial Conversion by *Paenibacillus macerans*

Chien Thang Doan [1,2], Thi Ngoc Tran [1,2], Van Bon Nguyen [2], Anh Dzung Nguyen [3] and San-Lang Wang [1,4,*]

1 Department of Chemistry, Tamkang University, New Taipei City 25137, Taiwan; doanthng@gmail.com (C.T.D.); tranngoctnu@gmail.com (T.N.T.)
2 Department of Science and Technology, Tay Nguyen University, Buon Ma Thuot 630000, Vietnam; bondhtn@gmail.com
3 Institute of Biotechnology and Environment, Tay Nguyen University, Buon Ma Thuot 630000, Vietnam; nadzungtaynguyenuni@yahoo.com.vn
4 Life Science Development Center, Tamkang University, New Taipei City 25137, Taiwan
* Correspondence: sabulo@mail.tku.edu.tw; Tel.: +886-2-2621-5656; Fax: +886-2-2620-9924

Received: 30 September 2018; Accepted: 31 October 2018; Published: 2 November 2018

Abstract: Chitinous materials from marine byproducts elicit great interest among biotechnologists for their potential biomedical or agricultural applications. In this study, four kinds of marine chitinous materials (squid pens, shrimp heads, demineralized shrimp shells, and demineralized crab shells) were used to screen the best source for producing chitosanase by *Paenibacillus macerans* TKU029. Among them, the chitosanase activity was found to be highest in the culture using the medium containing squid pens as the sole carbon/nitrogen (C/N) source. A chitosanase which showed molecular weights at 63 kDa was isolated from *P. macerans* cultured on a squid pens medium. The purified TKU029 chitosanase exhibited optimum activity at 60 °C and pH 7, and was stable at temperatures under 50 °C and pH 3-8. An analysis by MALDI-TOF MS revealed that the chitosan oligosaccharides (COS) obtained from the hydrolysis of water-soluble chitosan by TKU029 crude enzyme showed various degrees of polymerization (DP), varying from 3–6. The obtained COS enhanced the growth of four lactic acid bacteria strains but exhibited no effect on the growth of *E. coli*. By specialized growth enhancing effects, the COS produced from hydrolyzing water soluble chitosan with TKU029 chitinolytic enzymes could have potential for use in medicine or nutraceuticals.

Keywords: chitin; chitosan; protease; chitinase; chitosan oligomers

1. Introduction

Chitosan is a polysaccharide consisting of 1,4-ß-linked D-glucosamine residues, partially substituted with *N*-acetyl group. Recently, chitosan oligomer conversion has attracted attention among many researchers, because chitosan oligosaccharides are not only water-soluble, but also show various functional properties such as anti-inflammatory [1], anti-oxidative [2], anti-tumor [1,3], preservative [4], and prebiotic [5,6]. Chitosanase is a useful and environmentally-friendly tool for depolymerizing chitosan into oligosaccharides with various degrees of polymerization (DP). The major sources of chitosanase are bacteria, such as *Bacillus*, *Serratia*, *Aeromonas*, *Streptomyces*, *Pseudomonas*, and *Paenibacillus*. Almost all of these chitinolytic-producing bacteria were reported as using chitin or chitosan as the source of carbon/nitrogen (C/N). Commercialized chitin and chitosan products are mostly prepared from shrimp shells, crabs shells, or squid pens by chemical treatment to remove the mineral salts and proteins from these fishery processing by-products. In order to save on enzyme production cost, and in reutilizing the residual proteins, these chitin and protein-containing raw materials have been reported as the sole C/N source for enzyme production by *Bacillus* [7–10], *Pseudomonas* [11–13], and *Serratia* [14,15].

Until now, exopolysaccharides [16–18], α-glucosidase inhibitors [19,20], antioxidants [21], and biosurfactants [16] produced by *Paenibacillus* sp. growing on squid pens, shrimp shells, or crab shells have been reported; however, there have been few reports about chitinase production of *Paenibacillus* species on these low-cost chitinous materials. In the previous report [22], demineralized crab shells or squid pens have been used as the sole C/N source for comparing the activities of chitinase, chitosanases, proteases, and α-glucosidase inhibitors by 16 chitinolytic/proteolytic enzymes-producing strains, i.e., *Paenibacillus* sp. TKU029, *Paenibacillus* sp. TKU032, *Paenibacillus* sp. TKU037, *Paenibacillus* sp. TKU042 [22], *Bacillus licheniformis* [10], *Bacillus cereus* [2], *Serratia marcescens* [15], *Serratia ureilytica* [14], *Pseudomonas aeruginosa* [13]. Among these tested strains, *Paenibacillus* sp. TKU029 together with *Paenibacillus* sp. TKU042 produced the highest chitosanase activity when squid pens were used as the sole C/N source.

In this study, four kinds of the marine byproducts, i.e., squid pen powder (SPP), demineralized crab shell powder (deCSP), demineralized shrimp shell powder (deSSP), and shrimp head powder (SHP), were used as the sole C/N source to explore the production of chitosanase by *P. macerans* TKU029 via fermentation. The purification and characterization of these TKU029 chitosanase were performed. The oligomers obtained by hydrolyzing water-soluble chitosan with TKU029 chitosanase were analyzed by MALDI-TOF-MS, and their enhancing effect on the growth of lactic acid bacteria was also estimated.

2. Results and Discussion

2.1. Screening of Chitinous Materials as Sole C/N Source for Chitosanase Production

Chitinous materials have been proposed as an important factor for producing chitinase/chitosanase by fermentation [22]. Therefore, four containing-chitin marine byproducts (SHP, SPP, deCSP, and deSSP) were investigated for the production of chitinase by *P. macerans* TKU029 in this study. As shown in Figure 1, the highest chitosanase productivity by *P. macerans* TKU029 was observed with the C/N source of SPP (0.448 ± 0.022 U/mL, 2 day). These results were consistent with the research of Doan et al. [22], which showed that *Paenibacillus* sp. TKU042 produced the highest chitosanase activity on SPP (day 2).

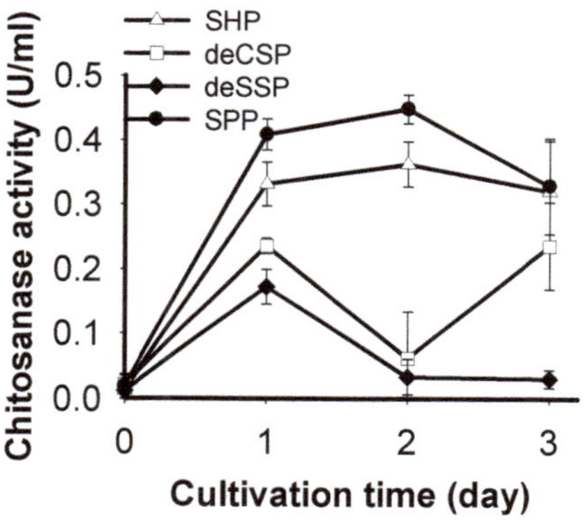

Figure 1. Production of chitosanase by *P. macerans* TKU029 using different chitin-containing materials as the C/N source. SHP, shrimp head powder; deCSP, demineralized crab shell powder; deSSP, demineralized shrimp shell powder; SPP, squid pen powder. The error bars represent standard deviations ($n = 3$).

SPP, with its high ratio of protein and low ratio of mineral salts, was claimed to be a good C/N source for producing exopolysaccharides and a bio surfactant by *P. macerans* TKU029 [16]. In this study, SPP was also found to be the best C/N source for chitinase production by *P. macerans* TKU029.

2.2. Purification and Characterization of Chitosanase

In order to explore the enzyme characterization and make a comparison with other reports, the chitosanase was purified from the culture supernatant (600 mL) of *P. macerans* TKU029 by ethanol precipitation and ion exchange chromatography of DEAE-Sepharose CL-6B. As shown in Figure 2, one chitosanase was eluted with a linear gradient of 0-1 M NaCl in the same buffer. The eluted fractions of chitosanasewas pooled for further purification by chromatography of Macro-Prep DEAE, respectively. Table 1 summarize the purification results of TKU029 chitosanase, respectively. TKU 029 chitosanase was purified from the culture supernatant with the weight recovery 1.43 mg, respectively. The final specific activity and recovery yields of TKU029 chitosanase were 24.19 U/mg and 10.51%, respectively (Table 1).

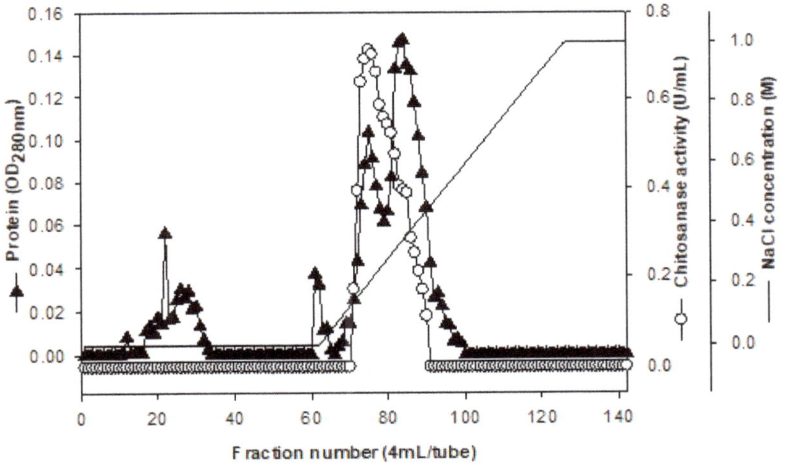

Figure 2. A typical elution profile of chitosanase on DEAE-Sepharose CL-6B column. The column was equilibrated with 50 mM phosphate buffer (pH 7) at a flow rate of 3 mL/min and 4 mL/fraction.

Table 1. Purification of the chitosanase from *P. macerans* TKU029.

Step	Total Protein (mg)	Total Activity (U)	Specific Activity (U/mg)	Recovery (%)	Purification (Fold)
Culture supernatant	1245.88	328.09	0.26	100.00	1.00
EtOH precipitation	60.31	83.90	1.39	25.57	5.28
DEAE-Sepharose CL-6B	10.45	63.17	6.04	19.25	22.95
Macro-Prep DEAE	1.43	34.48	24.19	10.51	91.87

Similar to most of the other chitinolytic enzymes-producing strains of *Paenibacillus* species, only one chitinase or chitosanase were purified from the culture supernatant [22–33]. However, the molecular mass of TKU029 chitosanase (63 kDa) estimated by SDS-PAGE (Figure 3) differed from the chitinases or chitosanases of the other *Paenibacillus* strains, for instance, *P. pasadenensis* NCIM5434 chitinase (35 kDa) [23], *Paenibacillus* sp. 1794 chitosanase (40 kDa) [24], *P. thermoaerophilus* TC22-2b chitinase (48 kDa) [25], *P. larvae* ATCC9545 (49 kDa) [26], *P. illinoisensis* KJA-424 chitinase (54 kDa) [33], *Paenibacillus* sp. D1 chitinase (56 kDa) [27], *P. barengoltzii* CAU904 chitinase (67 kDa) [28], *P. elgii* HOA73 chitinase (68 kDa) [29], *P. pasadenensis* CS0611 chitinase (69 kDa) [30], *Paenibacillus* sp. TKU042 chitosanase (70 kDa) [22], *Paenibacillus* sp. D2 chitosanase (85 kDa) [31], and *Paenibacillus* sp. FPU-7 (150 kDa) [32].

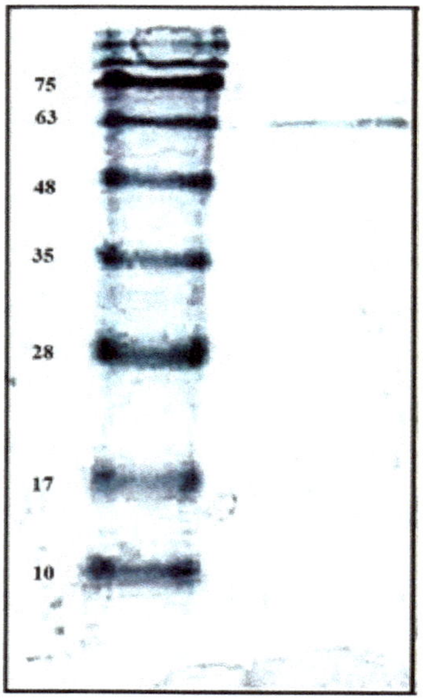

Figure 3. SDS-PAGE analysis of the chitosanase produced by TKU029.

Chitinolytic enzyme productions from *Paenibacillus* strains on a colloidal-containing chitin medium have been widely reported [23,25,27,33], but rarely on a containing-SPP medium [22]. By using squid pen, a marine byproduct, as the C/N source for microbial cultivation, the production cost of microbial chitosanase could be reduced. In this study, a chitosanase from *P. macerans* TKU029 were isolated by SPP conversion. To the best of our knowledge, this is the first report about chitosanase production from *P. macerans* species using the medium containing SPP.

2.3. Effects of pH and Temperature on Activity and Stability of Chitosanase

The effect of pH on the activities of TKU029 chitosanase was studied herein (Figure 4). The optimum pH for TKU029 chitosanase was pH 7. Compared to chitinase/chitosanase from other *Paenibacillus* strains, the optimum pH of TKU029 chitinase differed from most reports, which showed enzyme optimum activity on acid condition; for instance, *Paenibacillus* sp. D1 [27], *P. pasadenensis* CS0611 [30], and *P. illinoisensis* KJA-424 [33] were pH 5; *Paenibacillus* sp. 1794 was pH 4.8 [24]; *P. barengoltzii* was pH 3.5 [28]; *P. thermoaerophilus* TC22-2b was pH 4 [25]; and *Paenibacillus* sp. M4 was pH 6.5, but it was consistent with *P. elgii* HOA73 (pH 7) [29]. These results also observed TKU029 chitosanase to have broad pH stability (pH 3–8). Several *Paenibacillus* strains chitinases/chitosanases have broad pH stability close to that of TKU029 [28,29,34].

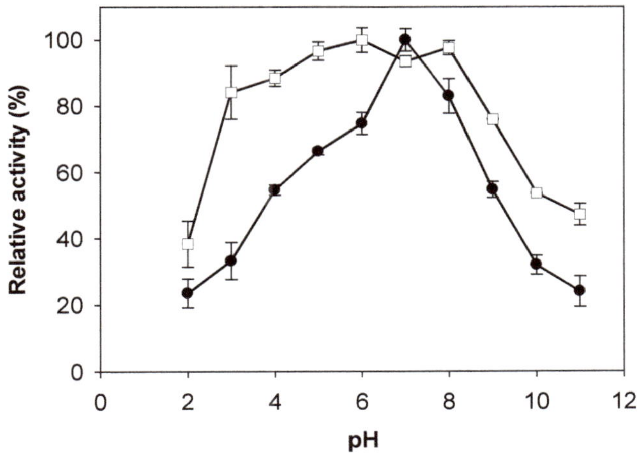

Figure 4. Effect of pH on activity and stability of TKU029 chitosanase. (●), enzyme activity; (□), enzyme stability. The error bars represent standard deviations ($n = 3$).

The optimum temperature and thermal stability of TKU 029 chitosanasewere also investigated (Figure 5). The optimum temperature of TKU029 chitosanase was 60 °C; it remained stable up to 50 °C. At the optimum temperature of 60 °C, the chitosanase still retained 76% activity. However, the activity was dramatically decreased to less than half of the highest activity when the temperature was above 60 °C. Generally, the optimum temperature of TKU029 chitosanase is higher than those of other *Paenibacillus* strains, such as *P. pasadenensis* NCIM 5434 [23], *Paenibacillus* sp. D1 [27], *P. elgii* HOA73 [29], *P. pasadenensis* CS0611 [30]. Due to the higher optimum temperature, it is suggested that TKU029 chitosanase may be suitable for industrial application.

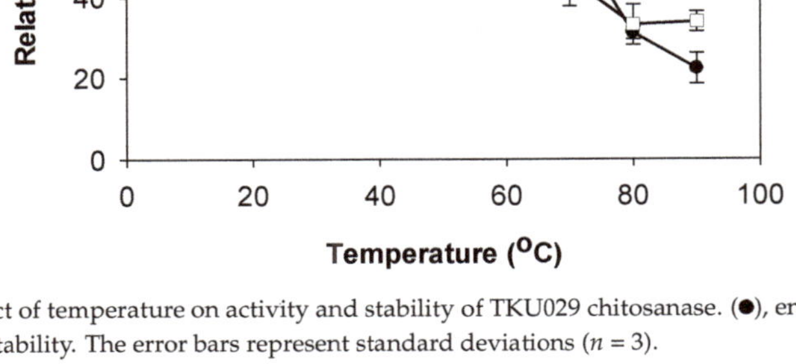

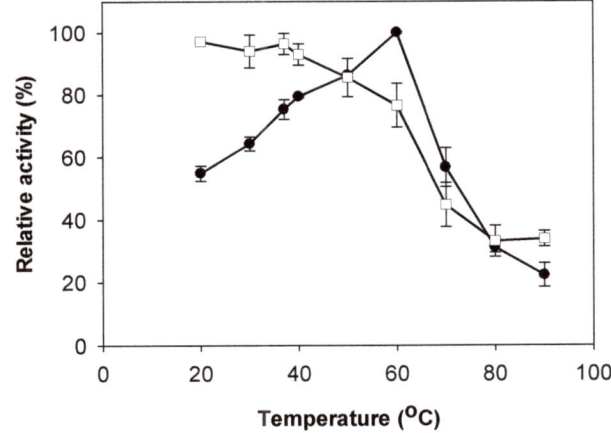

Figure 5. Effect of temperature on activity and stability of TKU029 chitosanase. (●), enzyme activity; (□), enzyme stability. The error bars represent standard deviations ($n = 3$).

2.4. Effect of Metal Ions on Activity of Chitosanase

To further explore the effect of some ion metals on their activities, TKU029 chitosanase were prepared in 50 mM phosphate buffer (pH 7) containing 5 mM of each chemical and incubated at 37 °C in 10 min. The mixtures were then examined for their residual activities. The results are summarized in

Table 2. TKU029 chitosanase activity was not affected by Zn^{2+} and Ca^{2+}, but other chemicals had clear effects on the enzyme. In the presence of Cu^{2+}, Mg^{2+}, Ba^{2+} and EDTA, the activity of TKU029 chitinase was dramatically reduced with 63.42%, 64.31%, 76.99%, and 68.10% residue activity. Interestingly, these results also showed that the addition of 5 mM Na^+ and Fe^{2+} into the enzyme solution could enhance chitinase activity (154.22% and 133.23%). Similarly, Meena et al. [34], also observed the increased activity with Fe^{2+} and Na^+ in *Paenibacillus* sp. BRSR-047 chitinase.

Table 2. Effect of metal ions on the activity of chitosanase.

	Relative Activity (%)
Control	100.00 ± 1.39
Cu^{2+}	63.42 ± 1.51
Zn^{2+}	99.75 ± 1.84
Mg^{2+}	64.31 ± 2.09
Na^+	154.22 ± 1.96
Ba^{2+}	76.99 ± 2.03
Ca^{2+}	108.81 ± 4.13
Fe^{2+}	133.23 ± 5.31
EDTA	68.10 ± 0.39

All data points were means ± standard deviations (n = 3).

2.5. Substrate Specificity of Chitosanase

The substrate specificity of TKU029 chitosanase was also investigated. As shown in Table 3, TKU029 chitosanase exhibited the most activity on water soluble chitosan, followed by chitosan, colloidal chitin and β-chitin, but with no activity on the α-chitin and non-chitin substrates. These results indicated that the rate of hydrolysis was strongly affected by the physical form of the substrate. In addition, since the enzyme expressed no activity on *p*-nitrophenyl-*N*-acetyl-*β*-D-glucosaminide (*p*NPG), a substrate used for analyzing exochitinase, TKU029 chitosanase could be initially classified as a endochitosanase.

Table 3. Substrate specificity of TKU029 chitosanase.

Substrate	**Relative Activity (%)**
Chitosan	100 ± 16.93
Water soluble chitosan	196.43 ± 15.55
α-Chitin	0
β-Chitin	12.30 ± 6.62
Colloidal Chitin	63.26 ± 4.08
*p*NPG	0
Cellulose	0
Dextran	0
Starch	0

All data points were means ± standard deviations (n = 3).

2.6. Chitosan Hydrolysis and COS Production

Since water soluble chitosan showed the most effect on TKU029 chitosanase activity, the hydrolysis products from this substrate were also studied. The course of chitosan sample degradation was conveniently studied by the measurement reducing sugar. Figure 6 shows the reducing sugar of the sample as a function of reaction time. The reducing sugar dramatically increased in the early stage of the reaction (after 1 h of reaction) and did not increase after 4 h.

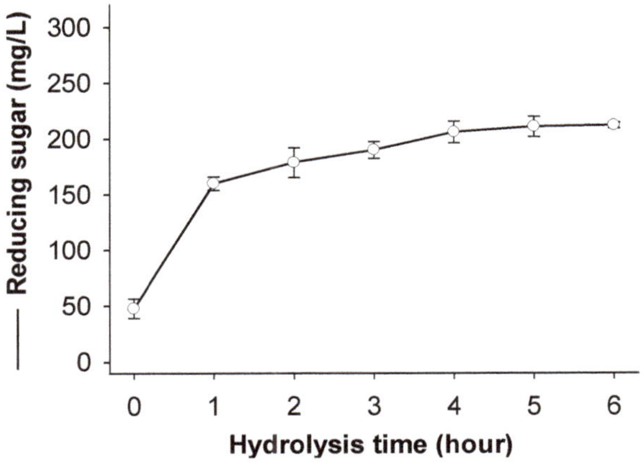

Figure 6. Hydrolysis time course measurement of reducing sugar with TKU029 chitosanase. The reaction mixture in a 250 mL Erlenmeyer flask containing 1% water soluble chitosan in 100 mL phosphate buffer (pH 7, 50 mM) and 10 mL of crude enzyme. The hydrolysis condition was carried at 50 °C in 6 h. The hydrolysis solution was then tested reducing sugar under the assay mentioned in the methods section. The error bars represent standard deviations ($n = 3$).

COS with low DP have been reported to exhibit several interesting bioactivities, for instance, antioxidant [2], antitumor [1,3], and prebiotic [5,6]. Thus, many studies have recently attracted interest for converting chitosan into chitooligosaccharides. Based on the obtained results, the chitosan hydrolysis by TKU029 crude enzyme was observed to possess great potential to produce chitosan oligosaccharide with low DP.

To obtain the low DP oligomers in the chitosan hydrolysis, selective precipitation in 90% methanol and acetone solutions was performed following the aforementioned method [2]. Since MALDI-TOF-MS analysis is limited to molecular masses higher than 500 Da, the DP < 2 oligomer could not be determined by this method. The product from the reaction with TKU029 crude enzyme is a mixture containing both homo-chitooligosaccharides, including $(GlcN)_4$ (Short form: G_4) (m/z 620, 701), G_5 (m/z 846), G_6 (m/z 927, 1040), $(GlcNAc)_4$ (Short form: A_4) (m/z 814), A_5 (m/z 1072) and herero-chitooligosacharides, including G_2A_1 (m/z 536, 566), G_2A_2 (m/z 733), G_4A_1 (m/z 905, 959), G_2A_4 (m/z 1153) (Figure 7). Compared to other reports, COS with different broad DP had been produced by various microoganism strains, for instance, *B. cereus* TKU027 (DP 4–9, 2–5) [35], *B. cereus* TKU031 (DP 3–8) [9], *Penicillium janthinellum* D4 (DP 3–9) [36], *Aspergillus fumigatus* S-26 (DP 2–7) [33], and *Bacillus* sp. KFB-C108 (DP 3–5) [37], while this study observed the DP up to 6 and it was only similar to *B. cereus* TKU022 (DP 2–6) [38]. On the other hand, differing chitosan hydrolysates from other *Bacillus* strains [9,35,38], the originally-classified genus of *Paenibacillus*, the hydrolysis products by TKU029 also contained homo-chitosaccharides with higher ratio than hetero-chitosaccharides (at the same DP) (Figure 7). These results indicated that TKU029 chitosanase may hydrolyze the water soluble chitosan by cleavage of glycosidic bonds of the type –G | A– and–A | G–, whereas the hyrolysis of –G | G– and –A | A– are slow. From these results, a quick and simple method to obtain chitosan oligosaccharide with low DP (3–6) could be performed by combining the TKU029 chitosanase hydrolysis reaction with water soluble chitosan at substrate and a selective methanol/acetone precipitation.

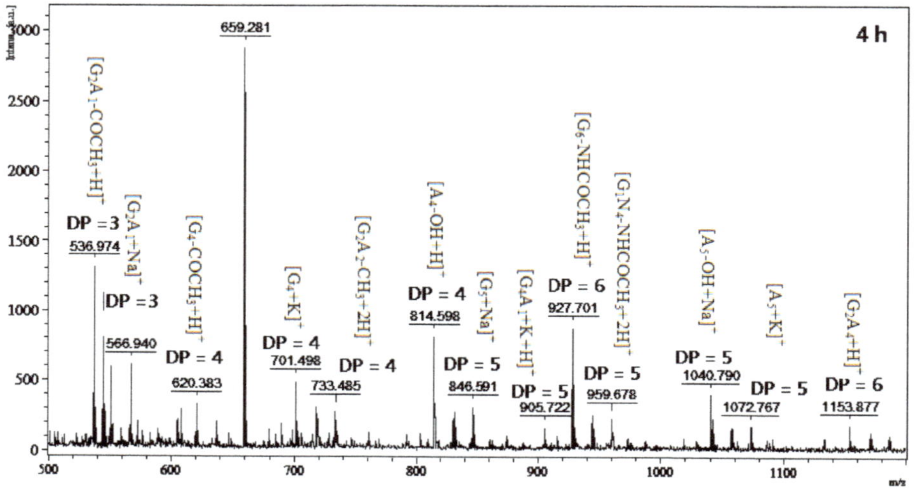

Figure 7. MALDI-TOF-MS of the oligomer mixtures obtained during water soluble chitosan hydrolysis. The proportion of low DP oligomer (DP < 7) was reduced by precipitation in the 90%methanol-soluble/90% acetone-insoluble fraction. The identified peaks are labeled with DP, in which DP indicates the degree of polymerization.

2.7. Evaluation of Growth Enhancing Effect of COS on Lactic Acid Bacteria

The effect of the chitosan oligosaccharides obtained from chitosan hydrolysis generated by TKU029 chitosanase on the growth of lactic acid bacteria were also studied. As shown in Figure 8, chitosan oligosaccharides, which were collected from different hydrolysis times, have a clear effect on the growth of lactic acid bacteria. The highest cell growth of *L. lactis* BCRC 10791 was found for the addition of 4-h hydrolyzed chitosan (136.59%), *L. paracasei* BCRC 14023 was 2 h (169.37%), *L. rhamnosus* BCRC 16,000 was 4 h (164.81%) and *L. rhamnosus* BCRC 10791 was 3 h (153.34%). Interestingly, adding 0.1% chitosan oligosaccharides into the medium did not increase the growth of *E. coli* BCRC 51950. These results differed to COS from other reports, which only showed the enhancing effect on lactic acid bacteria [5,6]. Due to a prebiotic requiring a selectivity effect on the growth of a limited group of bacteria, it is suggested that COS produced from TKU029 may have the potential to become a prebiotic candidate.

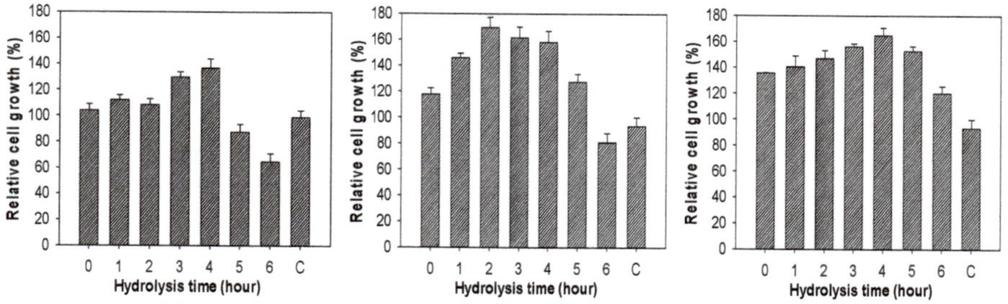

(a) (b) (c)

Figure 8. *Cont.*

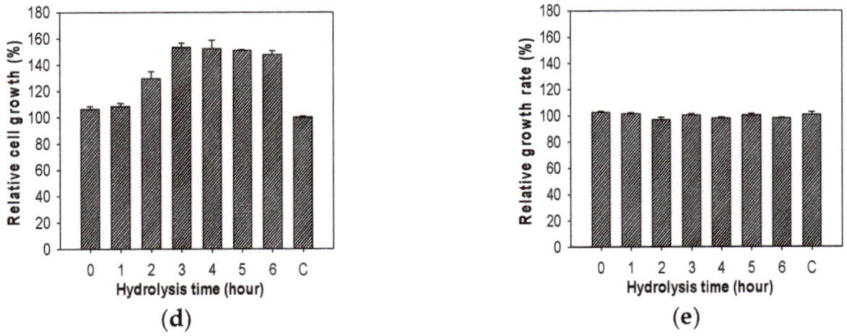

Figure 8. Effect of the chitosan hydrolysis on the growth of bacteria. (**a**), *L. lactis* BCRC 10791; (**b**), *L. paracasei* BCRC 14023; (**c**), *L. rhamnosus* BCRC 16000; (**d**), *L. rhamnosus* BCRC 10791; (**e**), *E. coli* BCRC 51,950. The error bars represent standard deviations ($n = 3$).

3. Materials and Methods

3.1. Materials

Squid pens, crab shells, and shrimp shells were collected from Shin-Ma Frozen Food Co. (I-Lan, Taiwan). Shrimp head powder (SHP) was gifted from Fwu-Sow Industry (Taichun, Taiwan). Demineralized shrimp shell powder (deSSP) and demineralized crab shell powder (deCSP) were prepared via acid treatment [22]. Chitin (from shrimp shell), tyrosine, D-glucosamine and the reagents (3,5-dinitrosalicylic acid and Folin-Ciocalteu) were all purchased from Sigma-Aldrich Corp. (Singapore). Macro-prep DEAE and Macro-Prep High S were bought from Bio-Rad (Hercules, CA, USA). All other reagents were the highest grade available. *P. macerans* TKU029 [16] was provided by Life Science Development Center, Tamkang University, Taiwan.

3.2. Measurement of Chitosanase Activity

The measurement of chitinase activity was performed according to a previously-described method [22], with modifications. Chitosan (1% in 50 mM phosphate buffer) was used as the substrate. The reaction was performed with 0.1 mL substrate and 0.1 mL enzyme solution, and kept at 37 °C for 30 min. The amount of reducing sugar produced in the supernatant was determined by DNS reagent, with D-glucosamine as the reference compound. One unit of enzyme activity was defined as the amount of enzyme that produced 1 μmol of reducing sugar per min.

3.3. Screening of Chitinous Materials as Sole C/N Source for Enzyme Activity

Four kinds of chitinous materials, i.e., crab shell powder (deCSP), squid pen powder (SPP), shrimp head powder (SHP), and demineralized shrimp shell powder (deSSP), were used as the sole sources of C/N (1%, *w*/*v*). *Paenibacillus macerans* TKU029 was grown in 100 mL of liquid medium in 250 mL Erlenmeyer flasks containing 1% of each chitinous material, 0.1% K_2HPO_4 and 0.05% $MgSO_4{\cdot}7H_2O$. The incubation was performed with 1% of seed culture, in 3 d at 37°C in a shaking incubator (150 rpm). During each of 24 h, the culture medium was collected for further measurements.

3.4. Purification of Chitosanae

P. macerans TKU029 was cultured in 100 mL of liquid medium in an Erlenmeyer flask (250 mL) containing 1% SPP, 0.1% K_2HPO_4 and 0.05% $MgSO_4.7H_2O$ in a shaking incubator for 3 days at 37 °C to collect culture supernatant. A protein precipitation step was performed by adding 1800 mL of cold ethanol (−20 °C) to 600 mL of culture supernatant and kept at 4 °C overnight. To collect the crude enzyme, the precipitate was centrifuged at 12,000× *g* for 30 min and then dissolved in a small amount of 50 mM phosphate buffer (pH 7). The obtained crude enzyme was loaded onto a DEAE-Sepharose

CL-6B column that had been equilibrated with 50 mM phosphate buffer. The obtained chitosanase (eluted by a linear gradient of 0–1 M NaCl in the same buffer) fractions were then further purified by A Macro-Prep DEAE column, respectively. The molecular mass of the purified enzymes was determined using the SDS-PAGE methods.

3.5. *Effects of pH and Temperature on Activity and Stability of Chitosanase*

The optimal temperature for the enzymatic reaction was performed at different points of temperature (20–100 °C) during 30 min. To assess the thermal stability, the enzyme solution was treated at a range of temperature during 15 min. The treated enzyme was then used to measure the residual activity.

The optimal pH of enzyme was measured in buffers of different pH values (pH 2–11). To determine the effect of pH on enzyme stability, the enzyme was incubated in buffer of different pH levels at 37 °C for 30 min, and the residual activity was measured at optimal pH value. The buffer systems used included glycine.HCl (50 mM, pH 2–3), acetate (50 mM, pH 4–5), phosphate (50 mM, pH 6–8) and Na_2CO_3-$NaHCO_3$ (50 mM, pH 9–11).

3.6. *Effect of Metal Ions on Chitosanase Activity*

Several metal ion salts (5 mM in final concentration) were used to investigate their effect on enzyme activity, i.e., $CuCl_2$, $ZnCl_2$, $MgCl_2$, NaCl, $BaCl_2$, $CaCl_2$, $FeCl_2$, and EDTA.

3.7. *Substrate Specificity*

Chitosanase was incubated in 50 mM phosphate buffer with various kinds of substrates at 60 °C for 30 min. α-chitin (from shrimp shell), β-chitin (from squid pen), chitosan (DD = 65.36% and MW = 350,000–500,000 Da), water soluble chitosan (DD = 66.66% and MW = 30,000 Da), colloidal chitin (from α-chitin), cellulose, dextran (70,000 Da), Starch (from potato) were included. The chitinase activity in colloidal chitin was used as a control to calculate the relative activity of enzyme in other substrates.

3.8. *MALDI-TOF MS Analysis*

A sample (1 μL) was prepared with 1 μL of 2,5-dihydroxybenzoic acid as a matrix in H_2O-CAN-TFA solution (50/50/0.1%, *v*/*v*/*v*). Positive ion mode of MALDI mass spectra was acquired with a MALDI-TOF instrument (Bruker Daltonics, Bremen, Germany) equipped with a nitrogen laser emitting at 337 nm operating in linear mode. Each mass spectrum was the accumulated data of approximately 30–50 laser shots. External 3-point calibration was used for mass assignment.

3.9. *Growth Enhancing Effect of COS on Lactic Acid Bacteria Test*

Four lactic acid strains were chosen for the experiment: *Lactobacillus lactis* BCRC 10791, *Lactobacillus paracasei* BCRC 14023, *Lactobacillus rhamnosus* BCRC 16,000, and *Lactobacillus rhamnosus* BCRC 10,791. The bacteria were cultured in MRS medium containing 0.1% (*w*/*v*) chitosan oligosaccharides for 24 h at 37 °C. To examine whether chitosan oligosaccharides could affect non-lactic acid bacteria, a strain of *E. coli* BCRC 51,950 was also cultured in LB medium containing 0.1% (*w*/*v*) chitosan oligosaccharides under the same condition with lactic acid bacteria. A measurement of optical density 600 nm of culture supernatant was used to calculate the cell growth of the bacteria.

4. Conclusions

Among the four marine chitinous materials, *Paenibacillus macerans* TKU029 achieved the best result for chitosanase production using squid pens as the sole carbon/nitrogen source. The molecular weight of the purified TKU029 chitosanase (63 kDa) was different from those of the other *Paenibacillus* strains. The oligomers obtained by hydrolyzing water soluble chitosan with TKU029 chitosanase possessed specifically enhancing effects on the growth of analyzed four lactic acid bacteria, and had no effect on *E. coli*. By the selective growth enhancing effect of COS, TKU029 chitosanase has potential to be used in the production of nutraceuticals.

Author Contributions: Conceptualization, S.-L.W. and C.T.D.; Methodology, C.T.D. and T.N.T.; Software, C.-T.D.; Validation, S.-L.W. and C.T.D.; Formal Analysis, C.T.D., T.N.T., V.B.N., and A.D.N.; Investigation, C.T.D., T.N.T.; Resources, S.-L.W.; Data Curation, C.T.D.; Writing—Original Draft Preparation, S.-L.W and C.T.D.; Writing—Review & Editing, S.-L.W. and C.T.D.; Visualization, S.-L.W. and C.T.D.; Supervision, S.-L.W.; Project Administration, S.-L.W.; Funding Acquisition, S.-L.W.

Funding: This work was supported in part by a grant from the Ministry of Sciences and Technology, Taiwan (MOST 106-2320-B-032-001-MY3).

Conflicts of Interest: The authors declare no conflict of interest.

References

1. Azuma, K.; Osaki, T.; Minami, S.; Okamoto, Y. Anticancer and anti-inflammatory properties of chitin and chitosan oligosaccharides. *J. Funct. Biomater.* **2015**, *6*, 33–49. [CrossRef] [PubMed]
2. Liang, T.W.; Chen, W.T.; Lin, Z.H.; Kuo, Y.H.; Nguyen, A.D.; Pan, P.S.; Wang, S.L. An amphiprotic novel chitosanase from *Bacillus mycoides* and its application in the production of chitooligomers with their antioxidant and anti-inflammatory evaluation. *Int. J. Mol. Sci.* **2017**, *17*, 1302. [CrossRef] [PubMed]
3. Liang, T.W.; Chen, Y.J.; Yen, Y.H.; Wang, S.L. The antitumor activity of the hydrolysates of chitinous materials hydrolyzed by crude enzyme from *Bacillus amyloliquefaciens* V656. *Process Biochem.* **2007**, *42*, 527–534. [CrossRef]
4. Sun, T.; Qin, Y.; Xu, H.; Xie, J.; Hu, D.; Xue, B.; Hua, X. Antibacterial activities and preservative effect of chitosan oligosaccharide Maillard reaction products on *Penaeus vannamei*. *Int. J. Biol. Macromol.* **2017**, *105*, 764–768. [CrossRef] [PubMed]
5. Liang, T.W.; Liu, C.P.; Wu, C.; Wang, S.L. Applied development of crude enzyme from *Bacillus cereus* in prebiotics and microbial community changes in soil. *Carbohydr. Polym.* **2013**, *92*, 2141–2148. [CrossRef] [PubMed]
6. Lee, H.W.; Park, Y.S.; Jung, J.S.; Shin, W.S. Chitosan oligosaccharides, dp 2–8, have prebiotic effect on the *Bifidobacterium bifidium* and *Lactobacillus* sp. *Anaerobe* **2002**, *8*, 319–324. [CrossRef]
7. Liang, T.W.; Chen, Y.Y.; Pan, P.S.; Wang, S.L. Purification of chitinase/chitosanase from *Bacillus cereus* and discovery of an enzyme inhibitor. *Int. J. Biol. Macromol.* **2014**, *63*, 8–14. [CrossRef] [PubMed]
8. Liang, T.W.; Lo, B.C.; Wang, S.L. Chitinolytic bacteria-assisted conversion of squid pen and its effect on dyes and adsorption. *Mar. Drugs* **2015**, *13*, 4576–4593. [CrossRef] [PubMed]
9. Wang, C.L.; Su, J.W.; Liang, T.W.; Nguyen, A.D.; Wang, S.L. Production, purification and characterization of a chitosanase from *Bacillus cereus*. *Res. Chem. Intermed.* **2014**, *40*, 2237–2248. [CrossRef]
10. Wang, S.L.; Wu, P.C.; Liang, T.W. Utilization of squid pen for the efficient production of chitosanase and antioxidants through prolonged autoclave treatment. *Carbohydr. Res.* **2009**, *244*, 979–984. [CrossRef] [PubMed]
11. Liang, T.W.; Jen, S.N.; Nguyen, A.D.; Wang, S.L. Application of chitinous materials in production and purification of a poly (L-lactic acid) depolymerase from *Pseudomonas tamsuii* TKU015. *Polymers* **2016**, *8*, 98. [CrossRef]
12. Wang, S.L.; Chen, S.J.; Liang, T.W.; Lin, Y.D. A novel nattokinase produced by *Pseudomonas* sp. TKU015 using shrimp shells as substrate. *Process Biochem.* **2009**, *44*, 70–76. [CrossRef]
13. Wang, S.L.; Hsu, W.H.; Liang, T.W. Conversion of squid pen by *Pseudomonas aeruginosa* K-187 fermentation for the production of *N*-acetyl chitooligosaccharides and biofertilizers. *Carbohydr. Res.* **2010**, *345*, 880–885. [CrossRef] [PubMed]
14. Kuo, Y.H.; Liang, T.W.; Liu, K.C.; Hsu, Y.W.; Hsu, H.; Wang, S.L. Isolation and identification of a novel antioxidant with antitumor activity from *Serratia ureilytica* using squid pen as fermentation substrate. *Mar. Biotechnol.* **2011**, *13*, 451–461. [CrossRef] [PubMed]
15. Wang, S.L.; Wang, C.Y.; Yen, Y.H.; Liang, T.W.; Chen, S.Y.; Chen, C.H. Enhanced production of insecticidal prodigiosin from *Serratia marcescens* TKU011 in media containing squid pen. *Process Biochem.* **2012**, *47*, 1684–1690. [CrossRef]

16. Liang, T.W.; Wu, C.C.; Cheng, W.T.; Chen, Y.C.; Wang, C.L.; Wang, I.L.; Wang, S.L. Exopolysaccharides and antimicrobial biosurfactants produced by *Paenibacillus macerans* TKU029. *Appl. Biochem. Biotechnol.* **2014**, *172*, 933–950. [CrossRef] [PubMed]
17. Liang, T.W.; Tseng, S.C.; Wang, S.L. Production and characterization of antioxidant properties of exopolysaccharides from *Paenibacillus mucilaginosus* TKU032. *Mar. Drugs* **2016**, *14*, 40. [CrossRef] [PubMed]
18. Liang, T.W.; Wang, S.L. Recent advances in exopolysaccharides from *Paenibacillus* spp.: Production, isolation, structure, and bioactivities. *Mar. Drugs* **2015**, *13*, 1847–1863. [CrossRef] [PubMed]
19. Nguyen, V.B.; Nguyen, A.D.; Wang, S.L. Utilization of fishery processing by product squid pens for *Paenibacillus* sp. fermentation on producing potent α-glucosidase inhibitors. *Mar. Drugs* **2017**, *15*, 274. [CrossRef] [PubMed]
20. Nguyen, V.B.; Wang, S.L. Reclamation of marine chitinous materials for the production of α-glucosidase inhibitors via microbial conversion. *Mar. Drugs* **2017**, *15*, 350. [CrossRef] [PubMed]
21. Wang, S.L.; Li, H.T.; Zhang, L.J.; Lin, Z.H.; Kuo, Y.H. Conversion of squid pen to homogentisic acid via *Paenibacillus* sp. TKU036 and the antioxidant and anti-inflammatory activities of homogentisic acid. *Mar. Drugs* **2016**, *14*, 183. [CrossRef] [PubMed]
22. Doan, C.T.; Tran, T.N.; Nguyen, V.B.; Nguyen, A.D.; Wang, S.L. Conversion of squid pens to chitosanases and proteases via *Paenibacillus* sp. TKU042. *Mar. Drugs* **2018**, *16*, 83. [CrossRef] [PubMed]
23. Loni, P.P.; Patil, J.U.; Phugare, S.S.; Bajekal, S.S. Purification and characterization of alkaline chitinase from *Paenibacillus pasadenensis* NCIM 5434. *J. Basic Microbiol.* **2014**, *54*, 1080–1089. [CrossRef] [PubMed]
24. Zitouni, M.; Fortin, M.; Scheerle, R.K.; Letzel, T.; Matteau, D.; Rodrigue, S.; Brzezinski, R. Biochemical and molecular characterization of a thermostable chitosanase produced by the strain *Paenibacillus* sp. 1794 newly isolated from compost. *Appl. Microbiol. Biotechnol.* **2013**, *97*, 5801–5813. [CrossRef] [PubMed]
25. Ueda, J.; Kurosawa, N. Characterization of an extracellular thermophilic chitinase from *Paenibacillus thermoaerophilus* strain TC22-2b isolated from compost. *World J. Microbiol. Biotechnol.* **2015**, *31*, 135–143. [CrossRef] [PubMed]
26. Garcia-Gonzalez, E.; Poppinga, L.; Fünfhaus, A.; Hertlein, G.; Hedtke, K.; Jakubowska, A.; Genersch, E. *Paenibacillus larvae* chitin-degrading protein PlCBP49 is a key virulence factor in American foulbrood of honey bees. *PLoS Pathogen.* **2014**, *10*, e1004284. [CrossRef] [PubMed]
27. Singh, A.K.; Chhatpar, H.S. Purification and characterization of chitinase from *Paenibacillus* sp. D1. *Appl. Biochem. Biotechnol.* **2011**, *164*, 77–88. [CrossRef] [PubMed]
28. Fu, X.; Yan, Q.; Wang, J.; Yang, S.; Jiang, Z. Purification and biochemical characterization of novel acidic chitinase from *Paenibacillus barengoltzii*. *Int. J. Biol. Macromol.* **2016**, *91*, 973–979. [CrossRef] [PubMed]
29. Kim, Y.H.; Park, S.K.; Hur, J.Y.; Kim, Y.C. Purification and characterization of a major extracellular chitinase from a biocontrol bacterium, *Paenibacillus elgii* HOA73. *Plant Pathol. J.* **2017**, *33*, 318–328. [CrossRef] [PubMed]
30. Guo, X.; Xu, P.; Zong, M.; Lou, W. Purification and characterization of alkaline chitinase from *Paenibacillus pasadenensis* CS0611. *Chin. J. Catalys.* **2017**, *38*, 665–672. [CrossRef]
31. Kimoto, H.; Kusaoke, H.; Yamamoto, I.; Fujii, Y.; Onodera, T.; Taketo, A. Biochemical and genetic properties of *Paenibacillus* glycosyl hydrolase having chitosanase activity and discoidin domain. *J. Biol. Chem.* **2002**, *277*, 14695–14702. [CrossRef] [PubMed]
32. Itoh, T.; Sugimoto, I.; Hibi, T.; Suzuki, F.; Matsuo, K.; Fujii, Y.; Taketo, A.; Kimoto, H. Overexpression, purification, and characterization of *Paenibacillus* cell surface-expressed chitinase ChiW with two catalytic domains. *Biosci. Biotechnol. Biochem.* **2014**, *78*, 624–634. [CrossRef] [PubMed]
33. Jung, W.J.; Kuk, J.K.; Kim, K.Y.; Kim, T.H.; Park, R.D. Purification and characterization of chitinase from *Paenibacillus illinoisensis* KJA-424. *J. Microbiol. Biotechnol.* **2005**, *15*, 274–280.
34. Meena, S.; Gothwal, R.K.; Saxena, J.; Nehra, S.; Mohan, M.K.; Ghosh, P. Effect of metal ions and chemical compounds on chitinase produced by a newly isolated thermotolerant *Paenibacillus* sp. BISR-047 and its shelf-life. *Int. J. Curr. Microbiol. Appl. Sci.* **2015**, *4*, 872–881.
35. Wang, S.L.; Liu, C.P.; Liang, T.W. Fermented and enzymatic production of chitin/chitosan oligosaccharides by extracellular chitinases from *Bacillus cereus* TKU027. *Carbohydr. Polym.* **2012**, *90*, 1305–1313. [CrossRef] [PubMed]

36. Nguyen, A.D.; Huang, C.C.; Liang, T.W.; Nguyen, V.B.; Pan, P.S.; Wang, S.L. Production and purification of a fungal chitosanase and chitooligomers from *Penicillium janthinellum* D4 and discovery of the enzyme activators. *Carbohydr. Polym.* **2014**, *108*, 331–337. [CrossRef] [PubMed]
37. Yoon, H.G.; Kim, H.Y.; Kim, H.K.; Kim, K.H.; Hwang, H.J.; Cho, H.Y. Cloning and expression of thermostable chitosanase gene from *Bacillus* sp. KFB-C108. *J. Microbiol. Biotechnol.* **1999**, *9*, 631–636.
38. Liang, T.W.; Hsieh, J.L.; Wang, S.L. Production and purification of a protease, a chitosanase, and chitin oligosaccharides by *Bacillus cereus* TKU022 fermentation. *Carbohydr. Res.* **2012**, *362*, 38–46. [CrossRef] [PubMed]

marine drugs

MDPI

Article

A Novel Complex of Chitosan–Sodium Carbonate and Its Properties

Jianying Qian [1], Xiaomeng Wang [1], Jie Shu [2], Chang Su [1], Jinsong Gong [1], Zhenghong Xu [1], Jian Jin [1,*] and Jinsong Shi [1,*]

[1] School of Pharmaceutical Science, Jiangnan University, Wuxi 214122, China; jackieqian@163.com (J.Q.); 17714542165@163.com (X.W.); emilysu1991@126.com (C.S.); gjs713@163.com (J.G.); zhenghxu@jiangnan.edu.cn (Z.X.)

[2] College of Chemistry, Chemical Engineering and Materials Science, Testing and Analysis Center, Soochow University, Suzhou 215123, China; shujie@suda.edu.cn

* Correspondence: jinjian31@126.com (J.J.); shijs@163.com (J.S.); Tel.: +86-510-8532-8177 (J.S.)

Received: 18 September 2018; Accepted: 26 October 2018; Published: 30 October 2018

Abstract: Chitosan has excellent properties, as it is nontoxic, mucoadhesive, biocompatible, and biodegradable. However, the poor water solubility of chitosan is a major disadvantage. Here, a novel chitosan-sodium carbonate complex was formed by adding a large amount of sodium carbonate to a chitosan/acetic acid solution, which is water-soluble. Fourier transform infrared spectroscopy, energy dispersive spectrometry, scanning electron microscopy, and solid-state nuclear magnetic resonance techniques were used to detect and characterize the aforementioned complex, which appeared to be a neat flake crystal. Solid-state nuclear magnetic resonance (SSNMR) was used to verify the connections between carbonate, sodium ions, and the protonated amino group in chitosan on the basis of ^{13}C signals at the chemical shift of 167.745 ppm and 164.743 ppm. Further confirmation was provided by the strong cross-polarization signals identified by the SSNMR 2D ^{13}C–^{1}H frequency-switched Lee–Goldberg heteronuclear correlation spectrum. The cytotoxicity of a film prepared using this complex was tested using rat fibroblasts. The results show that the film promoted cell proliferation, which provides evidence to support its nontoxicity. The ease of film-forming and the results of cytocompatibility testing suggest that the chitosan-sodium carbonate complex has the potential for use in tissue engineering.

Keywords: chitosan; cytotoxicity; polymer film; sodium carbonate; soluble chitosan complex

1. Introduction

Chitosan (chemical name: polyglucosamine(1-4)-2-amino-β-D-glucose) is obtained by the deacetylation of chitin, and it is widely found in the exoskeleton of crustaceans, e.g., crab shells, lobsters, and shrimp [1]. This natural polymer has excellent properties, as it is nontoxic, mucoadhesive, biocompatible, and biodegradable. Thus, it has received extensive attention from various industries [2–7].

The poor water solubility of chitosan is a major disadvantage [3,4]. It is slightly soluble in dimethyl sulfoxide and p-toluenesulfonic acid [5], and only dissolves in water under acidic conditions at pH < 6.5. Under acidic conditions, the amino groups on the chitosan chain are protonated and the positive charge is increased; thus, the polysaccharide chains repel each other to achieve a dissolution effect [6,7]. This is the main disadvantage of chitosan when used as a pharmaceutical excipient, especially when the drug is unstable under acidic conditions.

In order to solve this problem, researchers have chemically modified chitosan to improve its solubility. For example, *N,N,N*-trimethyl chitosan is a quaternized hydrophilic derivative of chitosan [8], sulfonated chitosan is prepared by using 1,3-propane sultone [9], and carboxymethyl chitosan is synthesized under conditions of basification by monochloroacetic acid [10]. Chemical modification can overcome the shortcoming of insolubility. However, the biosafety of the newly synthesized derivatives remains to be verified, as new groups may introduce unknown biological repellency to the compounds. The cytotoxicity, biocompatibility, and biodegradability of the derivatives need experimental verification [11,12].

Before the discovery of alkaline systems, chitosan was dissolved in organic acid solutions, such as acetic acid solutions. However, chitosan is unstable in acid solutions. The glycoside bonds and acetyl groups of chitosan can be hydrolyzed [13], though the rate of hydrolysis in dilute organic acids is fairly slow. In recent years, research has been carried out on the dissolution of chitosan in alkaline systems: in particular, alkali/urea solvents have been proposed. Using a LiOH/NaOH/KOH-urea system and a freeze-melt process, chitosan can be dissolved in an alkaline solvent system to form a uniform solution [14,15]. The intramolecular and intermolecular hydrogen bonds of chitosan are destroyed during the freezing process, and the recovery of hydrogen bonds is further hindered by the alkali and urea during the melting process, thus achieving dissolution [16]. However, this method involves a low temperature (at least −20 °C) and multiple freeze-thaw cycles.

Combinations of chitin/chitosan and inorganic salts are rarely reported. A novel hybrid material was prepared by the unidirectional crystal growth of $CaCO_3$ while the carbamation of chitin served as the template [17]. This chitin derivative was then converted to a gel film by soaking in methanol, immersing in calcium chloride solution, and adding ammonium carbonate vapor to form a chitin-$CaCO_3$ complex. A ternary complex between the ion pair $Si^{2+}CO_3{}^{2-}$ and the amino groups of chitosan was demonstrated [18]. Among these previous reports, the common point is that most of the reactants are carbonates. When the carbonates are salts of two valence metal ions, most of them are insoluble. In light of the LiOH/NaOH/KOH-urea system, it is possible that alkali carbonates can react with chitosan and form soluble complexes. Therefore, we tried to obtain a soluble chitosan complex by adding an alkali carbonate to a chitosan/acetic acid solution.

The main objective of this study was to provide a soluble chitosan-sodium carbonate complex, formed under alkaline conditions, which could be changed back to chitosan using simple treatments to maintain biocompatibility. By adding a large amount of sodium carbonate to a chitosan/acetic acid solution, this complex was obtained and had a pH of 10.1. We then focused our attention to its characteristics, structure, and cytotoxicity in order to gain information for its application in biomedicine.

2. Results and Discussion

The structures of the new compounds forming the chitosan (CS)-sodium carbonate (SC) complex are denoted as CS-SC-1 and CS-SC-2 (Figure 1b,c). A carbonate is bound to either two protonated amino groups to form a complex, or one protonated amino group and one sodium ion. In the figure, the connections between carbonate, ammonium, and sodium ions are highlighted in yellow.

2.1. Spectroscopic Investigations

Fourier transform infrared (FT-IR) spectrometry was used to monitor the structural changes in chitosan (A), the complex of chitosan-sodium carbonate (B), and restored chitosan (C). The obtained infrared spectra are shown in Figure 2. As the amino and hydroxyl groups formed intermolecular and intramolecular hydrogen bonds, the OH stretching vibration and NH stretching vibration, which were originally located around 3400 cm^{-1}, fused into a broad intense band at 3452–3365 cm^{-1} in the FT-IR spectrum of chitosan (A), whose characteristic absorption spectrum includes these peaks [19]. The spectrum of the complex (B) shows a completely different absorption peak at 3473 cm^{-1}, appearing as a sharp peak, which indicates that the hydrogen bonds between the amino and hydroxyl groups were destroyed, thus showing obvious OH or NH stretching vibrations. The two absorption peaks at 1655 cm^{-1} and 1593 cm^{-1}, which are peak I and peak II and represent amide bonds, are also characteristic peaks of chitosan (A) [20]. In the complex (B), these two characteristic peaks still exist but with a slight shift (1699 cm^{-1} and 1593 cm^{-1}), indicating the existence of a –NH–CO– structure in the complex. Thus, the residual acetamido in the main chain did not participate in the reaction. The IR spectrum of the complex (B) displayed additional peaks with respect to chitosan (A), which are characteristic peaks of the inserted carbonate group ($-CO_3^{2-}$) signals: 1466 cm^{-1} and 850 cm^{-1}. The strong absorption peaks at these two locations indicate carbonate signals [21].

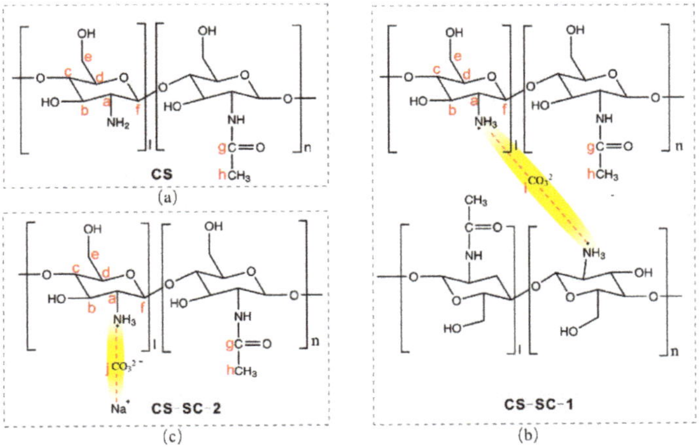

Figure 1. The chemical structural schemes of (**a**) chitosan (CS), (**b**) chitosan-sodium carbonate (CS-SC)-1, and (**c**) CS-SC-2. Carbon atoms are assigned using the alphabetical labels. The connections between carbonate, ammonium, and sodium ions are highlighted in yellow.

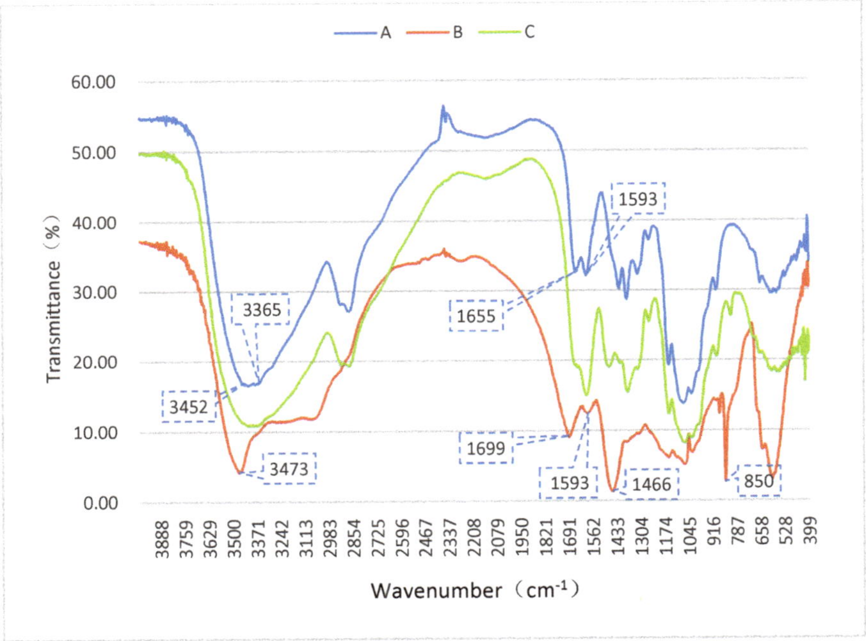

Figure 2. Fourier transform infrared (FT-IR) spectra of chitosan (A, blue), the complex of chitosan-sodium carbonate (B, red), and restored chitosan (C, green).

Other peaks, such as the CH_3 symmetrical stretching vibration, CH_2 asymmetric stretching vibration, CH stretching vibration, CH_2 bending vibration, CH_3 deformation vibration, and CO stretching vibration, were similar, proving that the basic structure of chitosan had not been changed, which was also confirmed by the solid-state nuclear magnetic resonance (SSNMR) spectra (in Figure 3). The peaks of C and A are nearly identical, indicating that chitosan could be converted back by adjusting the pH to neutral with hydrochloric acid.

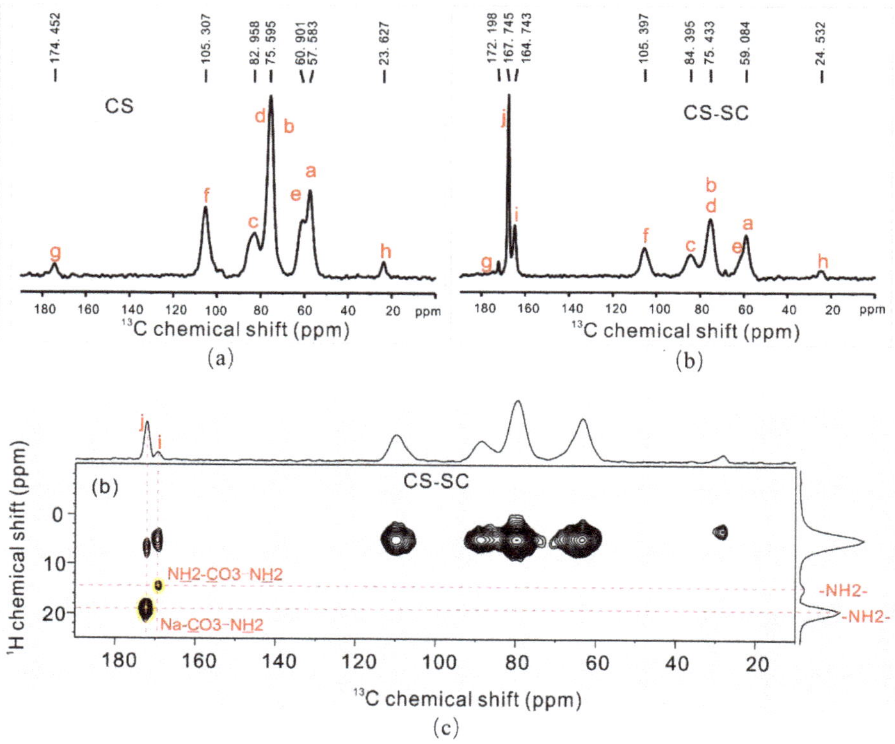

Figure 3. (**a**) Solid-state nuclear magnetic resonance (SSNMR) $^{13}C\{^{1}H\}$ cross-polarization (CP) spectrum of CS. (**b**) SSNMR $^{13}C\{^{1}H\}$ CP spectrum of CS-SC. Peaks are assigned using the alphabetical labels with respect to the structural schemes as shown in Figure 1. (**c**) SSNMR 2D ^{13}C–^{1}H frequency-switched Lee–Goldberg heteronuclear correlation (FSLG-HETCOR) spectrum of CS-SC, where correlations between CO_3 and NH_2 are highlighted in yellow.

Using a certain beam or monochromatic light (such as X-rays or ultraviolet light) to irradiate the sample, electrons in the atoms or in the molecules on the surface are emitted. The energy distribution of electrons, containing information on and characteristic energy of the surface of the sample, was studied to determine the features of the material surface. The count ratio is affected by the surface roughness of the sample, the angle of photoelectron detection, the X-ray power, and the passing energy; therefore, we could not identify the amount of each element by comparing the size of the peak area [22,23]. Atomic information of chitosan, the chitosan–sodium carbonate complex, and the restored chitosan was analyzed using an energy dispersive spectrometer (EDS) (Figure 4). The atomic percentages (Table 1) reflect the presence or absence of carbonate in the complex. Following the formation of the complex, the atomic percentage of the N atoms decreased significantly and the percentage of Na and O atoms increased, reflecting the addition of carbonate to the mixture. It can be speculated that the carbonate is associated with the amine, which is supported by ionic charges. When the complex was restored to chitosan, the atomic percentage of the N atoms increased because of the dissociation of sodium carbonate and the exposure of NH_2 to the surface.

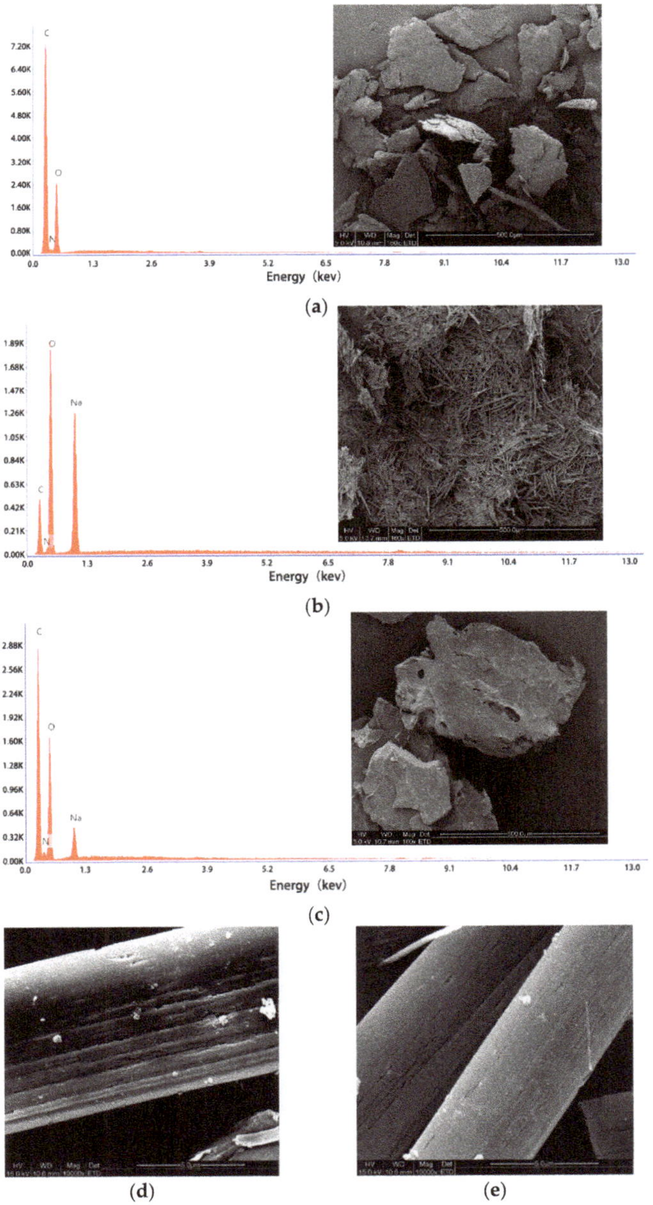

Figure 4. Energy dispersive spectrometry (EDS) spectra and microstructure (magnification 160×, scale bar 500 µm) of chitosan (**a**), the chitosan-sodium carbonate complex (**b**), and restored chitosan (**c**); microstructure (magnification 10,000×, scale bar 5 µm) of the chitosan–sodium carbonate complex (**d**,**e**).

Table 1. Atomic percentage of elements C, N, O, and Na.

Element	Atomic Percentage		
	A	B	C
C	61.99	33.87	53.62
N	7.92	2.14	9.66
O	30.09	48.91	34.24
Na	0.00	15.08	2.49

Chitosan can react with aldehydes (through the Schiff base reaction) by the condensation of amino and aldehyde groups. That is why chitosan can be crosslinked with glutaraldehyde to form a hydrogel [24,25]. The reaction formula is shown in Figure 5. We performed the Schiff base reaction with the chitosan-sodium carbonate complex and glutaraldehyde, adopting a typical preparation process. However, no gel was formed by crosslinking. We prepared restored chitosan by adjusting the solution to pH 5.0 with hydrochloric acid; then, the Schiff base reaction occurred successfully. Therefore, we suppose that the amine of chitosan combined with carbonate during the formation of the complex and dissociated during the restoration.

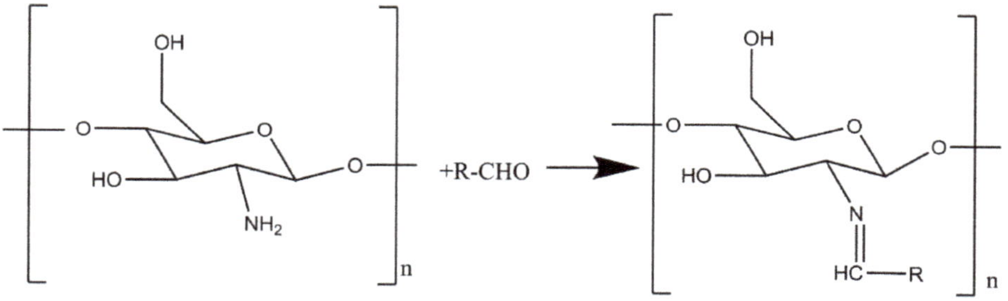

Figure 5. Schiff base reaction.

The microstructure of the three samples was observed by scanning electron microscopy (SEM). Chitosan appeared flake-like when magnified 160×, because the main polysaccharide chain was entangled. The complex formed a rod-like crystal and returned to a mass when adjusted to neutral pH (Figure 4a–c).

Biomacromolecules, such as polysaccharides, proteins, and glycoproteins, can serve as templates, control crystal growth, and thus result in the formation of highly organized complex structures [17]. When the chitosan-sodium carbonate complex was magnified 10,000×, it was observed that the crystalline structure was compact, which was obviously formed by the highly ordered arrangement of molecules (Figure 4d,e). Therefore, we suggest that the chitosan chain acted as a template, the sodium carbonate molecules inserted into it, and a neat crystal structure developed when the complex was formed.

We deduced that the structures of the new compounds that formed the chitosan complex were those of CS-SC-1 and CS-SC-2 in Figure 1b,c. A carbonate is bound to either two protonated amino groups to form a complex, or one protonated amino group and one sodium ion. The connections between carbonate and the sodium ions in the sodium carbonate with the protonated amino group in chitosan were verified by SSNMR (Figure 3), which is able to locally and selectively probe the chemical environment of each carbon nucleus. The identification of each ^{13}C peak corresponds with the alphabetical labels shown in Figures 1 and 3. Chitosan (Figures 1a and 3a) was identified by the ^{13}C resonances observed at carbon chemical shifts, δ~57.583 (Ca), 75.595 (Cb, Cd), 82.958 (Cc), 60.961 (Ce), 105.307 (Cf) ppm. Two additional ^{13}C resonances were observed at δ~174.452 (Cg) and 23.627 (Ch), which were assigned to the residual carbonyl (Cg) and methyl (Ch) typically present in the chitosan skeleton [26,27]. During the reaction of chitosan with sodium carbonate, a chitosan–sodium carbonate complex was obtained (Figure 1b,c), which was composed of CS-SC-1 and CS-SC-2. The structures of CS-SC-1 and CS-SC-2 were easily confirmed by the observation of two ^{13}C resonances corresponding to Ci and Cj at δ~164.743 (Ci) and 167.745 (Cj), respectively (Figure 3b). These structures are a consequence of the two possible reactions' dependence on the amount of sodium carbonate. When the amount of carbonate was insufficient, two ammonium ions bound to a carbonate; when the amount of carbonate was sufficient, one ammonium ion and one sodium ion each bound to carbonate, as shown in Figure 1b,c. It can be seen from the SSNMR 2D ^{13}C–^{1}H FSLG-HETCOR spectrum of CS-SC (Figure 3c) that the hydrogen on the amino group and the carbon in the carbonyl group had very strong cross-polarization signals, which proves the connection between them.

2.2. Cytotoxicity Results

Evaluation of cytotoxicity is an important cell viability method to validate the potential use of the chitosan-sodium carbonate complex in medical bioengineering. As the L929 fibroblast cell line is commonly used to determine the cell proliferation rate, the effect of the chitosan-sodium carbonate complex was assessed in this cell line by using the MTT assay [28,29].

Due to the porous film structure and biocompatibility, we believed that the film could promote cell proliferation [30]. The growth of a fibroblast cell culture was evaluated using the MTT assay [31] after 48 h exposure. Figure 6 shows the percentage of cell proliferation, determined as follows: (OD of experimental well/OD of blank well) × 100%.

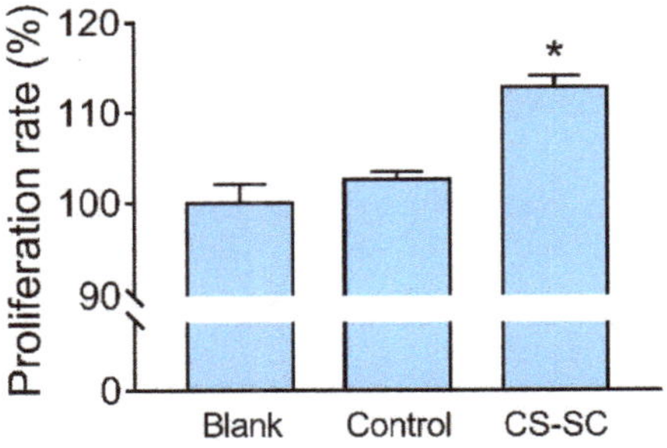

Figure 6. Percentage of cell proliferation after 48 h exposure. * Statistically significant differences were observed between the control film and CS-SC film wells (values are means ± s.e.m, $p < 0.05$, $n = 3$).

Cell viability was not significantly changed after exposure of L929 to the control film. As demonstrated in Figure 6, a statistically significant difference ($p < 0.05$) between the percentages of cell proliferation in the wells treated with CS-SC film relative to the control film was observed, indicating that the CS-SC film promoted cell proliferation.

The morphology of L929 fibroblast cells was observed by an inverted microscope. As shown in Figure 7a, the cells in the blank wells were tightly connected and had an irregular triangular or spindle shape. There were some non-adhesive cells in the wells containing control films suspended in the culture medium. The number of cells growing in the wells containing the complex films increased significantly, but the morphology of the cells changed slightly; the number of round cells was greater than that in the blank wells ($p < 0.05$) (Figure 7d).

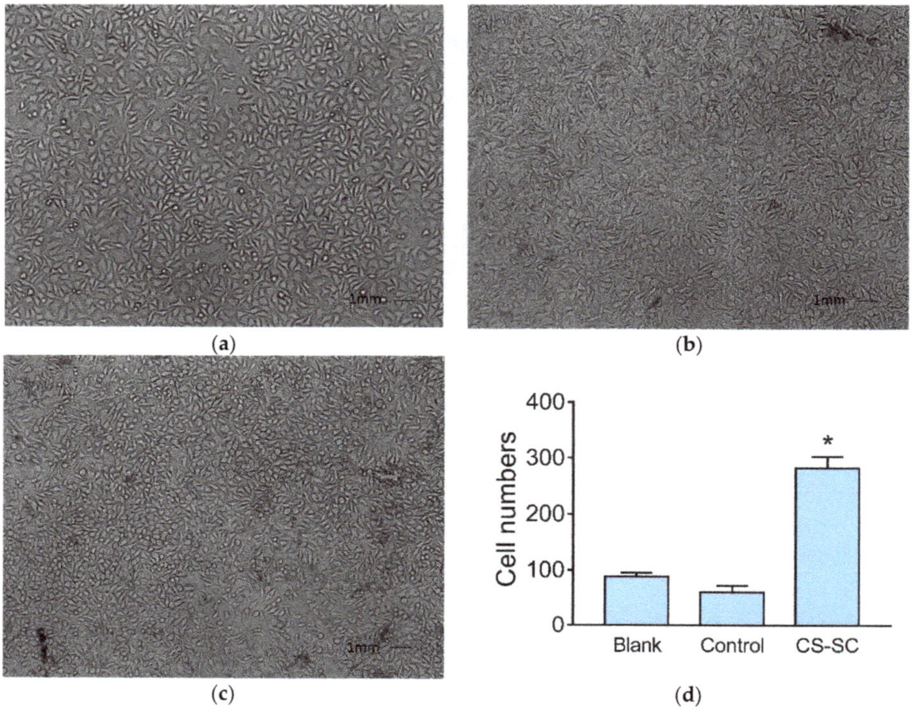

Figure 7. Morphology changes in L929 fibroblast cells in different wells and the statistical result of round cells. (**a**) Blank; (**b**) control; (**c**) CS-SC; (**d**) statistical result of round cells (values are means ± s.e.m, $p < 0.05$, $n = 3$).

3. Materials and Methods

3.1. Materials and Cell Line

Chitosan was purchased from Sinopharm Chemical Reagent Co., Ltd. (Shanghai, China). The degree of deacetylation was 90% and viscosity-average molecular weight was 5.3×10^4. Other reagents, such as sodium carbonate, acetic acid, ethanol, potassium bromide (KBr), and solvents, were analytical grade and were also supplied by Sinopharm Chemical Reagent Co., Ltd. (Shanghai, China). FBS (fetal bovine serum) and Dulbecco's Modified Eagle Medium (DMEM) culture medium were purchased from Gibco Company (Langley, OK, USA). Penicillin–streptomycin for the cell culture, as well as trypsin, were purchased from Beyotime Bio Technology Co., Ltd. (Shanghai, China). MTT (M2128) was supplied by Sigma Company (St. Louis, MO, USA).

Fibroblasts, NCTC clone 929 (mouse connective tissue), were purchased from Cell Resources Center (Shanghai Academy of Life Sciences, Chinese Academy of Sciences, Shanghai, China) and preserved in the School of Pharmaceutical Sciences, Jiangnan University. L929 cells were grown in DMEM supplemented with 10% (*v*/*v*) FBS and 100 IU/mL penicillin–streptomycin. The cells were maintained in a humid incubator (5% CO_2) at 37 °C [32].

3.2. Instruments

The structure of the complex was determined by FT-IR spectroscopy (Thermo Nicolet Corporation, NEXUS, Madison, WI, USA), SSNMR spectrometry with a superconducting magnet (Brook Corporation, Advance III/WB-400, Tübingen, Germany) and EDS (Ametek Corporation, TEAM Octane Super,

San Diego, CA, USA) equipped with SEM (Hitachi Corporation, S4800, Tokyo, Japan). The crystalline structure of the complex and morphology of the microporous films were studied by SEM (FEI Corporation, Quanta 200, Hillsboro, OR, USA). Cytotoxicity experiments were carried out using a microplate reader (MD Corporation, Spectra MAX M2e, San Jose, CA, USA) and an inverted microscope (Olympus Corporation, CKX 41, Tokyo, Japan).

3.3. Experimental Procedure

3.3.1. Preparation of the Chitosan-Sodium Carbonate Complex

One gram of chitosan was added to 100 mL of water in a beaker and stirred for 1 min. One milliliter of glacial acetic acid (CAS:64-19-7) was added and stirred until completely dissolved. Sodium carbonate solution (50 mL of 0.5 mol/L) was rapidly added, which produced a large number of bubbles, and the solution was stirred until most of the bubbles vanished. The solution was viscous and was used to prepare the films (Section 3.3.2).

The chitosan-sodium carbonate complex was obtained by adding absolute ethanol to the beaker, which produced a white floc. The volume of absolute ethanol was 3× (*v*/*v*) that of the aforementioned solution. Then, the floc was vacuum-filtered and freeze-dried.

The chitosan-sodium carbonate complex can be returned to chitosan by treatments such as dialysis, using acid to adjust the pH to neutral, and washing with a certain concentration of ethanol. In this study, we prepared the restored chitosan by adjusting the complex solution pH to neutral with hydrochloric acid, and then freeze-dried the gelatinous precipitate.

3.3.2. Preparation of the Polymer Films

To each well of a 96-well plate, 100 μL of the complex solution was added, spread evenly, and washed with 50% ethanol (*v*/*v*), thus forming a layer of film. The solvent was evaporated in the oven at 80 °C for 1 h. The film was then soaked in 75% ethanol (*v*/*v*) for 12 h and washed with phosphate buffered saline (PBS) three times.

The control film was prepared as follows: 1 g of chitosan was dissolved in 1% acetic acid solution (*v*/*v*). A total of 100 μL of the chitosan/acetic acid solution was added to the well, spread evenly, and soaked in a 0.1 mol/L sodium hydroxide solution until a layer of film was formed [14]. The solvent was evaporated in the oven at 80 °C for 1 h. The film was then soaked in 75% ethanol (*v*/*v*) for 12 h and washed with PBS three times.

3.3.3. Schiff Base Reaction

A total of 1 g of the chitosan-sodium carbonate complex was dissolved in 50 mL of deionized water, and 1.0 mL of glutaraldehyde (50% *v*/*v*) was dissolved in 20 mL of deionized water. The two solutions were mixed under vigorous stirring for 10 min [25].

3.3.4. FT-IR

The KBr method was used [20]. The scanning range was 400–4000 cm^{-1}, with step length 1 cm^{-1}, and scanning was performed 32 times.

3.3.5. NMR

SSNMR experiments were performed on a Bruker Advance III HD 400 spectrometer (Tübingen, Germany) operating at a Larmor frequency of 400.25 MHz for 1H and 100.64 MHz for ^{13}C; the spectrometer was equipped with an H/F/X triple-resonance magic-angle spinning (MAS) probe, supporting MAS rotors with an outer diameter of 3.2 mm. The rf-nutation frequency for ^{1}H and ^{13}C was 78.1 kHz, corresponding to 3.2 μs and a 90° pulse. 1D $^{13}C\{^{1}H\}$ cross-polarization/magic-angle spinning (CP/MAS) spectra were recorded using a CP contact time of 2 ms, a recycle delay of 5 s, and 1024 scans, with SPINAL-64 decoupling applied during acquisition [33]. The 2D ^{13}C–^{1}H FSLG-HECTOR [34] experiments used a MAS frequency of 10.0 kHz, a recycle delay of 3 s, and a cross-polarization (CP) time of 0.5 ms at 100 scans for a total of 70 t1 increments. Each t1 increment had a span of one basic FSLG block (30.21 μs), [35], and high-power ^{1}H SPINAL-64 decoupling was used during acquisition. A scaling factor of 0.570 was determined by recording a 2D spectrum for adamantane using identical experimental conditions to rescale the indirect dimension for the investigated samples. The chemical shifts are referenced with respect to tetramethyl silane (TMS), using adamantane as the second standard (^{1}H, δ = 1.85 ppm; ^{13}C, δ = 38.49 ppm).

3.3.6. SEM

The prepared film was freeze-dried, cut into strips, or torn off from the surface to observe the internal structure. After surface sputtering, the morphology and structure were observed by SEM [36].

3.3.7. Cytotoxicity Study

The MTT method was used to analyze the effect of the film formed by the novel complex on the relative cell proliferation ratio of L929 rat fibroblasts and cytotoxicity. The preparation of the films was the same as that detailed in Section 3.3.2. Briefly, L929 cells were seeded into 96-well plates (1×10^5 cells per well) and incubated for 48 h. To each well, 20 μL of 5 mg/mL MTT in PBS was added and then cultured for 4 h. Finally, 100 μL of DMSO was added instead of the above medium to dissolve the formazan crystals. OD was determined at 570 nm by using a microplate reader [37]. Cell growth and viability were observed and photographed using an inverted microscope.

3.3.8. Statistical Analysis

The results are expressed as means ± s.e.m. Statistical analysis was performed using one-way ANOVA followed by Newman–Keuls post hoc tests. All the analyses were conducted using GraphPad Prism 5 (GraphPad Software, Inc., La jolla, CA, USA), and, if $p < 0.05$, results were considered statistically significant.

4. Conclusions

A water-soluble complex of chitosan–sodium carbonate is reported, which was obtained by adding a large amount of sodium carbonate to chitosan/acetic acid solution. FT-IR, EDS, and SEM findings support the formation of carbonate crystallization in the complex. Furthermore, SSNMR ^{13}C{^{1}H} CP confirmed the association between the ammonium cation and carbonate anions. The complex could be returned to chitosan by soaking in an alcohol solution, and the film maintained good biocompatibility. We showed, for the first time, that this new CS-SC film may promote cell proliferation, making it a candidate material for tissue engineering. Furthermore, greater focus should be directed toward the principle of dissolution and the solubility of the chitosan–sodium carbonate complex at different degrees of deacetylation and from different sources.

Author Contributions: J.J., J.S. (Jingsong Shi), Z.X. and J.Q. conceived and designed the experiments; J.Q., X.W., and C.S. performed the experiments; J.Q. and J.G. analyzed the data; J.S. (Jie Shu) contributed reagents/materials/analysis tools; J.Q. and J.S. (Jingsong Shi) wrote the paper.

Acknowledgments: This work was supported by the National first-class discipline program of Light Industry Technology and Engineering (LITE2018-18), Top-notch Academic Programs Project of Jiangsu Higher Education Institutions (PPZY2015B146), Research subjects on teaching reform of higher education in Jiangsu Province (2017jsjg146), 2018 college students' innovation training program of Jiangnan University.

Conflicts of Interest: The authors declare no conflict of interest.

References

1. Wu, Q.-X.; Lin, D.-Q.; Yao, S.-J. Design of Chitosan and Its Water Soluble Derivatives-Based Drug Carriers with Polyelectrolyte Complexes. *Mar. Drugs* **2014**, *12*, 6236–6253. [CrossRef] [PubMed]

2. Yang, S.; Shao, D.; Wang, X.; Hou, G.; Nagatsu, M.; Tan, X.; Ren, X.; Yu, J. Design of Chitosan-Grafted Carbon Nanotubes: Evaluation of How the –OH Functional Group Affects Cs^+ Adsorption. *Mar. Drugs* **2015**, *13*, 3116–3131. [CrossRef] [PubMed]
3. Younes, I.; Rinaudo, M. Chitin and Chitosan Preparation from Marine Sources. Structure, Properties and Applications. *Mar. Drugs* **2015**, *13*, 1133–1174. [CrossRef] [PubMed]
4. Jiang, Y.; Fu, C.; Wu, S.; Liu, G.; Guo, J.; Su, Z. Determination of the Deacetylation Degree of Chitooligosaccharides. *Mar. Drugs* **2017**, *15*, 332. [CrossRef] [PubMed]
5. Mourya, V.K.; Inamdar, N.N. Chitosan-modifications and applications: Opportunities galore. *React. Funct. Polym.* **2008**, *68*, 1013–1051. [CrossRef]
6. Riva, R.; Ragelle, H.; des Rieux, A.; Duhem, N.; Jérôme, C.; Véronique Préat, V. Chitosan and chitosan derivatives in drug delivery and tissue engineering. In *Chitosan for Biomaterials II.*; Jayakumar, R., Prabaharan, M., Muzzarelli, R.A.A., Eds.; Springer: Berlin, Germany, 2011; pp. 19–44.
7. de Queiroz Antonino, R.S.C.M.; Lia Fook, B.R.P.; de Oliveira Lima, V.A.; de Farias Rached, R.Í.; Lima, E.P.N.; da Silva Lima, R.J.; Peniche Covas, C.A.; Lia Fook, M.V. Preparation and Characterization of Chitosan Obtained from Shells of Shrimp (*Litopenaeus vannamei* Boone). *Mar. Drugs* **2017**, *15*, 141. [CrossRef] [PubMed]
8. Kulkarni, A.D.; Patel, H.M.; Surana, S.J.; Vanjari, Y.H.; Belgamwar, V.S.; Pardeshi, C.V. *N,N,N*-Trimethyl chitosan: An advanced polymer with myriad of opportunities in nanomedicine. *Carbohydr. Polym.* **2017**, *157*, 875–902. [CrossRef] [PubMed]
9. Sun, Z.; Shi, C.; Wang, X.; Fang, Q.; Huang, J. Synthesis, characterization, and antimicrobial activities of sulfonated chitosan. *Carbohydr. Polym.* **2017**, *155*, 321–328. [CrossRef] [PubMed]
10. Kamari, A.; Aljafree, N.F.A.; Yusoff, S.N.M. *N,N*-dimethylhexadecyl carboxymethyl chitosan as a potential carrier agent for rotenone. *Int. J. Biol. Macromol.* **2016**, *88*, 263–272. [CrossRef] [PubMed]
11. Straccia, M.C.; d'Ayala, G.G.; Romano, I.; Oliva, A.; Laurienzo, P. Alginate Hydrogels Coated with Chitosan for Wound Dressing. *Mar. Drugs* **2015**, *13*, 2890–2908. [CrossRef] [PubMed]
12. Bellich, B.; D'Agostino, I.; Semeraro, S.; Gamini, A.; Cesàro, A. "The Good, the Bad and the Ugly" of Chitosans. *Mar. Drugs* **2016**, *14*, 99. [CrossRef] [PubMed]
13. Varum, K.M.; Ottoy, M.H.; Smidsrod, O. Acid hydrolysis of chitosans. *Carbohydr. Polym.* **2001**, *46*, 89–98. [CrossRef]
14. Duan, J.; Liang, X.; Cao, Y.; Wang, S.; Zhang, L. High strength chitosan hydrogels with biocompatibility via new avenue based on constructing nanofibrous architecture. *Macromolecules* **2015**, *48*, 2706–2714. [CrossRef]
15. Fang, Y.; Zhang, R.; Duan, B.; Liu, M.; Lu, A.; Zhang, L. Recyclable universal solvents for chitin to chitosan with various degrees of acetylation and construction of robust hydrogels. *ACS Sustain. Chem. Eng.* **2017**, *5*, 2725–2733. [CrossRef]
16. Fang, Y.; Duan, B.; Lu, A.; Liu, M.; Liu, H.; Xu, X.; Zhang, L. Intermolecular interaction and the extended wormlike chain conformation of chitin in naoh/urea aqueous solution. *Biomacromolecules* **2015**, *16*, 1410–1417. [CrossRef] [PubMed]
17. Nishimura, T.; Ito, T.; Yamamoto, Y.; Yoshio, M.; Kato, T. Macroscopically ordered polymer/CaCO3 hybrids prepared by using a liquid-crystalline template. *Angew. Chem. Int. Ed.* **2008**, *47*, 2800–2803. [CrossRef] [PubMed]
18. Piron, E.; Domard, A. Formation of a ternary complex between chitosan and ion pairs of strontium carbonate. *Int. J. Biol. Macromol.* **1998**, *23*, 113–120. [CrossRef]
19. Fu, R.; Ji, X.; Ren, Y.; Wang, G.; Cheng, B. Antibacterial blend films of cellulose and chitosan prepared from binary ionic liquid system. *Fibers Polym.* **2017**, *18*, 852–858. [CrossRef]
20. Silva, D.S.; Almeida, A.; Prezotti, F.; Cury, B.; Campana-Filho, S.P.; Sarmento, B. Synthesis and characterization of 3,6-O,O′-dimyristoyl chitosan micelles for oral delivery of paclitaxel. *Colloids Surf. B* **2017**, *152*, 220–228. [CrossRef] [PubMed]
21. Taleb, M.F.; Alkahtani, A.; Mohamed, S.K. Radiation synthesis and characterization of sodium alginate/chitosan/hydroxyapatite nanocomposite hydrogels: A drug delivery system for liver cancer. *K. Mohamed, Polym. Bull.* **2015**, *72*, 725–742.
22. Roomans, G.M.; Dragomir, A. X-ray microanalysis in the scanning electron microscope. *J. Electron Microsc.* **2014**, *1117*, 639–661.
23. Xing, Q. Information or resolution: Which is required from an SEM to study bulk inorganic materials? *Scanning* **2016**, *38*, 864–879. [CrossRef] [PubMed]

24. Peng, S.; Meng, H.-C.; Zhou, L.; Chang, J. Synthesis of Novel Magnetic Cellulose-Chitosan Composite Microspheres and Their Application in Laccase Immobilization. *J. Nanosci. Nanotechnol.* **2014**, *14*, 7010–7014. [CrossRef] [PubMed]
25. Chang, X.H.; Chen, D.R.; Jiao, X.L. Chitosan-based aerogels with high adsorption performance. *J. Phys. Chem. B* **2008**, *112*, 7721–7725. [CrossRef] [PubMed]
26. King, C.; Stein, R.S.; Shamshina, J.L.; Rogers, R.D. Measuring the Purity of Chitin with a Clean, Quantitative Solid-State NMR Method. *ACS Sustain. Chem. Eng.* **2017**, *5*, 8011–8016. [CrossRef]
27. Oliveira, J.R.; Martins, M.C.L.; Mafra, L.; Gomes, P. Synthesis of an O-alkynyl-chitosan and its chemoselective conjugation with a PEG-like amino-azide through click chemistry. *Carbohydr. Polym.* **2012**, *87*, 240–249. [CrossRef]
28. Zhao, Y.; Wang, Z.; Zhang, Q.; Chen, F.; Yue, Z.; Zhang, T.; Deng, H.; Huselstein, C.; Anderson, D.P.; Chang, P.R.; et al. Accelerated skin wound healing by soy protein isolate-modified hydroxypropyl chitosan composite films. *Int. J. Biol. Macromol.* **2018**, *118*, 1293–1302. [CrossRef] [PubMed]
29. Shanmugapriya, K.; Kim, H.; Saravana, P.S.; Chun, B.-S.; Kang, H.W. Fabrication of multifunctional chitosan-based nanocomposite film with rapid healing and antibacterial effect for wound management. *Int. J. Biol. Macromol.* **2018**, *118*, 1713–1725. [CrossRef] [PubMed]
30. Gómez Chabala, L.F.; Cuartas, C.E.E.; López, M.E.L. Release Behavior and Antibacterial Activity of Chitosan/Alginate Blends with *Aloe vera* and Silver Nanoparticles. *Mar. Drugs* **2017**, *15*, 328. [CrossRef] [PubMed]
31. Zhang, Q.C.; Luo, H.; Zhang, Y.; Zhou, Y.; Ye, Z.; Tan, W.; Lang, M. Fabrication of three-dimensional poly(epsilon-caprolactone) scaffolds with hierarchical pore structures for tissue engineering. *Mater. Sci. Eng. C* **2013**, *33*, 2094–2103. [CrossRef] [PubMed]
32. Kanimozhi, K.; Basha, S.K.; Kumari, V.S.; Kaviyarasu, K.; Maaza, M. In vitro cytocompatibility of chitosan/PVA/methylcellulose - Nanocellulose nanocomposites scaffolds using L929 fibroblast cells. *Appl. Surf. Sci.* **2018**, *449*, 574–583. [CrossRef]
33. Fung, B.M.; Khitrin, A.K.; Ermolaev, K. An improved broadband decoupling sequence for liquid crystals and solids. *J. Magn. Reson.* **2000**, *142*, 97–101. [CrossRef] [PubMed]
34. Van Rossum, B.J.; Forster, H.; de Groot, H.J.M. High-field and high-speed CP-MAS C-13 NMR heteronuclear dipolar-correlation spectroscopy of solids with frequency-switched Lee-Goldburg homonuclear decoupling. *J. Magn. Reson.* **1997**, *124*, 516–519. [CrossRef]
35. Ladizhansky, V.; Vega, S. Polarization transfer dynamics in Lee-Goldburg cross polarization nuclear magnetic resonance experiments on rotating solids. *J. Chem. Phys.* **2000**, *112*, 7158–7168. [CrossRef]
36. Szymańska, E.; Szekalska, M.; Czarnomysy, R.; Lavrič, Z.; Srčič, S.; Miltyk, W.; Winnicka, K. Novel Spray Dried Glycerol 2-Phosphate Cross-Linked Chitosan Microparticulate Vaginal Delivery System—Development, Characterization and Cytotoxicity Studies. *Mar. Drugs* **2016**, *14*, 174. [CrossRef] [PubMed]
37. Magesh, G.; Bhoopathi, G.; Nithya, N.; Arun, A.P.; Ranjith Kumar, E. Structural, morphological, optical and biological properties of pure ZnO and agar/zinc oxide nanocomposites. *Int. J. Biol. Macromol.* **2018**, *117*, 959–966. [CrossRef] [PubMed]

marine drugs

Review

Enzymatic Modification of Native Chitin and Conversion to Specialty Chemical Products

Nathanael D. Arnold [1], Wolfram M. Brück [2], Daniel Garbe [1] and Thomas B. Brück [1,*]

[1] Werner Siemens Chair of Synthetic Biotechnology, Dept. of Chemistry, Technical University of Munich (TUM), 85748 Garching, Germany; nathanael.arnold@tum.de (N.D.A.); daniel.garbe@tum.de (D.G.)

[2] Institute for Life Technologies, University of Applied Sciences Western Switzerland Valais-Wallis, 1950 Sion 2, Switzerland; wolfram.bruck@hevs.ch

* Correspondence: brueck@tum.de

Received: 14 December 2019; Accepted: 28 January 2020; Published: 30 January 2020

Abstract: Chitin is one of the most abundant biomolecules on earth, occurring in crustacean shells and cell walls of fungi. While the polysaccharide is threatening to pollute coastal ecosystems in the form of accumulating shell-waste, it has the potential to be converted into highly profitable derivatives with applications in medicine, biotechnology, and wastewater treatment, among others. Traditionally this is still mostly done by the employment of aggressive chemicals, yielding low quality while producing toxic by-products. In the last decades, the enzymatic conversion of chitin has been on the rise, albeit still not on the same level of cost-effectiveness compared to the traditional methods due to its multi-step character. Another severe drawback of the biotechnological approach is the highly ordered structure of chitin, which renders it nigh impossible for most glycosidic hydrolases to act upon. So far, only the Auxiliary Activity 10 family (AA10), including lytic polysaccharide monooxygenases (LPMOs), is known to hydrolyse native recalcitrant chitin, which spares the expensive first step of chemical or mechanical pre-treatment to enlarge the substrate surface. The main advantages of enzymatic conversion of chitin over conventional chemical methods are the biocompability and, more strikingly, the higher product specificity, product quality, and yield of the process. Products with a higher M_w due to no unspecific depolymerisation besides an exactly defined degree and pattern of acetylation can be yielded. This provides a new toolset of thousands of new chitin and chitosan derivatives, as the physio-chemical properties can be modified according to the desired application. This review aims to provide an overview of the biotechnological tools currently at hand, as well as challenges and crucial steps to achieve the long-term goal of enzymatic conversion of native chitin into specialty chemical products.

Keywords: chitin; chitosan; chitooligosaccharides; enzymatic modification; biotechnology; chitinase; chitosanase; lytic polysaccharide monooxygenase; chitin deacetylase

1. Introduction

Since the first International Conference on Chitin/Chitosan (ICCC) was held in 1977, the interest in chitin-derived products has increased substantially. It is one of the most abundant biopolymers on our planet, second only to cellulose, occurring in the exoskeletons of crustaceans and insects, the radulae of molluscs, as well as in fungi and algae cell walls, rendering it a readily available resource. The amount of chitin produced every year by living organisms on a global scale is estimated to be in the magnitude of 10^{10}–10^{11} tons, of which 10^6 tons are produced solely by the seafood processing industry in the form of crustacean shell wastes originating from shrimps, prawn, crabs, and lobsters [1]. These secondary products are composites of a stabilizing chitin scaffold interfaced with calcium carbonate, protein, carotenoids, hereby predominantly astaxanthin, and small amounts of lipids. The relation of the respective components is dependent on the source species and seasonal changes. This can be exemplified by sclerotin, the tanned proteinaceous matrix constituting most of the insects' exoskeletons.

As the global demand for luxury foods increases, large amounts of crustacean shell wastes are generated that are disposed into either the ocean or landfills. Although chitin itself is biodegradable, its natural composites are recalcitrant and barely accessible for naturally occurring enzymes, therefore accumulating over time and threatening coastal ecosystems [2].

2. Conventional and Biotechnological Methods of Chitin Extraction and Conversion

2.1. Chemical Chitin Extraction

The conventional extraction of chitin is performed chemically by demineralising the ground crustacean shells by means of strong acids, favourably HCl, and subsequently removing residual protein through incubation with a strong base, whereby NaOH is the alkali of choice [3,4]. If so desired, the chitin flakes can be bleached by H_2O_2, $KMnO_4$, or equally strong oxidizing agents in an additional step to remove remaining dyes. The whole process generates hazardous by-products while rendering valuable minerals and amino acids hardly recyclable, yielding chitin with a low M_w (molecular weight), since the aggressive chemicals attack the crystalline structure and therefore randomly degrade the co-polymer chains [5] (Figure 1, left side).

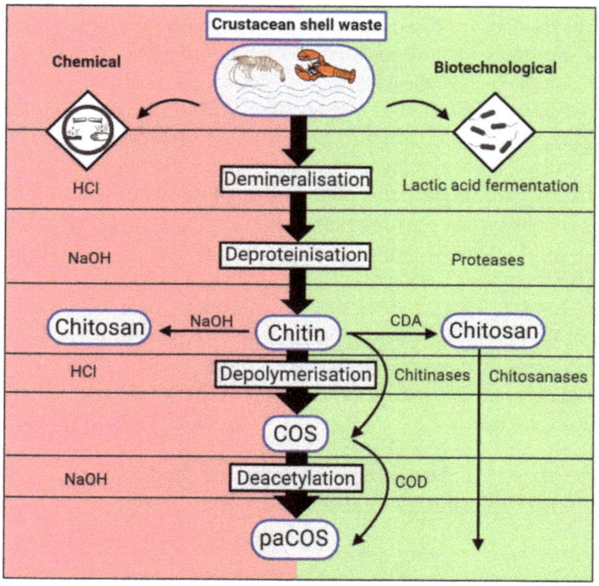

Figure 1. Chemical and biotechnological chitin extraction methods from crustacean shell waste. Since native chitin from marine sources is a composite of calcium carbonate, protein, carotenoids, and small amounts of lipids, it has to be processed for industrial applications. After mincing and cleaning of the crustacean shell waste, it has to be freed of minerals and proteins. This can be achieved chemically (red, left side) by the employment of HCl and NaOH, respectively, while biotechnological approaches (green, right side) utilise lactic acid bacteria fermentation for mineral removal and protease cocktails for the excision of residual protein. To obtain the industrially relevant end products of chitosan and its partially acetylated chitooligosaccharides (paCOS), chitin is depolymerised by acid-hydrolysis or chitinases in a first step. Afterwards, the obtained chitooligosaccharides (COS) are N-deacetylated with 50% NaOH at room temperature or 120 °C, conventionally, or through chitin oligosaccharide deacetylases (COD), enzymatically. If high M_w chitosan is desired, the isolated chitin can be converted directly through incubation with hot alkali or chitin deacetylases. The figure was created with BioRender.

2.2. Chemical Processing of Chitin into Chitosan

After obtaining mineral- and protein-free chitin from crustacean wastes, with the help of strong mineral acids and NaOH, respectively, the chitin is converted into chitosan by means of 25–50% NaOH-assisted de-N-acetylation. This can be done at room temperature (homogeneous deacetylation) or at elevated temperatures (heterogeneous deacetylation) depending on the desired product, with the latter being the preferred method for industrial needs [1,6]. Afterwards the product is washed to remove the alkali and dried to obtain chitosan flakes. The whole process harnesses randomly deacetylated chitosan chains with varying M_w and an unspecific P_A (pattern of acetylation), which have to be fractionated according to their physiochemical properties with elaborate, time-consuming methods [7]. Complementing the thermochemical approach, microwave irradiation was successfully used to increase the speed, yield, and degree of deacetylation (D_D) of chitosan obtained from shrimp shells [8]. El Knidri et al. took this method a step further, utilising microwave irradiation exclusively to produce chitosan, which accelerated the whole process 16-fold [9]. The obtained chitosan had a higher M_w with an equal D_D of about 80% as that of thermochemically yielded chitosan.

2.3. Biotechnological Chitin Extraction

Biotechnological methods to obtain chitin from crustacean shell wastes comprise demineralisation through lactic acid bacteria fermentation and deproteinisation by means of proteolytic bacteria or protease cocktails [10–13]. Alternatively, protease activity may simply be induced passively by pH reduction in lactic acid fermentation due to conversion of glucose, leading to accumulation of calcium lactate and removal of residual protein [14]. As a consequence, chitin with demineralisation degrees up to 99% and deproteinsation degrees around 95% can be achieved [15], retracting the protein and minerals in a liquid phase without environmentally harming by-products. Both successive two-step fermentations and one-batch co-fermentations have been tried hereby, while the latter approach would reduce costs in an industrial scale significantly [16–18]. While the succession of the demineralisation and deproteinisation steps does not negatively affect the quality or yield of chemically processed crustacean shells, it is of importance to perform the demineralisation prior to protein removal, since the minerals can inhibit protease activity [4,19]. The majority of research projects have focused on aerobic fermentation as instrument of choice, requiring aeration and careful monitoring of batch O_2 contents, which represents an additional cost factor. Bajaj and colleagues demonstrated the efficiency of anaerobic fermentation of shrimp shell waste with simple tools, e.g., minced meat and bio-yoghurt as sources for proteolytic- and lactic-acid bacteria, respectively (Figure 1, right side).

In their outstanding study they were not only able to reuse their fermentation liquor for another large-scale fermentation (300 L), attaining chitin with comparable degrees of deproteinisation, but also produced chitosan with a higher viscosity than commercially available products [20].

Despite the grievous disadvantages of chemical chitin extraction, it still remains the standard procedure in the industry to date, probably due to the faster extraction times.

2.4. Biotechnological Chitin Conversion

Biotechnological chitin processing be achieved by applying several enzymes, either to cleave chitin into smaller fragments, the chitooligosaccharides (COS), through chitinases (EC 3.2.1.14) and β-N-acetylhexosaminidases (EC 3.2.1.52), or by conversion into chitosan via chitin-deacetylases, catalysing the hydrolysis of the acetamido group (EC 3.5.1.41). As auxiliary enzymes, lytic chitin monooxygenases (LPMOs, EC 1.14.99.53) may be deployed, as they are able to hydrolyse native crystalline chitin by oxidation. This increases the accessibility for regular chitinases. Chitosan can also be cleaved enzymatically by chitosanases (EC 3.2.1.132) to produce prevalently deacetylated COS.

3. Characterisation of Chitin, Chitosan, and Chitooligosaccharides

3.1. Chitin

The homo-polymer chitin is assembled by units of N-acetyl-D-glucosamine (GlcNAc) covalently bound through β-(1-4)-glycosidic links, possessing a high M_W (Figure 2a). The polysaccharide has a lot in common with cellulose structurally, the difference is due to acetamido groups substituting for the hydroxyl groups at position 2 of the respective 2-deoxy-D-glucopyranose-subunits. In nature, chitin exists as a co-polymer comprised of randomly distributed GlcNAc and D-glucosamine (GlcN) subunits, in which the acetylated D-glucosamines prevail. Chitin is not soluble in aqueous solutions due to its high hydrophobicity and resembles a rigid, inflexible crystalline structure, since the acetamido groups form strong hydrogen bonds between adjacent polymer chains, which again are ordered in micro-fibrils. The polysaccharide is primarily found as part of composite materials, where it acts as a stabilizing scaffold interfaced with minerals like calcium carbonate, protein, or both.

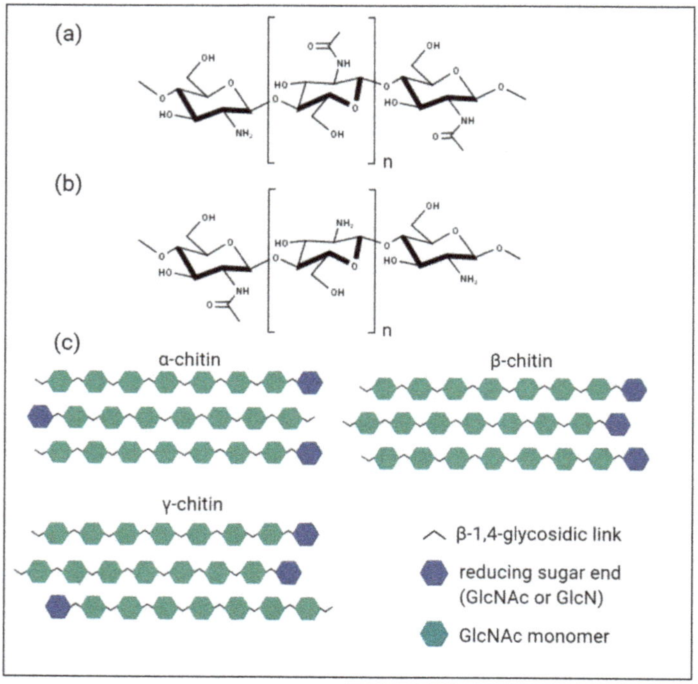

Figure 2. Chemical structures of chitin and chitosan. (**a**) Chitin is a homo-polymer assembled of N-acetyl-D-glucosamine monomers (GlcNAc), covalently bound through β-(1-4)-glycosidic linkages. In nature, it occurs as a co-polymer comprised of both GlcNAc and non-acetylated D-glucosamine (GlcN) subunits, with a molar GlcNAc fraction > 50%. (**b**) Chitosan is the deacetylated derivative of chitin, defined by a ratio of GlcN to GlcNAc monomers of > 1,0. It exhibits solubility in aqueous acetic solvents. (**c**) Chitin has three different allomorphs, which differ in the orientation of the respective polymer chains within the micro-fibril macro structure. The most abundant and resilient α-chitin is formed by antiparallel aligned polysaccharide chains. In β-chitin, the sugar chains are ordered in a parallel manner, therefore exhibiting weaker intramolecular interactions. The γ-allomorph of chitin is characterized by a mixture of both antiparallel and parallel aligned chains, which leads to a polymer with fractions of higher and lower levels of crystallinity. The figure was created with BioRender.

The strength of the inter- and intramolecular interactions within the chitin micro-fibrils is dependent on the orientation of the polymer chains, which is manifested in the three naturally occurring allomorphs of α-, β-, and γ-chitin [1] (Figure 2c). The most abundant and resilient α-form of chitin is characterized by the antiparallel alignment of the polymer chains; it occurs in all exoskeletons of arthropoda. In contrast, within β-chitin the polymer chains are lining up in a parallel manner, exhibiting weaker intramolecular interactions and therefore projecting more accessibility for enzymes. The most prominent source would be squid pens, although the β-allomorph is also present in other molluscs like krill. Structurally γ-chitin differs through a mixture of both parallel and antiparallel alignment of interspersed polymer chains, leading to fractions with higher or lower crystallinity levels, respectively, and it naturally occurs in beetle larvae and cephalopods.

Due to these inherent chemical and physical characteristics of chitin its commercial applications in the native form are currently rather limited. Commonly native chitin is utilised as fertilizer in agriculture, as it contains nitrogen, or as an inducer of plant defence mechanisms, enhancing the resistance against fungi by the promotion of chitinases [21–23]. Furthermore, chitin is employed as a food additive [24] as well as a packaging material for affinity chromatography columns to purify proteins with a carbohydrate-binding domain, or as sorbent to pre-concentrate phenol and chlorophenols by means of solid phase extraction, as validated by HPLC [25,26].

3.2. Chitosan

The abundant polysaccharide chitin finds an increased number of applications once it is converted into its deacetylated form chitosan, which is defined by a ratio of GlcN to GlcNAc units > 1.0 in the random copolymer [4] (Figure 2b). This transfers into the molar fraction of N-acetylated glucosamine monomers, which represents the degree of acetylation (D_A), also commonly expressed in percentage (%D_A).

In research the term chitosan is defined more loosely and comprises hetero-polymer chains with a minimal degree of deacetylation (D_D) of about 10%, while only fully acetylated chains, exclusively assembled from GlcNAc, are being referred to as chitin. Generally, chitosan is less abundant in nature compared to chitin, occurring only in cell walls of *Zygomycetes* fungi species [27].

The conventional conversion of chitin into its functionalised form chitosan is realised by means of 50% w/w NaOH at high temperatures (80–120 °C) with a 1:10 solid to liquid ratio to hydrolyse the acetamido groups [6]. This yields a chitosan product with a low degree of polymerisation (DP), an undefined D_A, in addition to an unspecific pattern of acetylation (P_A). All of the aforementioned factors combined are critical for the physio-chemical properties and bioactivity of chitosan.

Chitosan is soluble in weakly acetic solutions and demonstrates antibacterial, antifungal, antioxidant, anti-inflammatory, and antitumoral activities, besides being physiologically inert and biodegradable [28–30]. Moreover, it exhibits a cationic nature in acetic solution, which is unique among polysaccharides, therefore having the ability to bind to negatively charged surfaces [31,32]. This feature is assumed to be responsible for its antibacterial appeal, either binding to the surface of bacteria, therefore blocking their metabolism or alternatively through attachment of smaller chitosan fragments to the negatively charged DNA, effecting the inhibition of RNA translation [30,33].

3.3. Chitooligosaccharides

Correspondingly to chitin, the high M_w and viscosity of chitosan, in addition to its low solubility in water, hinder easy processing for industrial applications. Therefore, chitin or chitosan are generally depolymerised either chemically, mechanically, or by means of enzyme degradation to obtain smaller fragments, so-called chitooligosaccharides (COS) or partially acetylated chitooligosaccharides (paCOS), which are soluble in water while exhibiting the same positive traits as their highly polymerised source materials [34]. These COS possess a DP between 2–20 and varying D_A, P_A, and F_A (fraction of acetylation), which determine their respective biological activity [35,36]. The degree of solubility increases with the D_D and is higher for chitooligosaccharides (COS) with a relatively lower DP and a

M_w up to 3.9 kDa [37]. Chitooligomers with a high DP above 6 and low M_w are thought to be more biologically active than COS with a low DP and high M_w. As are all sugars, chitooligosaccharides are sensitive to autooxidation and thus should be stored at preferably -20 °C under dry and inert conditions. Their shelf life can be increased significantly when antioxidants are added prior to storage [38].

Hence it is a highly attractive biomolecule for various industry segments, from cosmetics and biomedicine to wastewater treatment, textile and paper production, biotechnology as well as the food and agricultural industries. We refer to several excellent reviews that address possible applications of chitin and its derivatives extensively [22,39–43].

To support the increased interest in chitosan derivatives with numbers: its global market is expected to grow at a CAGR (Compound Annual Growth Rate) of 6.3% over the next five years, while exceeding 118,000 tons [44,45]. Also taking into account that the traditional ways of extracting and converting native chitin into its functionalized derivatives are done chemically under toxic waste production, it becomes clear that there exists an urgent necessity to find a suitable biotechnological approach to process crustacean shells by means of enzymes. Not only does this ameliorate the disposal issues for seafood processing companies, but, in doing so, the unused potential of basically free industrial feedstock can be exploited to create specialty chemical products in a more sustainable way with a higher degree of quality [46].

4. Characterization of Enzymes Acting on Chitin and its Derivatives

4.1. Chitinases

Chitinases (EC 3.2.1.14) belong to the group of glycosyl hydrolases (GHs) and are spread across the GH families 18 and 19, while the family of GH20 contains additional chitinolytic enzymes. These include β-N-acetylhexosaminidases (EC 3.2.1.52), usually referred to as chitobiases, which catalyse the breakdown of dimeric GlcNAc-units (chitobiose) into monomers from terminal-reducing or non-reducing ends of chitin or chitindextrin. Although they all hydrolyse glycosidic β-(1,4)-links of acetylated D-glucosamine units, substantial differences in the mode of action, the amino acid sequence and catalytic sites do exist. While the catalytic regions of GH18 and GH20 glycosidases are characterized through a triosephosphate isomerase (TIM) barrel $(\beta/\alpha)_8$ domain, chitinases from GH19 have a α-helix rich lysozyme-like domain. The family of GH18 is divided into the subfamilies A and B, of which the first additionally possesses a chitinase insertion domain (α + β), or CID, inserted between the seventh α and β-strand of the TIM barrel. The CID consists of five or six anti-parallel β-strands and one α-helix and is putatively responsible for the tunnel-like catalytic cleft and the processive mode of action of the subfamily A chitinases of GH18.

Both enzyme families share a conserved DxDxE motif on the fourth β-strand and catalyse the hydrolytic reaction by a substrate-assisted mechanism [47].

4.1.1. Processive and Non-Processive Chitinases

A chitinase is described as acting processively if it does not release its substrate after hydrolysing a glycosidic link but rather catalyses several cycles in succession while remaining attached to the solid substrate. This is possible by the threading of single chitin chains through the tunnel-like catalytic cleft, while cleaving off disaccharides simultaneously [48]. Non-processive chitinases, on the other hand, detach after every single hydrolysis round, subsequently reattaching to another GlcNAc–GlcNAc link located elsewhere, in a random fashion [49]. Processivity is important to hydrolyse crystalline chitin, maneuvering the enzyme close to a free polysaccharide chain end at the cost of reaction speed [49,50]. Moreover, through the permanent attachment of enzyme and substrate, reattachment of hydrolysed chitobioses is prevented, therefore increasing efficiency.

4.1.2. Endo- and Exo-Chitinases

Chitinases can be specified by their endo- or exo-modus operandi on chitin. The determining factor hereby is the product length formed through chitin hydrolysis. Endo-chitinases cleave glycosidic bonds randomly along the polymer chain in a non-processive manner, producing predominantly chitiobioses, but also other low-M_W multimers like chitotrioses $(GlcNAc)_2$ or chitotetraoses $(GlcNAc)_4$. Exo-chitinases catalyse the degradation of crystalline chitin from the reducing or non-reducing end processively, releasing N, N′-diacetylchitobioses successively, while remaining attached to the substrate. Interestingly, it is always the second and not the first glycosidic β-(1,4)-link that is attacked by exo-chitinases, thereby releasing chitobiose blocks. Another type of exo-acting enzyme would be the β-N-acetylhexosaminidases, which hydrolyse soluble oligomeric degradation products of endo-chitinases into monomeric GlcNAc, targeting the non-reducing end [51]. As their name implies, they catalyse the hydrolysis of hexoses in both gluco- and galacto-configurations [52]. Data suggest that the exo-processing manner of some chitinases is connected to the inaccessibility of crystalline chitin micro-fibrils rather than the enzyme architecture per se, potentially making obsolete the definition by means of product length. Sikorski et al. showed with the example of *Serratia marcescens* chitinases A and B (*sm*ChiA and *sm*ChiB)—two enzymes thought to be exo-chitinases—how, through repositioning of the 'roof' in the tunnel-like substrate binding groove, the substrate chitosan could be processed in endo-fashion by the same enzymes [53].

4.1.3. Chitinases with Transglycosylation Capabilities

Intriguingly, several chitinases of family 18 were discovered in the recent past that are capable of not only breaking glycosidic bonds in chitin but likewise of creating new links between small polysaccharide fragments, thus producing longer COS with a DP of up to 13. Enzymatically producing COS with DPs > 4 resembles one of the major limitations currently, since the main products of chitinases are prevalently either dimeric or monomeric, given that the incubation time is long enough. However, these higher polymeric COS hold more value for biomedical and other advanced applications (such as antioxidants with antimicrobial activity in the food and cosmetics industry [30,41,54], biofungicides [55,56], wound healing-agents [57–59], in gene therapy [60–62], as immuno-stimulants in tumour therapy [63–65] etc.), while shorter COS can be harnessed for low value products like fish feed or fertilizer exclusively. The transglycosylation (TG) reaction takes place when a retaining enzyme induces the transfer of a glycosidic residue instead of a nucleophilic water molecule from a donor to an acceptor sugar molecule [51,66]. Madhuprakash et al. solved the crystal structure for *Sp*ChiD of *Serratia proteamaculans*, a chitinase exhibiting both hydrolysis and TG activity. They unravelled how a 13-residue protruding loop in the deep active binding cleft blocked a large number of subsites and suggested this structural characteristic to be responsible for the TG aptitude [67]. Furthermore, the majority of dual action mode chitinases seem to exhibit aromatic amino residues in their catalytic site, suggesting a processive mechanism [67,68]. The exact mechanism of TG events is not fully understood, however for the catalysis of disaccharides it could be shown that the TG is autocondensation-driven and has to happen faster than the glycosidic hydrolysis [69]. Consistent evidence from several studies illustrates how the transfer of COS is dependent on the amount and length of substrate and the proportion and nature of the enzyme. Hereby an excess amount of substrate appears to be beneficial for a TG activity, while a surplus of the glycosidase seems to push the reaction equilibrium towards a predominant hydrolysis agitation [66,68,70].

4.2. Chitosanases

Chitosanases (EC 3.2.1.132) are distributed among the families GH5, GH7, GH8, GH46, GH75, and GH80, illustrating their extensive sequence diversities. Another relevant family when talking about chitosan active enzymes would be GH2 with its exo-1,4-β-D-glucosaminidases, which hydrolyse D-glucosamine residues of chitosan and chitosanoligosaccharides from the non-reducing termini successively [71,72]. The endochitosanase family members of GH46 have been studied the most thoroughly, with four crystal structures available and various expression and site-directed mutagenesis studies to encode their mechanism [73–75]. To generalize, GH46 chitosanases are mainly built out of α-helices with two globular domains, a minor and major lobe, divided by a deep substrate binding cleft [76,77]. Hereby their core structure resembles that of the well-studied *Escherichia coli* bacteriophage T4 lysozyme (GH24) and to a lesser extent lysozymes belonging to the families GH22,23 and barley chitinases of GH19, in spite of low sequence homology. This catalytic and substrate binding site is constituted of two α-helices and a three-stranded β-sheet and has presumably developed from divergent evolution [78]. Hence, these five aforementioned families are also referred to as the lysozyme superfamily.

While the families of GH5, 7, and 8 comprise enzymes with several other activities like cellulases, xylanases, and glucanases, the families of GH46, 75, and 80 consist of chitosanases exclusively, which are thought to act by an inverting mechanism [79,80]. The inverting reaction mechanism describes a one-step, single-displacement hydrolysis of a glycosidic bond, which results in the net inversion of the anomeric configuration, assisted by a general base and general acid in the form of amino acid side chains [81]. The retaining reaction mechanism on the other hand comprises a two-step, double-displacement hydrolysis of a glycosidic bond, which results in the net retention of the anomeric configuration. Analogously, it is also assisted by two amino acid side chains, which act as both acid/base respectively and nucleophiles to catalyse the process [82]. Both pathways involve oxocarbenium ion-like transition states, whilst the retaining reaction mechanism also includes an additional covalent glycosyl–enzyme intermediate.

Chitosanases are further classified into the subclasses I, III, and IV based on their substrate specificity [83]. All chitosanases share the ability to hydrolyse glycosidic β-(1,4)-linked GlcN-GlcN, although the majority are able to recognize either GlcN-GlcNAc (subclass III) or GlcNAc-GlcN (subclass I) bonds as well, but not both [84,85]. Subclass II chitosanases are restricted to solely recognising and cleaving GlcN–GlcN links. Only chitosanases of the subclass IV are by definition able to cleave both GlcNAc–GlcN and GlcN–GlcNAc, as well as GlcN–GlcN [86]. Moreover, chitosanases have in common an inability to recognize GlcNAc–GlcNAc links in partially acetylated chitosan, although evidence against the strict distinction between chitinases and chitosanases has been unravelled. Hegsett et al. found a glycoside hydrolysing enzyme in *Streptomyces coelicolor*, which they referred to as A3(2), that was able to cleave GlcN–GlcN, GlcNAc–GlcN links and—untypically for chitosanases—GlcNAc–GlcNac, albeit at a much slower rate [87]. Since GlcNAc–GlcNAc and GlcN–GlcNAc dimer products, both of which had to be the result of two independent cleavage events of the hexamer substrate, were not detected after prolonged incubation time, two possible explanations persist. Either A3(2) has an absolute specificity for GlcN subunits at the subsite -2 or it cannot cleave GlcN–GlcNAC links at all.

4.3. Chitin Deacetylases

Chitin deacetylases (CDAs, EC 3.5.1.41) and chitooligosaccharides deacetylases (CODs, EC 3.5.1.105) are able to de-N-acetylate chitin and COS respectively, hydrolysing their acetamido groups. They belong to the carbohydrate esterase family 4 (CE4), which also comprises acetyl xylan esterase, peptidoglycan GlcNAc deacetylase, and peptidoglycan N-acetylmuramic acid deacetylase. Structurally, these enzymes share a NodB homology domain, named after the NodB oligosaccharide esterase. The latter is one of the first enzymes to be discovered in the CE4 family, being involved in the nod factor biosynthesis of synergistic *Rhizobium* bacteria. The de-N-acetylation reaction mechanism is proposed to be a nucleophile attack by the conserved Asp–His–His catalytic triad of the CDA on the carbonyl carbon. To date, five different catalytic motifs of CDAs are known, each containing conserved histidine and aspartic acid residues [88]. To elucidate in detail, a catalytic water molecule is at first bound through the metal cofactor Zn^{2+} (in rare cases also Cu^{2+}). Secondly, a proton from this water molecule is withdrawn by the catalytic base aspartic acid, therefore creating a nucleophile to attack the carbonyl carbon in the substrate. This results in the intermediate tetrahedral oxyanion, whose negative charge is stabilized by the metal cofactor, which is then protonized by the catalytic acid histidine on the nitrogen [89]. Thereby the free amine group is released alongside an acetate molecule on the zinc.

Living organisms take advantage of CDAs both intracellularly, for instance, fungi like *Mucor rouxii* for cell wall morphogenesis or to protect themselves from hostile chitinases [90]; or extracellularly, as observed in maritime bacteria which secrete the enzymes to convert and hydrolyse crustacean shell wastes in succession [91]. Interestingly, the CDAs and CODs are not only highly substrate specific, relying on different recognition patterns, but additionally generate products with specific D_A and P_A [88]. The resulting D_A is hereby dependent on the mechanism of the respective CDA, which can be one of the following three:

1. Enzymes with the multiple attack mechanism bind to their respective recognition site in the polysaccharide chain and process a number of sequential deacetylations, after which they detach and bind to a different region. In the case of high M_W substrate so-called block–copolymer structures arise, in which several adjacent, consecutive GlcN subunits alternate with regions of ambiguous D_A or GlcNAc, where the CDA is not active. Shorter polymer chains or COS become deacetylated entirely [92].
2. Enzymes following the multiple chain mechanism tightly bind to their recognition site of the substrate, resulting in an enzyme–polymer complex. In contrast to the multiple attack mechanism, the complex already dissociates after a single deacetylation reaction, with the enzyme binding to another recognition site afterwards [93]. For polymeric substrates this results in random distribution of deacetylated subunits and therefore P_A. For COS no obvious proposition can be made, depending on the specific substrate length and involved enzyme; either a full deacetylation or a specific pattern can be generated. It is of peculiar interest to discover CDAs with new and unique patterns of deacetylation, since the influence of P_A on the physio-chemical properties of paCOS remains to be further elucidated in detail. Furthermore, the discovery of more CDAs might also benefit our understanding of their modes of action and in doing so, our ability to tailor chitin- and chitosan oligomers with defined D_A and P_A.
3. Ultimately, single-chain-acting CDAs are processive enzymes that deacetylate a single substrate molecule sequentially by means of several catalytic events. Some bacterial CODs, which are specific for a single position, resulting in mono-deacetylated products (e.g., *Rhizobium* sp. NodB or *Vibrio* sp. CDA and COD) also belong to this group [94]. See Figure 3 for an overview of enzymatic activities of chitinases, LPMO, CDA and chitosanases towards chitin and chitosan polymer chains.

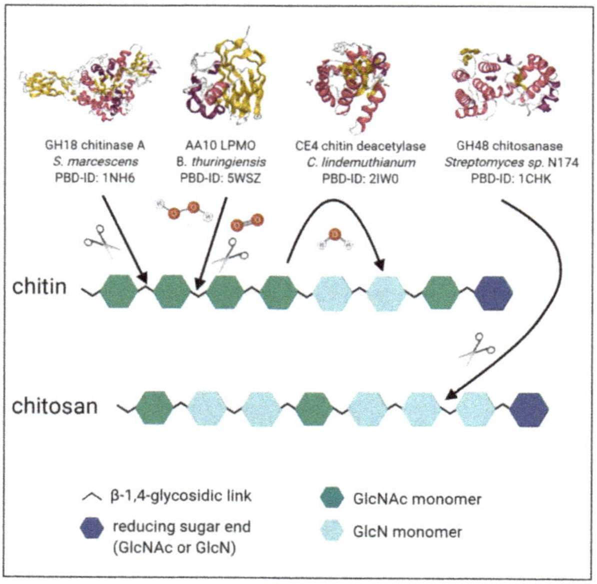

Figure 3. Enzymes with catalytic activity towards chitin and chitosan. The crystal structures of the chitinase A from *Serratia marcescens* [95], the lytic polysaccharide monooxygenase (LPMO) from *Bacillus thuringiensis* [96], the chitin deacetylase (CDA) from *Colletotrichum lindemuthianum* [97] and the chitosanase from *Streptomyces* sp. N174 [77], derived from the RCSB protein data bank (PDB), are illustrated as exemplary enzymes of their respective catalytic activity. Red coloured parts are α-helices, while β-sheets are indicated by yellow. Chitinases generally hydrolyse the β-(1,4)-glycosidic links between two GlcNAc monomers. Their modes of action, amino sequence, and catalytic sites can vary substantially. LPMOs are copper-dependent enzymes, which cleave chitin by oxidation of C1 or C4. They can recruit either H_2O_2 or O_2 as co-substrate and need an external reducing agent. The NodB-related CDAs hydrolyse the acetamido groups of GlcNAc monomers with a catalytic water molecule. Each enzyme exhibits specificity for target substrate sequences and creates unique deacetylation patterns. Chitosanases generally hydrolyse the β-(1,4)-glycosidic links between two GlcN monomers with a retaining or inverting mechanism. The specificity towards an additional substrate besides GlcN-GlcN is common. The figure was created with BioRender.

The fact that carbohydrate esterases are highly inactive on crystalline substrates, preferring soluble derivatives like glycol chitin, chitosan, or COS/paCOS, represents a significant drawback to their applicability in the biotechnological conversion of crustacean shell wastes. Interestingly, this can be counteracted by the co-application of LPMOs, which cleave polymer chain ends on the surface of crystalline chitin, as a result enhancing the activity of CDAs [98]. Moreover, several CDAs and CODs are known to possess a carbohydrate binding module (CBM) fused to their catalytic domain, therefore increasing the accessibility of the recalcitrant substrate to the active site [99].

4.4. Lytic Polysaccharide Monooxygenases

Lytic polysaccharide monooxygenases (LPMOs, EC 1.14.99.53) are classified into the six auxiliary activity enzyme AA families 9–16 based on sequence, while chitin-processing LPMOs are distributed to the groups 10, 11, and 15. These copper enzymes are characterized by the ability to disrupt the crystalline structure of polymeric polysaccharide substrates by oxidation of the glycosidic link, thus creating new chain ends for common hydrolases to act upon recalcitrant carbohydrates. They are the only enzymes known to date to act on recalcitrant polysaccharide, which confers them a key role in the utilisation of crustacean shell wastes as a chitin source. Furthermore, all LPMOs share a unique histidine–brace motif inside the catalytic region, which is located close to the surface, allowing them to tightly bind a single copper ion by two conserved histidine residues [100,101]. The solvent-exposed flat architecture of the active site is the reason for the ability of some LPMOs to oxidize the crystalline lattice structure of insoluble substrates like chitin or cellulose. The structure of the catalytic region hereby differs amongst different LPMOs, since loops that shape the substrate contact surface are responsible for conferring substrate specificity and regioselectivity. Both single catalytic domain- and multidomain proteins have been discovered, mirroring the high substrate promiscuity of LPMOs. Similar to CDAs, some LPMOs are known to have a C-terminal CBM fused to their catalytic domain with a short linker, further boosting the substrate specificity and binding affinity [102,103]. Since LPMOs do not actively cleave glycosidic linkages inside polysaccharide chains, the nomenclature may be misleading concerning its function, and therefore several researchers proposed the name polysaccharide monooxygenases (PMOs) instead. The cleavage of the glycosidic bond happens rather spontaneously, after the strong C–H bond of either C1 or C4 is deprived of one hydrogen atom and subsequently hydroxylated by the LPMO with O_2 or H_2O_2 as co-substrate. To increase the binding affinity to the polysaccharide and to activate the co-substrate, reduction of the active site Cu(II) to Cu(I) is required [104]. Depending on the co-substrate and the attacked carbon atom, different reaction mechanisms occur. Given that the C1-positioned carbon atom of the glycosidic bond is oxidized, aldonolactone products occur that hydrate to aldonic acids, while C4 oxidation leads to the formation of 4-ketoaldose products that hydrate to *gem*-diol [105–107].

4.4.1. LPMO Mechanisms with O_2 as Co-substrate

When O_2 is utilized to produce an oxidizing species strong enough to hydroxylate the glycosidic bond, the oxygenase reaction happens regioselectively without inactivation of the enzyme itself [108]. Under absence of substrate and H_2O_2, the Cu(I) active state LPMO readily reduces dioxygen, thus generating H_2O_2 while transferring the enzyme in its Cu(II) resting state; this is also referred to as futile cycle [109]. The addition of polysaccharide influences the reaction kinetics fundamentally, leading to a coupled hydroxylation reaction of the polysaccharide with O_2. Hereby two reaction mechanisms are proposed: in the first one, the Cu(I) active state LPMO reacts with O_2 and an additional electron as well as two additional protons provided by external reductants, ending in the Cu(II) oxidation state after every cycle. Since the hydrogen atom has to be abstracted before the delivery of the electron and two protons for this mechanism to work, Cu(II)-$O_2^{\bullet-}$ is most likely the oxidizing species [110,111]. In the second mechanism, one external electron donor is necessary again to render the LPMO in its Cu(I) catalytic state initially. Thereafter, two electrons and protons have to be provided, which leads to the heterolytical cleavage of the O–O bond in the dioxygen co-substrate and as a consequence, the formation of a Cu(II)-oxyl oxidizing species (Cu(II)-$O^{\bullet}$). Following the hydroxylation of the polysaccharide, the Cu(I)-state enzyme is regenerated, ready for another monooxygenase reaction cycle [112].

4.4.2. LPMO Mechanisms with H_2O_2 as Co-substrate

A study indicated that H_2O_2, and not molecular oxygen, is the preferred co-substrate of LPMOs in a peroxidase reaction with polysaccharides [113], with a 26-fold faster reaction speed and the ability to outcompete O_2 in the presence of chitin substrate. Contradictive arguments would be the non-regioselective oxidation mode of polysaccharide chains in presence of H_2O_2 in addition to the inactivation of the enzyme itself as result of detrimental self-oxidation events [108,114]. Moreover, when peroxide was applied to abduct H_2O_2 as co-substrate in an experimental setup of the *Neurospora crassa* secretome and a commercial cellulose gel, no negative effect on the hydrolysation could be observed, thus impeaching its physiological contribution [108]. Interestingly enough, carbohydrates possess the ability to scavenge H_2O_2, which could explain the undirected oxidation of glycosidic bonds, while at the same time ameliorating self-inactivation of the LPMO when exposed to higher than micro-molar concentrations of H_2O_2, which they can resist. Hereby the correct ratio of H_2O_2 to saturating amounts of substrate are of utmost importance to guarantee a sustainable processivity, since the LPMOs are protected of self-oxidation as long as substrate is bound to the active site [114].

Analogously to the O_2-utilizing reaction mechanism, the LPMO catalytic centre has to be pre-reduced into its Cu(I) oxidation state when harnessing H_2O_2 as co-substrate. Promising candidates for external electron donors of bacterial PMSOs are oxidoreductases or other redox-active enzymes [115]. Since H_2O_2 constitutes a two-electron reduced O_2 species, no additional external electron source is required after the initial priming reduction to regenerate the Cu(I)-LPMO after each catalytic cycle. The reactivity of H_2O_2 might rely on the same Cu-oxyl oxidizing species as that with O_2, omitting a Cu(II)-OOH intermediate. Computational evidence supports a Fenton chemistry-like production of $^{\bullet}OH$ radicals as means of Cu-oxyl intermediate formation [116], while the heterolytic cleavage of the O–O bond of a Cu(I)-OOH intermediate has also been proposed as alternative pathway [108]. Recently a copper-dependent particulate methane monooxygenase (pMMO), involved in the methane-to-methanol oxidation, was found to have a similar active site architecture and potential mechanism as LPMOs [117], representing another stepping stone in deciphering the highly interesting class of auxiliary enzymes.

5. Pretreatment of Native Chitin and COS Synthesis

The central constriction of straightforward COS synthesis from native chitin is its crystalline tertiary structure, resulting from the parallel or anti-parallel packaging of single saccharide chains, which again are ordered as a micro-fibril superstructure. As a consequence, most chitinolytic enzymes can barely access and thus catalyse the recalcitrant substrate, making a pretreatment inevitable. For research purposes, e.g., screening for chitinolytic microorganisms or enzymatic activity assays, it is a common practice to prepare either so-called colloidal chitin (CC) or swollen chitin by means of hydrochloric acid or phosphoric acid treatment, respectively, to increase the substrate surface and solubility. For large-scale industrial purposes on the other hand, this is neither economically nor environmentally feasible. Several endeavours have been undertaken to overcome this hurdle, ranging from physical and mechanical to chemical and lastly, biotechnological pathways.

5.1. Physical Pretreatment Methods and COS Synthesis

The most obvious method would be the mechanical grinding of crustacean shell wastes, which as a matter of fact represents the starting point of processing, whether it is chemical or biotechnological. In doing so, reliable removal of minerals and meat residues is ensured. However, experience has shown that this method alone is not sufficient for common chitinases to hydrolyse the rigid substrate flakes. To advance the general idea of a mechano-chemical breakdown, Nakagawa et al. developed a "converge" ball mill, generating fine chitin particles with reduced crystallinity, which they could convert afterwards into GlcNAc or $GlcNAc_2$ by means of commercial enzyme mixes with high efficiency [118]. When chitosan is depolymerised in aqueous solution to obtain paCOS, salt formation is inevitable, diminishing the range of applications. This particular drawback can be circumvented by mechano-chemical grinding prior to enzymatic conversion [119].

Other studies examined the effects of gamma irradiation, microwaving, steam explosion, and low ultra-frequency sonification on the structures of chitin and chitosan. These physical approaches predominantly lead to partially depolymerised polysaccharide chains with a hardly controllable range of product M_w, herein often times short COS with low DP (1-4), while consuming large amounts of energy or right-out damaging the structural integrity of chitin oligomers, rendering them inconvenient for industrial mass production [120–125] chemical chitin pretreatment.

Since the chemicals, which are deployed to both extract and successively convert chitin into chitosan (50% NaOH at high temperatures for several hours) and lastly process it into paCOS (35% HCl at 80 °C for short amount of time), are very strong bases and acids, no additional pretreatment is applied on an industrial level. In a chemoenzymatic approach, chitin will be processed with phosphoric acid into swollen chitin or hydrochloric acid into colloidal chitin to increase the accessibility and solubility for a following enzymatic degradation into COS.

Recent studies investigated the chemical pretreatment of chitin by means of so-called ionic liquids (ILs), salts with a melting point below 100 °C and natural deep eutectic solvents (NADES), which consist of quaternary ammonium salts with a hydrogen bond donor-like amines or carboxylic acids. Both of these solvents have a low vapour pressure, rendering them inflammable, and are chemically inert, reusable, and stable. However, IL are more expensive and toxic in comparison to the biologically degradable NADES, which are assembled of primary plant metabolites (amino acids, sugars, and carboxylic acids) occurring in the tissue of living organisms [126–129]. Interestingly enough, ILs can solubilise polysaccharides into a hydrogel-like amorphous substance without decreasing the DP, therefore increasing the amount of enzyme binding sites presented and overall conversion rate up to 90-fold as shown for cellulose [130]. Zhu et al could extract chitin directly from lobster shells catalysed by NADES consisting of mixtures of choline chloride (vitamin B_4) and mild carboxylic acids like malonic and lactic acid in different ratios, obtaining a 20% yield [131,132]. Two subgroups with different degrees of crystallinity of the resulting chitin could be distinguished, both of which projected a porous structure. These results are promising, albeit no further investigations have been conducted so far to our knowledge into what extent chitinase activity is enhanced on NADES-pretreated substrate.

5.2. Chemical COS Synthesis

The chemical hydrolysis of chitin and chitosan has been examined thoroughly with various acids, among them hydrochloric acid, nitrous acid, phosphorous acid, sulphuric acid, lactic acid, formic acid, and trichloroacetic acid [35,133–136]. Additionally, reductive oxidants like hydrogen peroxide and potassium persulfate were applied to obtain water-soluble chitin derivatives [137,138].

Einbu and colleagues unraveled the acidic hydrolysis mechanism of HCl in detail, distinguishing between three general steps of depolymerisation, monomer production, and deacetylation, eventually yielding GlcN and acetic acid. Hydrochloric acid breaks GlcNAc–GlcN and GlcNAc–GlcNAc glycosidic bonds two to three orders of magnitudes faster compared to GlcN–GlcNAc and GlcN–GlcN links [34,133]. Possible explanations involve (a) the protective effect of the positively charged amino-group of GlcN against the protonation of the glycosidic oxygen and (b) the stabilisation of the oxocarbenium transition state by the N-acetyl group of GlcNAc. The initial enzyme hydrolysis rate is furthermore highly dependent on the substrate D_A and increases proportionally to a higher F_A, while decreasing at longer reaction times due to deacetylation. The same study revealed how the degradation and accompanying N-deacetylation of chitosan took place in comparable rates in a diluted 3 M HCl solution, while the hydrolysis rate of glycosidic linkages was ten-fold faster than the rate of deacetylation in highly concentrated 12 M HCl. Trombotto et al. [139] were able to produce a homogenous series of chitosan-oligomers with a DP of 2-12 and a D_A between 0–90% by a two-step procedure: (i) the acid hydrolysis of fully de-N-acetylated chitosan (D_A 0) into COS of various DP and, after selective precipitations, (ii) the partial re-N-acetylation of those well-defined chito-oligomers dissolved in H_2O/MeOH (50% each) with the addition of stoichiometric amounts of acetic anhydride (Ac_2O) to obtain the expected D_A.

Nonetheless, severe drawbacks for the chemical processing of COS remain, such as a wide DP range of resulting COS, including secondary compounds that are cumbersome to isolate, low yields, prevalent monomeric (low quality) products, residual acidity, and resulting toxicity of waste products, potential structural alterations of products, and high costs [35,36,140].

5.3. Biotechnological Chitin Pretreatment

To meet the challenge of the recalcitrant 3-D structure of chitin fibrils in a more sustainable way, enzymatic and fermentation pretreatments are the techniques of choice.

As alluded above, LPMOs may facilitate chitin hydrolysis through oxidation of crystalline chitin, therefore increasing the accessibility for chitinases. This synergistic effect represents untapped potential as a chitin pretreatment method for COS production, preferably in a one-pot approach. The focus of most studies was to discover new enzymes and to understand the mechanisms involved in LPMO substrate oxidation, rather than applying the AA family members in large-scale chitin conversion experiments. For lignocellulose containing substrates like wheat straw, corn stover, poplar, and wood, several research groups illustrated how the addition of LPMOs to commercial cellulolytic cocktails increased the saccharification yield by around 20–30% in average, given that oxygen and sufficient reducing agents to drive the reaction were present [109,141,142].

Wang and colleagues pretreated crab shells mechanically, on the one hand obtaining crude (600 μm) and ultramicro grinded (100 μm) particles, and on the other hand with an additional Alcalase 2.4L FG commercial protease mix [143]. Unfortunately, only the fine particles hereby received this treatment. Further enzymatic hydrolysis with the heterologously expressed *Bacillus subtilis* subsp. *Niger* chitinase *Bs*Chi were shown to be enhanced by 242%, in comparison to untreated substrate and mechanically treated crab shells (only 81% improvement).

Zhang et al. fermented chitin powder with *Chitinolyticbacter meiyuanensis* SYBC-H1 prior to hydrolysis and observed a transformation of the crystalline substrate towards a fleecy, fiber-like structure with diameters ranging from 10–200 nm [144]. Moreover, the reduction of the M_W and crystallinity was supported by X-ray diffraction and size exclusion chromatography analysis. When applying 8 U of purified *Chitinolyticbacter meiyuanensis* SYBC-H1 chitinase to a 50 mL reaction system with 20 g L^{-1} of the amorphous, self-proclaimed CBF chitin, 19.2 g L^{-1} of monomeric GlcNAc was obtained with a yield of 96% within 6 h.

5.4. Biotechnological COS Synthesis

Biologically active COS or paCOS can be produced enzymatically through (1) depolymerisation of pretreated chitin or regular chitosan with the corresponding glycosidic hydrolases chitinase and chitosanase. This yields mainly trimeric to monomeric glucosamines eventually, while statistical mixtures of higher DP product are obtained through the modulation of incubation time in the case of chitin [80]. Enzymatic degradation of partially acetylated chitosan polymers, however, tends to attain longer paCOS with mixed P_A, D_A, and DP and a higher likelihood of bioactivity [34,145]. (2) In vitro polymerisation of chito-oligomers using hydrolases with transglycosylating activity, resulting in high DP COS [146,147]. (3) De- or re-N-acetylation of chitooligosaccharides, deploying chitin- or chitooligosaccharide-deacetylases to introduce specific P_A and D_A of choice [94,145], or (4) in-vitro synthesis of defined chito-oligomers with a heterologous system, expressing chitinsynthases and CDA from fungi [148].

Chitinolytic enzymes have a high substrate subsite specificity and clearly defined catalytic activity, yielding partially defined products in a controlled reaction with less undesired by-products, contrary to acidic hydrolysis. Glycosyl hydrolases of the family 18, for instance, need an acetylated GlcNAc unit at the -1 subsite of the enzyme in order for them to break the glycosidic linkage of a GlcNAc but not GlcN unit, always resulting in a paCOS product with a GlcNAc at its reducing end [47,80]. A whole cluster of amino residues is involved in binding the long substrate polymers to the active enzyme site. The enzymatic cleavage of the glycosidic bond is defined to happen between the amino residues -1 and +1 of the active site, -n indicates the non-reducing end, whereas +n marks the reducing sugar end [149].

Pantaleone et al. showed furthermore, that chitosan is susceptible to a broad range of unspecific hydrolases, among them glycanases, proteases, lipases, and a tannase derived from various sources [150]. Other studies have successfully employed papain, pectinases, β-glucosidase, and cocktails containg α-amylase, proteinase, and protease [151–154]. Although hydrolytic activities towards chitosan might be caused by contaminations with chitosanases, and a rather large range of paCOS is obtained that way, crude enzyme mixes might represent economically feasible tools to produce chitosan-oligomers.

6. Quantitative and Qualitative Separation of COS Mixtures

The biological activity of COS is the sum of their structural properties, like M_W, DP, D_A, F_A, and P_A. Hence, the separation of hetero-chitooligomer mixtures according to their DP and single COS content are mandatory when trying to meet the high-quality standards necessary for biomedical applications and research. Additional qualitative analysis methods determining the secondary structural properties of COS, like D_D and P_A, are key in understanding their effect mechanism.

Various procedures have been employed to recover and purify COS of common DP, amongst them gelfitration [155], ultrafiltration [156], and capillary electrophoresis (CE) with a laser-induced fluorescence detector [157]. The underlying principle of CE is that the amount of COS monomers present in acidic aqueous solution has an impact on the electrophoretic mobility. Although only small amounts of samples (5 μM) are required for high resolution analysis, the high material costs and the time-consuming process of derivatization with the fluorescence marker limit its large scale application severely. Nanofiltration has moreover been reported to distinguish between COS with a DP of 6–8 [158].

Chromatographic methods comprise immobilised metal anion chromatography for short COS with a DP of up to 4 (IMAC) [159], high-performance liquid chromatography (HPLC) with various detectors [157,160,161], and hydrophilic interaction chromatography (HILIC) coupled with an evaporative light-scattering detector (ELSD) [162]. Size-exclusion chromatography was successfully used to separate COS with a similar DP of -20 according to their length, independent from their D_D and P_A, chaining SuperDex30 (GE Healthcare) columns and is typically the method of choice [163]. Aside from that, Ion-exchange chromatography (IEX) or cation-exchange chromatography can be applied to separate COS because the positively charged amino groups of deacetylated sugars interact with the negatively charged ion-exchange column packing material [164]. Further, hydrophilic interaction/weak cation-exchange mixed-mode chromatography (HILIC/WCX) [165] and mass spectroscopy coupled with a hybrid Q-TOF analyser [166] have been deployed. An immobilized lysozyme affinity chromatography, targeting the acetyl-group, proved useful in separating fully de-N-acetylated chitosan fragments with an average DP of 22 [167]. Continuous chromatography application or up-scaling is restricted by the necessity of column packing cleaning in between measurements, small analyte amounts at a time, and high production costs.

HPLC is probably the most frequently applied analysis method to gain structural insights of COS. Due to the acetyl group, a UV-light detector can be used to quantify GlcNAc units through monitoring of the absorbance rate at around 210 nm with an amino column [168], a reversed-phase column [169], or a carbohydrate column [170,171]. Chitosan-derived COS with a high D_D can only be analysed by this method if the analytes are derivatized with a chromophore in a strenuous process, since an absorbing element would be missing otherwise [172]. Alternatively to UV-light detectors, refractive index (RI) detectors typically coupled to amino columns [155] or size-exclusion columns [133] are resorted to, since they are able to identify both GlcN and GlcNAc subunits. Drawbacks of this methods are a low sensitivity and the inability to be employed for gradient-chromatography; furthermore, due to the high polarity of COS, the retention interaction with column material is rather weak and expensive equipment and solvents are generally required for HPLC. Further, the resolution decreases with the increase of COS chain length.

HILIC represents a method to separate compounds according to their polarity and is especially suitable for carbohydrates. Jiang et al developed an effective COS separation method with a stationary maltose-bond HILIC phase but recognized the impracticability of this method for large-scale applications due to the low solubility of high M_W COS in organic solvents [173]. Dong et al. developed a mixed HILIC/WCX approach, however, especially when analysing COS with high DP, the resolution of cation-exchange columns became increasingly inaccurate [165,173].

High performance anionic exchange chromatography with pulsed amperometric detection (HAPAEC PAD) was validated as a sensitive tool to distinguish de-N-acetylated glucosamines with

DP 1–6 rapidly and with low sample concentrations [171]. Nevertheless, no reliable predictions can be made for acetylated glucosamines or COS above DP 6 with this technique.

Hamer et al. introduced novel P_A into $(GlcNAc)_5$ with two deacetylases and were able to illustrate this by means of UHPLC coupled to an evaporative light-scattering detector (ELSD) and an electrospray ionization mass spectrometry (ESI–MS detector) [174].

To confirm the existence of an acetyl group or rather, a lack thereof, at the reducing and non-reducing sugar ends, as well as neighbouring variants, nuclear magnetic resonance (NMR) is employed. Studies have made use of both ^1H NMR [92,133] and ^{13}C NMR [7,175] to obtain sequence information of short COS of up to DP 5. Since the acquired information is merely limited to the average frequency of diads and triads, no definitive structure for COS mixtures can be obtained.

The matrix-assisted laser desorption/ionization time-of-flight mass spectrometry (MALDI-TOF MS) is another common method to identify COS according to their mass and charge of ions [139,176,177]. Besides the DP itself, information about the residue distribution within chito-oligomers of consistent DP can be derived as a function of D_A [139,177].

Recently Jiang et al. reported the development of two inexpensive, accurate, and easy to perform methods to determine the D_D, namely an acid-base titration with bromocresol green in addition to a first-order derivative UV spectroscopy. The viability of their methods was supported furthermore by the comparison with ^1H NMR [178].

An overview of both the preparative and analytical methods is provided in Table S1 and Table S2, respectively.

7. Perspectives and Conclusions

Despite substantial advancements in the field of biotechnological conversion of chitin in the last decades, chemical approaches reign supreme over enzymatic approaches on an industrial level. Green technologies are held back by excessive production costs of high-quality enzymes and the lower yields in comparison to chemical means of processing. The high crystallinity levels of native chitin in aqueous solution pose an addition challenge that requires a more sustainable pretreatment strategy in the long term. While some processive-acting chitinases, e.g., from the well-understood model organism *S. marcescens*, can depolymerise crystalline chitin, this ability comes with the cost of low conversion rates [50].

To overcome low yields, one promising route is to genetically engineer and thus optimize chitinolytic enzymes. Limón et al. illustrated how the fusion of a cellulose-binding domain to the fungal *Trichoderma harzianum* chitinases Chit33 and Chit42, respectively, increased the substrate-binding capacities which led to higher depolymerisation rates and anti-fungal activities [179,180]. Following studies deepened our understanding of the importance of carbohydrate-binding domains and enzyme–substrate interaction strength for the conversion of recalcitrant chitin [181–183].

Directed evolution has also been identified as an efficient method to generate chitinases with enhanced properties. Through error-prone PCR and DNA shuffling, mutant gene libraries are assembled and sequentially screened for chitinolytic activity. Fan et al. targeted the fungal *Beauveria bassiana* chitinase Bbchit1 using this method. Unexpectedly, they observed higher conversion rates for two Bbchit1 variants with point mutations outside the enzymatic substrate binding site [184]. Songsiriritthigul et al. proceeded similarly by mutant library construction and DNA shuffling of two chitinase genes from *B. licheniformis* with 99% identical sequence, obtaining one mutant with up to 2.7-fold improved activity towards colloidal chitin in comparison to wild-type variants, depending on pH [185].

A successful COS in vitro synthesis will most likely consist of several different enzymes combined, yet the complex enzymatic interactions of such a multi-step approach is still poorly understood and has to be further elucidated. Mekasha et al. examined the optimal enzyme ratios of a five mono-component cocktail for the complete saccharification of shrimp and crab chitins in their pioneering work. The cocktail incorporated the *S. marcescens* chitinases *Sm*ChitA, *Sm*ChitB, and

*Sm*ChitC, a LPMO, and a β-N-acetylhexosaminidase [186]. The optimised cocktail yielded significantly higher chitin saccharification yields (70%) in comparison to a minimal *Sm*ChitA and *Sm*ChitB cocktail (40%). Moreover, different *Sm*ChitB to SmChitC ratios turned out to be beneficial for effective hydrolysation of the respective shrimp or crab chitins, while the *Sm*ChitA content of 40% was shared between both optimised cocktails. Further investigations into synergistic kinetics of chitin-targeting enzymes will be critical in developing a method to produce COS directly from crustacean shell wastes. One cannot emphasize enough the utmost importance of LPMOs for the degradation of crystalline chitin sources in the future, as they might represent the key protein class to solve both issues of recalcitrant substrate pretreatment and low efficiency of chitinases at the same time in a sustainable manner.

Intensive research efforts of the recent past allowed discovery of more chitinolytic enzymes, which also led to an increased understanding of their modes of action. As a result a new sort of novel class of chitinases has emerged—broad-specificity chitinases, which might contribute a lot to the cost reduction [187]. At present, only eight enzymes are reported to exhibit two to three different modes of chitin processing at the same time (with exochitinase, endochitinase, and β-N-acetylhexosaminidase activity being the different options). These can be categorised into single catalytic domain and multi-catalytic domain chitinases. Hence, either one catalytic site is able to perform multiple catalytic activities or several catalytic regions with distinct action modes toward chitin exist. In line with these findings, Hegsett et al. reported the *Streptomyces coelicolor* chitosanase A3(2) with potential activity towards all β-1,4-O-glycosidic linkages [87]. Further understanding of the mechanisms of broad-specificity glycosyl hydrolases like these might render the application of several abundant enzymes obsolete, therefore reducing production costs dramatically. To complicate things even more, chitinases of the GH18 family with secondary transglycosylating activities have been unravelled. Since COS production with the support of crude enzyme mixes or chitinases results in mostly small DP 1–3 fragments, TG-chitinases coupled with chitin deacetylases (CDA) might pose the missing link in recovering paCOS with higher M_w and a P_A and D_D of choice out of GlcNAc. Martinez et al. were able to supress the chitinolytic activity of a fungal *Trichoderma atroviride* chitinase with TG capabilities through site-directed mutagenesis [188]. This effort solved the persistent issue of product self-hydrolysation and represents an interesting new tool for COS engineering, as the in vitro polymerisation of longer chitin- and chitosan-oligomers circumvents the complex high DP COS production through hydrolases.

Another method, which was largely neglected with few exceptions [189,190], is the solid state fermentation. A recent study indicated that nearly dry conditions might be beneficial for the enzyme activity of chitinases, as this mirrors natural conditions for terrestrial chitinolytic organisms [189]. Therien and colleagues developed a self-proclaimed RAging method, in which they alternated between ball-mill grinding of shrimp and crab shells already containing a commercial chitinase mix, with resting periods at 45 °C for 20 times. Only those with diluted acetic-acid-pretreated chitin sources could be converted into GlcNAc with a conversion rate of at least 40% without the necessity of solvents.

Lastly, the center of attention has revolved around aerobic glycosyl hydrolase producers for a long time, while anaerobic organisms represent mainly unknown territory to date. This is despite the fact that aeration in industrial large-scale fermentations has to be carefully monitored and represents a cost factor, while very promising studies with anaerobic fermentations have been conducted [20] and the role of maritime organisms for the natural recycling of crustacean wastes is undisputed [191].

With the recent findings of more and more chitin-directed enzyme classes like TG-chitinases, broad specificity chitinases and chitosanases, LMPO, CDA, and COD, paired with an increased understanding of their mechanisms in addition to the development of cheap and easy analysis methods for COS [178], all parts of the puzzle seem to be complete. The last stepping stone for the sustainable conversion of natural chitin waste streams is to piece all these puzzles pieces together into a method that is suitable for large-scale applications. Regarding product specificity and quality, enzymatic approaches surpassed chemical means of chitin processing years ago, and the economic reasons that prevent the prevalent application of biotechnological methods in the industry might be resolved in the near future.

Supplementary Materials: The following are available online at http://www.mdpi.com/1660-3397/18/2/93/s1.

Author Contributions: N.D.A., T.B.B., W.M.B., and D.G. developed the concept for the manuscript; N.D.A. drafted the manuscript and figures, T.B.B., W.M.B., and D.G. corrected and finalized the manuscript together with N.D.A. All authors have read and agreed to the published version of the manuscript.

Funding: This research was funded by the German Ministry for Education and Research with the grant number 031B0838B. T.B.B. gratefully acknowledges funding of the Werner Siemens Foundation for the opportunity to establish the new research field of Synthetic Biotechnology at TUM.

Conflicts of Interest: The authors do not declare any conflict of interest.

References

1. Tharanathan, R.N.; Kittur, F.S. Chitin–the undisputed biomolecule of great potential. *Crit. Rev. Food Sci. Nutr.* **2003**, *43*, 61–87. [CrossRef]
2. Shirai, K.; Guerrero, I.; Huerta, S.; Saucedo, G.; Castillo, A.; Gonzalez, R.O.; Hall, G.M. Effect of initial glucose concentration and inoculation level of lactic acid bacteria in shrimp waste ensilation. *Enzym. Microb. Technol.* **2001**, *28*, 446–452. [CrossRef]
3. Dhillon, G.S.; Kaur, S.; Brar, S.K.; Verma, M. Green synthesis approach: Extraction of chitosan from fungus mycelia. *Crit. Rev. Biotechnol.* **2013**, *33*, 379–403. [CrossRef] [PubMed]
4. Younes, I.; Rinaudo, M. Chitin and Chitosan Preparation from Marine Sources. Structure, Properties and Applications. *Mar. Drugs* **2015**, *13*, 1133–1174. [CrossRef] [PubMed]
5. Beaney, P.; Lizardi-Mendoza, J.; Healy, M. Comparison of chitins produced by chemical and bioprocessing methods. *J. Chem. Technol. Biotechnol.* **2005**, *80*, 145–150. [CrossRef]
6. Blair, H.S.; Ho, T.-C. Studies in the adsorption and diffusion of ions in chitosan. *J. Chem. Technol. Biotechnol. Biotechnol.* **2007**, *31*, 6–10. [CrossRef]
7. Weinhold, M.X.; Sauvageau, J.C.; Kumirska, J.; Thöming, J. Studies on acetylation patterns of different chitosan preparations. *Carbohydr. Polym.* **2009**, *78*, 678–684. [CrossRef]
8. Omara, N.; Elsebaie, E.; Kassab, H.; Salama, A. Production of chitosan from shrimp shells by microwave technique and its use in minced beef preservation. *Slov. Veter. Res.* **2019**, *56*, 773–780. [CrossRef]
9. El Knidri, H.; El Khalfaouy, R.; Laajeb, A.; Addaou, A.; Lahsini, A. Eco-friendly extraction and characterization of chitin and chitosan from the shrimp shell waste via microwave irradiation. *Process. Saf. Environ. Prot.* **2016**, *104*, 395–405. [CrossRef]
10. Healy, M.; Green, A.; Healy, A. Bioprocessing of Marine Crustacean Shell Waste. *Acta Biotechnol.* **2003**, *23*, 151–160. [CrossRef]
11. Hajji, S.; Ghorbel-Bellaaj, O.; Younes, I.; Jellouli, K.; Nasri, M. Chitin extraction from crab shells by Bacillus bacteria. Biological activities of fermented crab supernatants. *Int. J. Boil. Macromol.* **2015**, *79*, 167–173. [CrossRef] [PubMed]
12. A Cira, L.; Huerta, S.; Hall, G.M.; Shirai, K. Pilot scale lactic acid fermentation of shrimp wastes for chitin recovery. *Process. Biochem.* **2002**, *37*, 1359–1366. [CrossRef]
13. Harkin, C.; Lynch, C.; Brück, W. Isolation & identification of bacteria for the treatment of brown crab (Cancer pagurus) waste to produce chitinous material. *J. Appl. Microbiol.* **2015**, *118*, 954–965. [PubMed]
14. Xu, Y.; Gallert, C.; Winter, J. Chitin purification from shrimp wastes by microbial deproteination and decalcification. *Appl. Microbiol. Biotechnol.* **2008**, *79*, 687–697. [CrossRef]
15. Castro, R.; Guerrero-Legarreta, I.; Bórquez, R. Chitin extraction from Allopetrolisthes punctatus crab using lactic fermentation. *Biotechnol. Rep.* **2018**, *20*, e00287. [CrossRef]
16. Jung, W.J.; Jo, G.H.; Kuk, J.H.; Kim, K.Y.; Park, R.D. Extraction of chitin from red crab shell waste by cofermentation with Lactobacillus paracasei subsp. tolerans KCTC-3074 and Serratia marcescens FS-3. *Appl. Microbiol. Biotechnol.* **2006**, *71*, 234–237. [CrossRef]
17. Zhang, H.; Jin, Y.; Deng, Y.; Wang, D.; Zhao, Y. Production of chitin from shrimp shell powders using Serratia marcescens B742 and Lactobacillus plantarum ATCC 8014 successive two-step fermentation. *Carbohydr. Res.* **2012**, *362*, 13–20. [CrossRef]

18. Liu, P.; Liu, S.; Guo, N.; Mao, X.; Lin, H.; Xue, C.; Wei, D. Cofermentation of Bacillus licheniformis and Gluconobacter oxydans for chitin extraction from shrimp waste. *Biochem. Eng. J.* **2014**, *91*, 10–15. [CrossRef]
19. Kaur, S.; Dhillon, G.S. Recent trends in biological extraction of chitin from marine shell wastes: A review. *Crit. Rev. Biotechnol.* **2013**, *35*, 44–61. [CrossRef]
20. Bajaj, M.; Freiberg, A.; Winter, J.; Xu, Y.; Gallert, C. Pilot-scale chitin extraction from shrimp shell waste by deproteination and decalcification with bacterial enrichment cultures. *Appl. Microbiol. Biotechnol.* **2015**, *99*, 9835–9846. [CrossRef]
21. Sarai, S.; Ram, A.; Peña-chora, G.; Hern, M. Enhanced Tolerance against a Fungal Pathogen and Insect Resistance in Transgenic Tobacco Plants Overexpressing an Endochitinase Gene from Serratia marcescens. *Int. J. Mol. Sci.* **2019**, *20*. [CrossRef]
22. Park, B.K.; Kim, M.-M. Applications of Chitin and Its Derivatives in Biological Medicine. *Int. J. Mol. Sci.* **2010**, *11*, 5152–5164. [CrossRef]
23. Dutta, P.K.; Duta, J.; Tripathi, V.S. Chitin and Chitosan: Chemistry, properties and applications. *J. Sci. Ind. Res.* **2004**, *63*, 20–31.
24. Harikrishnan, R.; Kim, J.-S.; Balasundaram, C.; Heo, M.-S. Dietary supplementation with chitin and chitosan on haematology and innate immune response in Epinephelus bruneus against Philasterides dicentrarchi. *Exp. Parasitol.* **2012**, *131*, 116–124. [CrossRef] [PubMed]
25. Rhee, J.-S.; Jung, M.-W.; Paeng, K.-J. Evaluation of Chitin and Chitosan as a Sorbent for the Preconcentration of Phenol and Chlorophenols in Water. *Anal. Sci.* **1998**, *14*, 1089–1092. [CrossRef]
26. Bloch, R.; Burger, M.M. Purification of wheat germ agglutinin using affinity chromatography on chitin. *Biochem. Biophys. Res. Commun.* **1974**, *58*, 13–19. [CrossRef]
27. Bartnicki-Garcia, S.; Nickerson, W.J. Isolation, composition, and structure of cell walls of filamentous and yeast-like forms of Mucor rouxii. *Biochim. Biophys. Acta* **1962**, *58*, 102–119. [CrossRef]
28. Younes, I.; Hajji, S.; Frachet, V.; Rinaudo, M.; Jellouli, K.; Nasri, M. Chitin extraction from shrimp shell using enzymatic treatment. Antitumor, antioxidant and antimicrobial activities of chitosan. *Int. J. Boil. Macromol.* **2014**, *69*, 489–498. [CrossRef]
29. Xia, W.; Liu, P.; Zhang, J.; Chen, J. Biological activities of chitosan and chitooligosaccharides. *Food Hydrocoll.* **2011**, *25*, 170–179. [CrossRef]
30. Goy, R.C.; De Britto, D.; Assis, O.B.G. A review of the antimicrobial activity of chitosan. *Polímeros* **2009**, *19*, 241–247. [CrossRef]
31. Rinaudo, M. Chitin and chitosan: Properties and applications. *Prog. Polym. Sci.* **2006**, *31*, 603–632. [CrossRef]
32. Sorlier, P.; Denuzière, A.; Viton, C.; Domard, A. Relation between the degree of acetylation and the electrostatic properties of chitin and chitosan. *Biomacromolecules* **2001**, *2*, 765–772. [CrossRef] [PubMed]
33. Chung, Y.-C.; Su, Y.-P.; Chen, C.-C.; Jia, G.; Wang, H.-L.; Wu, J.C.G.; Lin, J.-G. Relationship between antibacterial activity of chitosan and surface characteristics of cell wall. *Acta Pharmacol. Sin.* **2004**, *25*, 932–936. [PubMed]
34. Aam, B.B.; Heggset, E.B.; Norberg, A.L.; Sørlie, M.; Vårum, K.M.; Eijsink, V.G.H. Production of Chitooligosaccharides and Their Potential Applications in Medicine. *Mar. Drugs* **2010**, *8*, 1482–1517. [CrossRef] [PubMed]
35. Lodhi, G.; Kim, Y.-S.; Hwang, J.-W.; Kim, S.-K.; Jeon, Y.-J.; Je, J.-Y.; Ahn, C.-B.; Moon, S.-H.; Jeon, B.-T.; Park, P.-J. Chitooligosaccharide and Its Derivatives: Preparation and Biological Applications. *BioMed Res. Int.* **2014**, *2014*, 1–13. [CrossRef] [PubMed]
36. Liaqat, F.; Eltem, R. Chitooligosaccharides and their biological activities: A comprehensive review. *Carbohydr. Polym.* **2018**, *184*, 243–259. [CrossRef]
37. Kim, S.-K.; Rajapakse, N. Enzymatic production and biological activities of chitosan oligosaccharides (COS): A review. *Carbohydr. Polym.* **2005**, *62*, 357–368. [CrossRef]
38. Bahrke, S. Mass Spectrometric Analysis of Chitooligosachharides and their Interaction with proteins. Ph.D. Thesis, Universität Potsdam, Potsdam, Germany, 2008; pp. 1–232.
39. Elieh-Ali-Komi, D.; Hamblin, M.R. Chitin and Chitosan: Production and Application of Versatile Biomedical Nanomaterials. *Int. J. Adv. Res.* **2016**, *4*, 411–427.
40. Hamed, I.; Özogul, F.; Regenstein, J.M. Industrial applications of crustacean by-products (chitin, chitosan, and chitooligosaccharides): A review. *Trends Food Sci. Technol.* **2016**, *48*, 40–50. [CrossRef]

41. Casadidio, C.; Peregrina, D.V.; Gigliobianco, M.R.; Deng, S.; Censi, R.; Di Martino, P. Chitin and Chitosans: Characteristics, Eco-Friendly Processes, and Applications in Cosmetic Science. *Mar. Drugs* **2019**, *17*, 369. [CrossRef]
42. Malerba, M.; Cerana, R. Recent Advances of Chitosan Applications in Plants. *Polym.* **2018**, *10*, 118. [CrossRef] [PubMed]
43. Thadathil, N.; Velappan, S.P. Recent developments in chitosanase research and its biotechnological applications: A review. *Food Chem.* **2014**, *150*, 392–399. [CrossRef] [PubMed]
44. Kaczmarek, M.B.; Struszczyk-Swita, K.; Li, X.; Szczęsna-Antczak, M.; Daroch, M. Enzymatic Modifications of Chitin, Chitosan, and Chitooligosaccharides. *Front. Bioeng. Biotechnol.* **2019**, *7*, 243. [CrossRef] [PubMed]
45. Gómez-Ríos, D.; Barrera-Zapata, R.; Ríos-Estepa, R. Comparison of process technologies for chitosan production from shrimp shell waste: A techno-economic approach using Aspen Plus ®. *Food Bioprod. Process.* **2017**, *103*, 49–57. [CrossRef]
46. Yan, N.; Chen, X. Sustainability: Don't waste seafood waste. *Nature* **2015**, *524*, 155–157. [CrossRef] [PubMed]
47. Van Aalten, D.M.F.; Komander, D.; Synstad, B.; Gåseidnes, S.; Peter, M.G.; Eijsink, V.G.H. Structural insights into the catalytic mechanism of a family 18 exo-chitinase. *Proc. Natl. Acad. Sci. USA* **2001**, *98*, 8979–8984. [CrossRef]
48. Hamre, A.G.; Frøberg, E.E.; Eijsink, V.G.; Sørlie, M. Thermodynamics of tunnel formation upon substrate binding in a processive glycoside hydrolase. *Arch. Biochem. Biophys.* **2017**, *620*, 35–42. [CrossRef]
49. Davies, G.; Henrissat, B. Structures and mechanisms of glycosyl hydrolases. *Structure* **1995**, *3*, 853–859. [CrossRef]
50. Zakariassen, H.; Aam, B.B.; Horn, S.J.; Vårum, K.M.; Sørlie, M.; Eijsink, V.G.H. Aromatic Residues in the Catalytic Center of Chitinase A from Serratia marcescens Affect Processivity, Enzyme Activity, and Biomass Converting Efficiency. *J. Boil. Chem.* **2009**, *284*, 10610–10617. [CrossRef]
51. Oyeleye, A.; Normi, Y.M. Chitinase: Diversity, limitations, and trends in engineering for suitable applications. *Biosci. Rep.* **2018**, *38*, 1–21. [CrossRef]
52. Slámová, K.; Bojarová, P.; Petrásková, L.; Křen, V. β-N-Acetylhexosaminidase: What's in a name...? *Biotechnol. Adv.* **2010**, *28*, 682–693. [CrossRef] [PubMed]
53. Sikorski, P.; Sørbotten, A.; Horn, S.J.; Eijsink, V.G.H.; Vårum, K.M. Serratia marcescens chitinases with tunnel-shaped substrate-binding grooves show endo activity and different degrees of processivity during enzymatic hydrolysis of chitosan. *Biochemistry* **2006**, *45*, 9566–9574. [CrossRef] [PubMed]
54. Lin, S.B.; Chen, S.H.; Peng, K.C. Preparation of antibacterial chito-oligosaccharide by altering the degree of deacetylation of β-chitosan in a Trichoderma harzianum chitinase-hydrolysing process. *J. Sci. Food Agric.* **2009**, *89*, 238–244. [CrossRef]
55. Eweis, M.; Elkholy, S.; Elsabee, M. Antifungal efficacy of chitosan and its thiourea derivatives upon the growth of some sugar-beet pathogens. *Int. J. Boil. Macromol.* **2006**, *38*, 1–8. [CrossRef]
56. Tikhonov, V.E.; Stepnova, E.A.; Babak, V.G.; Yamskov, I.A.; Palma-Guerrero, J.; Jansson, H.-B.; Lopez-Llorca, L.V.; Salinas, J.; Gerasimenko, D.V.; Avdienko, I.D.; et al. Bactericidal and antifungal activities of a low molecular weight chitosan and its N-/2(3)-(dodec-2-enyl)succinoyl/-derivatives. *Carbohydr. Polym.* **2006**, *64*, 66–72. [CrossRef]
57. Ribeiro, M.P.; Espiga, A.; Silva, D.; Henriques, J.; Ferreira, C.; Silva, J.C.; Pires, E.; Chaves, P. Development of a new chitosan hydrogel for wound dressing. *Wound Repair Regen.* **2009**, *17*, 817–824. [CrossRef] [PubMed]
58. You, Y.; Park, W.H.; Ko, B.M.; Min, B.-M. Effects of PVA sponge containing chitooligosaccharide in the early stage of wound healing. *J. Mater. Sci. Mater. Electron.* **2004**, *15*, 297–301. [CrossRef]
59. Dai, T.; Tanaka, M.; Huang, Y.-Y.; Hamblin, M.R. Chitosan preparations for wounds and burns: antimicrobial and wound-healing effects. *Expert Rev. Anti-Infect. Ther.* **2011**, *9*, 857–879. [CrossRef]
60. Köping-Höggård, M.; Mel'nikova, Y.S.; Vårum, K.M.; Lindman, B.; Artursson, P. Relationship between the physical shape and the efficiency of oligomeric chitosan as a gene delivery system in vitro and in vivo. *J. Gene Med.* **2003**, *5*, 130–141. [CrossRef]
61. Köping-Höggård, M.; Tubulekas, I.; Guan, H.; Edwards, K.; Nilsson, M.; Vårum, K.M.; Artursson, P. Chitosan as a nonviral gene delivery system. Structure–property relationships and characteristics compared with polyethylenimine in vitro and after lung administration in vivo. *Gene Ther.* **2001**, *8*, 1108–1121. [CrossRef]

62. Strand, S.P.; Lélu, S.; Reitan, N.K.; Davies, C.D.L.; Artursson, P.; Vårum, K.M. Molecular design of chitosan gene delivery systems with an optimized balance between polyplex stability and polyplex unpacking. *Biomaterials* **2010**, *31*, 975–987. [CrossRef] [PubMed]
63. Wang, Z.; Zheng, L.; Yang, S.; Niu, R.; Chu, E.; Lin, X. N-Acetylchitooligosaccharide is a potent angiogenic inhibitor both in vivo and in vitro. *Biochem. Biophys. Res. Commun.* **2007**, *357*, 26–31. [CrossRef] [PubMed]
64. Xiong, C.; Wu, H.; Wei, P.; Pan, M.; Tuo, Y.; Kusakabe, I.; Du, Y. Potent angiogenic inhibition effects of deacetylated chitohexaose separated from chitooligosaccharides and its mechanism of action in vitro. *Carbohydr. Res.* **2009**, *344*, 1975–1983. [CrossRef] [PubMed]
65. Li, X.; Min, M.; Du, N.; Gu, Y.; Hode, T.; Naylor, M.; Chen, D.; Nordquist, R.E.; Chen, W.R. Chitin, Chitosan, and Glycated Chitosan Regulate Immune Responses: The Novel Adjuvants for Cancer Vaccine. *Clin. Dev. Immunol.* **2013**, *2013*, 1–8. [CrossRef]
66. Purushotham, P.; Podile, A.R. Synthesis of Long-Chain Chitooligosaccharides by a Hypertransglycosylating Processive Endochitinase of Serratia proteamaculans 568. *J. Bacteriol.* **2012**, *194*, 4260–4271. [CrossRef]
67. Madhuprakash, J.; Singh, A.; Kumar, S.; Sinha, M.; Kaur, P.; Sharma, S.; Podile, A.R.; Singh, T.P. Structure of chitinase D from Serratia proteamaculans reveals the structural basis of its dual action of hydrolysis and transglycosylation. *Int. J. Biochem. Mol. Boil.* **2013**, *4*, 166–178.
68. Mallakuntla, M.K.; Vaikuntapu, P.R.; Bhuvanachandra, B.; Das, S.N.; Podile, A.R. Transglycosylation by a chitinase from Enterobacter cloacae subsp. cloacae generates longer chitin oligosaccharides. *Sci. Rep.* **2017**, *7*, 5113. [CrossRef]
69. Bojarová, P.; Kren, V. Glycosidases: A key to tailored carbohydrates. *Trends Biotechnol.* **2009**, *27*, 199–209. [CrossRef]
70. Mangas-Sanchez, J.; Adlercreutz, P. Enzymatic preparation of oligosaccharides by transglycosylation: A comparative study of glucosidases. *J. Mol. Catal. B Enzym.* **2015**, *122*, 51–55. [CrossRef]
71. Tanaka, T.; Fukui, T.; Atomi, H.; Imanaka, T. Characterization of an Exo-ß-D-Glucosaminidase Involved in a Novel Chitnolytic Pathway from the Hyperthermophilic Archaeon Thermococcus kodakaraensis KOD1. *J. Bacteriol.* **2003**, *185*, 5175–5181. [CrossRef]
72. Fukamizo, T.; Fleury, A.; Côté, N.; Mitsutomi, M.; Brzezinski, R. Exo-β-d-glucosaminidase from Amycolatopsis orientalis: catalytic residues, sugar recognition specificity, kinetics, and synergism. *Glycobiology* **2006**, *16*, 1064–1072. [CrossRef] [PubMed]
73. Viens, P.; Lacombe-Harvey, M.-È.; Brzezinski, R. Chitosanases from Family 46 of Glycoside Hydrolases: From Proteins to Phenotypes. *Mar. Drugs* **2015**, *13*, 6566–6587. [CrossRef] [PubMed]
74. Tremblay, H.; Yamaguchi, T.; Fukamizo, T.; Brzezinski, R. Mechanism of chitosanase-oligosaccharide interaction: Subsite structure of Streptomyces sp. N174 chitosanase and the role of Asp57 carboxylate. *J. Biochem.* **2001**, *130*, 679–686. [CrossRef] [PubMed]
75. Fukamizo, T.; Amano, S.; Yamaguchi, K.; Yoshikawa, T.; Katsumi, T.; Saito, J.-I.; Suzuki, M.; Miki, K.; Nagata, Y.; Ando, A. Bacillus circulans MH-K1 Chitosanase: Amino Acid Residues Responsible for Substrate Binding. *J. Biochem.* **2005**, *138*, 563–569. [CrossRef] [PubMed]
76. Saito, J.-I.; Kita, A.; Higuchi, Y.; Nagata, Y.; Ando, A.; Miki, K. Crystal structure of chitosanase from Bacillus circulans MH-K1 at 1.6-A resolution and its substrate recognition mechanism. *J. Boil. Chem.* **1999**, *274*, 30818–30825. [CrossRef] [PubMed]
77. Marcotte, E.M.; Monzingo, A.F.; Ernst, S.R.; Brzezinski, R.; Robertas, J.D. X-ray structure of an anti-fungal chitosanase from streptomyces N174. *Nat. Genet.* **1996**, *3*, 155–162. [CrossRef]
78. Monzingo, A.F.; Marcotte, E.M.; Hart, P.J.; Robertas, J.D. Chitinases, chitosanases, and lysozymes can be divided into procaryotic and eucaryotic families sharing a conserved core. *Nat. Genet.* **1996**, *3*, 133–140. [CrossRef]
79. Cheng, C.Y.; Chang, C.H.; Wu, Y.J.; Li, Y.K. Exploration of glycosyl hydrolase family 75, a chitosanase from Aspergillus fumigatus. *J. Biol. Chem.* **2006**, *281*, 3137–3144. [CrossRef]
80. Hoell, I.A.; Vaaje-Kolstad, G.; Eijsink, V.G. Structure and function of enzymes acting on chitin and chitosan. *Biotechnol. Genet. Eng. Rev.* **2010**, *27*, 331–366. [CrossRef]
81. McCarter, J.D.; Withers, G.S. Mechanisms of enzymatic glycoside hydrolysis. *Curr. Opin. Struct. Boil.* **1994**, *4*, 885–892. [CrossRef]

82. McIntosh, L.P.; Hand, G.; Johnson, P.E.; Joshi, M.D.; Körner, M.; Plesniak, L.A.; Ziser, L.; Wakarchuk, W.W.; Withers, S.G. The pK(a) of the general acid/base carboxyl group of a glycosidase cycles during catalysis: A 13C-NMR study of Bacillus circulans xylanase. *Biochemistry* **1996**, *35*, 9958–9966. [CrossRef] [PubMed]
83. Fukamizo, T.; Ohkawa, T.; Ikeda, Y.; Goto, S. Specificity of chitosanase from Bacillus pumilus. *Biochim. Biophys. Acta (BBA) Protein Struct. Mol. Enzym.* **1994**, *1205*, 183–188. [CrossRef]
84. Mitsutomi, M.; Isono, M.; Uchiyama, A.; Nikaidou, N.; Ikegami, T.; Watanabe, T. Chitosanase activity of the enzyme previously reported as β-1,3-1,4-glucanase from Bacillus circulans WL-12. *Biosci. Biotechnol. Biochem.* **1998**, *62*, 2107–2114. [CrossRef] [PubMed]
85. Fenton, D.M.; Eveleigh, D.E. Purification and Mode of Action of a Chitosanase from Penicillium islandicum. *Microbiology* **1981**, *126*, 151–165. [CrossRef]
86. Hirano, K.; Watanabe, M.; Seki, K.; Ando, A.; Saito, A.; Mitsutomi, M. Classification of Chitosanases by Hydrolytic Specificity towardN1,N4-Diacetylchitohexaose. *Biosci. Biotechnol. Biochem.* **2012**, *76*, 1932–1937. [CrossRef]
87. Heggset, E.B.; Dybvik, A.I.; Hoell, I.A.; Norberg, A.L.; Sørlie, M.; Eijsink, V.G.H.; Vårum, K.M. Degradation of Chitosans with a Family 46 Chitosanase fromStreptomyces coelicolorA3(2). *Biomacromolecules* **2010**, *11*, 2487–2497. [CrossRef]
88. Zhao, Y.; Park, R.-D.; Muzzarelli, R.A.A. Chitin Deacetylases: Properties and Applications. *Mar. Drugs* **2010**, *8*, 24–46. [CrossRef]
89. Blair, D.E.; Schüttelkopf, A.W.; Macrae, J.I.; Van Aalten, D.M.F. Structure and metal-dependent mechanism of peptidoglycan deacetylase, a streptococcal virulence factor. *Proc. Natl. Acad. Sci. USA* **2005**, *102*, 15429–15434. [CrossRef]
90. Araki, Y.; Ito, E. A Pathway of Chitosan Formation in Mucor rouxii. Enzymatic Deacetylation of Chitin. *JBIC J. Boil. Inorg. Chem.* **1975**, *55*, 71–78. [CrossRef]
91. Tsigos, I.; Martinou, A.; Kafetzopoulos, D.; Bouriotis, V. Chitin deacetylases: New, versatile tools in biotechnology. *Trends Biotechnol.* **2000**, *18*, 305–312. [CrossRef]
92. Martinou, A.; Bouriotis, V.; Stokke, B.T.; Vårum, K.M. Mode of action of chitin deacetylase from Mucor rouxii on partially N-acetylated chitosans. *Carbohydr. Res.* **1998**, *311*, 71–78. [CrossRef]
93. Hekmat, O.; Tokuyasu, K.; Withers, S.G. Subsite structure of the endo-type chitin deacetylase from a Deuteromycete, Colletotrichum lindemuthianum: An investigation using steady-state kinetic analysis and MS. *Biochem. J.* **2003**, *374*, 369–380. [CrossRef]
94. Grifoll-Romero, L.; Pascual, S.; Aragunde, H.; Biarnés, X.; Planas, A. Chitin Deacetylases: Structures, Specificities, and Biotech Applications. *Polymers* **2018**, *10*, 352. [CrossRef]
95. Aronson, N.N.; Halloran, B.A.; Alexyev, M.F.; Amable, L.; Madura, J.D.; Pasupulati, L.; Worth, C.; Van Roey, P. Family 18 chitinase–oligosaccharide substrate interaction: Subsite preference and anomer selectivity of Serratia marcescens chitinase A. *Biochem. J.* **2003**, *376*, 87–95. [CrossRef]
96. Zhang, H.; Zhao, Y.; Cao, H.; Mou, G.; Yin, H. Expression and characterization of a lytic polysaccharide monooxygenase from Bacillus thuringiensis. *Int. J. Boil. Macromol.* **2015**, *79*, 72–75. [CrossRef]
97. Blair, D.E.; Hekmat, O.; Schüttelkopf, A.W.; Shrestha, B.; Tokuyasu, K.; Withers, S.G.; Van Aalten, D.M.F. Structure and Mechanism of Chitin Deacetylase from the Fungal PathogenColletotrichum lindemuthianum. *Biochemistry* **2006**, *45*, 9416–9426. [CrossRef]
98. Liu, Z.; Gay, L.M.; Tuveng, T.R.; Agger, J.W.; Westereng, B.; Mathiesen, G.; Horn, S.J.; Vaaje-Kolstad, G.; Van Aalten, D.M.F.; Eijsink, V.G.H. Structure and function of a broad-specificity chitin deacetylase from Aspergillus nidulans FGSC A4. *Sci. Rep.* **2017**, *7*, 1746. [CrossRef] [PubMed]
99. Hoßbach, J.; Bußwinkel, F.; Kranz, A.; Wattjes, J.; Cord-Landwehr, S.; Moerschbacher, B.M. A chitin deacetylase of Podospora anserina has two functional chitin binding domains and a unique mode of action. *Carbohydr. Polym.* **2018**, *183*, 1–10. [CrossRef] [PubMed]
100. Vaaje-Kolstad, G.; Forsberg, Z.; Loose, J.S.; Bissaro, B.; Eijsink, V.G. Structural diversity of lytic polysaccharide monooxygenases. *Curr. Opin. Struct. Boil.* **2017**, *44*, 67–76. [CrossRef] [PubMed]
101. Tandrup, T.; Frandsen, K.E.H.; Johansen, K.S.; Berrin, J.-G.; Leggio, L.L. Recent insights into lytic polysaccharide monooxygenases (LPMOs). *Biochem. Soc. Trans.* **2018**, *46*, 1431–1447. [CrossRef] [PubMed]
102. Crouch, L.I.; Labourel, A.; Walton, P.H.; Davies, G.J.; Gilbert, H.J. The Contribution of Non-catalytic Carbohydrate Binding Modules to the Activity of Lytic Polysaccharide Monooxygenases. *J. Boil. Chem.* **2016**, *291*, 7439–7449. [CrossRef]

103. Hansson, H.; Karkehabadi, S.; Mikkelsen, N.; Douglas, N.R.; Kim, S.; Lam, A.; Kaper, T.; Kelemen, B.; Meier, K.K.; Jones, S.M.; et al. High-resolution structure of a lytic polysaccharide monooxygenase from Hypocrea jecorina reveals a predicted linker as an integral part of the catalytic domain. *J. Boil. Chem.* **2017**, *292*, 19099–19109. [CrossRef] [PubMed]
104. Hangasky, J.A.; Marletta, M.A. A Random-Sequential Kinetic Mechanism for Polysaccharide Monooxygenases. *Biochemistry* **2018**, *57*, 3191–3199. [CrossRef] [PubMed]
105. Isaksen, T.; Westereng, B.; Aachmann, F.L.; Agger, J.W.; Kracher, D.; Kittl, R.; Ludwig, R.; Haltrich, D.; Eijsink, V.G.; Horn, S.J. A C4-oxidizing lytic polysaccharide monooxygenase cleaving both cellulose and cello-oligosaccharides. *J. Biol. Chem.* **2014**, *289*, 2632–2642. [CrossRef]
106. Vaaje-Kolstad, G.; Westereng, B.; Horn, S.J.; Liu, Z.; Zhai, H.; Sørlie, M.; Eijsink, V.G.H. An Oxidative Enzyme Boosting the Enzymatic Conversion of Recalcitrant Polysaccharides. *Science* **2010**, *330*, 219–222. [CrossRef]
107. Beeson, W.T.; Phillips, C.M.; Cate, J.H.D.; Marletta, M.A. Oxidative cleavage of cellulose by fungal copper-dependent polysaccharide monooxygenases. *J. Am. Chem. Soc.* **2012**, *134*, 890–892. [CrossRef]
108. Hangasky, J.A.; Iavarone, A.T.; Marletta, M.A. Reactivity of O2 versus H2O2 with polysaccharide monooxygenases. *Proc. Natl. Acad. Sci. USA* **2018**, *115*, 4915–4920. [CrossRef]
109. Bissaro, B.; Várnai, A.; Røhr, A.K.; Eijsink, V.G.H. Oxidoreductases and Reactive Oxygen Species in Conversion of Lignocellulosic Biomass. *Microbiol. Mol. Boil. Rev.* **2018**, *82*, e00029-18.
110. Hedegård, E.D.; Ryde, U. Molecular mechanism of lytic polysaccharide monooxygenases†. †Electronic supplementary information (ESI) available: Detailed description of the employed computational methods and protein setup. QM and MM energy components and B3LYP energies for most reaction paths. *Chem. Sci.* **2018**, *9*, 3866–3880. [CrossRef]
111. Bertini, L.; Breglia, R.; Lambrughi, M.; Fantucci, P.; De Gioia, L.; Borsari, M.; Sola, M.; Bortolotti, C.A.; Bruschi, M. Catalytic Mechanism of Fungal Lytic Polysaccharide Monooxygenases Investigated by First-Principles Calculations. *Inorg. Chem.* **2018**, *57*, 86–97. [CrossRef]
112. Hemsworth, G.R.; Davies, G.J.; Walton, P.H. Recent insights into copper-containing lytic polysaccharide mono-oxygenases. *Curr. Opin. Struct. Boil.* **2013**, *23*, 660–668. [CrossRef] [PubMed]
113. Bissaro, B.; Røhr, Å.K.; Müller, G.; Chylenski, P.; Skaugen, M.; Forsberg, Z.; Horn, S.J.; Vaaje-Kolstad, G.; Eijsink, V.G.H. Oxidative cleavage of polysaccharides by monocopper enzymes depends on H2O2. *Nat. Methods* **2017**, *13*, 1123–1128. [CrossRef] [PubMed]
114. Kuusk, S.; Bissaro, B.; Kuusk, P.; Forsberg, Z.; Eijsink, V.G.H.; Sørlie, M.; Väljamäe, P. Kinetics of H2O2-driven degradation of chitin by a bacterial lytic polysaccharide monooxygenase. *J. Boil. Chem.* **2018**, *293*, 12284. [CrossRef] [PubMed]
115. Gardner, J.G.; Crouch, L.; Labourel, A.; Forsberg, Z.; Bukhman, Y.V.; Gilbert, H.J.; Keating, D.H.; Vaaje-Kolstad, G. Systems biology defines the biological significance of redox-active proteins during cellulose degradation in an aerobic bacterium. *Mol. Microbiol.* **2014**, *94*, 1121–1133. [CrossRef] [PubMed]
116. Wang, B.; Johnston, E.M.; Li, P.; Shaik, S.; Davies, G.J.; Walton, P.H.H.; Rovira, C. QM/MM Studies into the H2O2-Dependent Activity of Lytic Polysaccharide Monooxygenases: Evidence for the Formation of a Caged Hydroxyl Radical Intermediate. *ACS Catal.* **2018**, *8*, 1346–1351. [CrossRef]
117. Cao, L.; Caladararu, O.; Rosenzweig, A.C.; Ryde, U. Quantum Refinement Does Not Support Dinuclear Copper Sites in Crystal Structures of Particulate Methane Monooxygenase. *Angew. Chem. Int. Ed. Engl.* **2018**, *57*, 162–166. [CrossRef]
118. Nakagawa, Y.S.; Oyama, Y.; Kon, N.; Nikaido, M.; Tanno, K.; Kogawa, J.; Inomata, S.; Masui, A.; Yamamura, A.; Kawaguchi, M.; et al. Development of innovative technologies to decrease the environmental burdens associated with using chitin as a biomass resource: Mechanochemical grinding and enzymatic degradation. *Carbohydr. Polym.* **2011**, *83*, 1843–1849. [CrossRef]
119. Jung, W.-J.; Park, R.-D. Bioproduction of Chitooligosaccharides: Present and Perspectives. *Mar. Drugs* **2014**, *12*, 5328–5356. [CrossRef]
120. Li, K.; Xing, R.; Liu, S.; Qin, Y.; Meng, X.; Li, P. Microwave-assisted degradation of chitosan for a possible use in inhibiting crop pathogenic fungi. *Int. J. Boil. Macromol.* **2012**, *51*, 767–773. [CrossRef]
121. Sahu, A.; Goswami, P.; Bora, U. Microwave mediated rapid synthesis of chitosan. *J. Mater. Sci. Mater. Med.* **2009**, *20*, 171–175. [CrossRef]

122. Hai, L.; Diep, T.B.; Nagasawa, N.; Yoshii, F.; Kume, T. Radiation depolymerization of chitosan to prepare oligomers. *Nucl. Instruments Methods Phys. Res. Sect. B Beam Interactions Mater. Atoms* **2003**, *208*, 466–470. [CrossRef]
123. Yoksan, R.; Akashi, M.; Miyata, M.; Chirachanchai, S. Optimal γ-Ray Dose and Irradiation Conditions for Producing Low-Molecular-Weight Chitosan that Retains its Chemical Structure. *Radiat. Res.* **2004**, *161*, 471–480. [CrossRef] [PubMed]
124. Xing, R.; Liu, S.; Yu, H.; Guo, Z.; Wang, P.; Li, C.; Li, Z.; Li, P. Salt-assisted acid hydrolysis of chitosan to oligomers under microwave irradiation. *Carbohydr. Res.* **2005**, *340*, 2150–2153. [CrossRef] [PubMed]
125. Villa-Lerma, G.; González-Márquez, H.; Gimeno, M.; López-Luna, A.; Bárzana, E.; Shirai, K. Ultrasonication and steam-explosion as chitin pretreatments for chitin oligosaccharide production by chitinases of Lecanicillium lecanii. *Bioresour. Technol.* **2013**, *146*, 794–798. [CrossRef]
126. Husson, E.; Hadad, C.; Huet, G.; Laclef, S.; Lesur, D.; Lambertyn, V.; Jamali, A.; Gottis, S.; Sarazin, C.; Van Nhien, A.N. The effect of room temperature ionic liquids on the selective biocatalytic hydrolysis of chitin via sequential or simultaneous strategies. *Green Chem.* **2017**, *19*, 4122–4131. [CrossRef]
127. Berton, P.; Shamshina, J.L.; Ostadjoo, S.; King, C.A.; Rogers, R.D. Enzymatic hydrolysis of ionic liquid-extracted chitin. *Carbohydr. Polym.* **2018**, *199*, 228–235. [CrossRef]
128. Zdanowicz, M.; Wilpiszewska, K.; Spychaj, T. Deep eutectic solvents for polysaccharides processing. A review. *Carbohydr. Polym.* **2018**, *200*, 361–380. [CrossRef]
129. Roda, A.; Matias, A.A.; Paiva, A.; Duarte, A.R.C. Polymer Science and Engineering Using Deep Eutectic Solvents. *Polymers* **2019**, *11*, 912. [CrossRef]
130. Dadi, A.P.; Schall, C.A.; Varanasi, S. Mitigation of cellulose recalcitrance to enzymatic hydrolysis by ionic liquid pretreatment. *Appl. Biochem. Biotechnol.* **2007**, *137*, 407–421.
131. Zhu, P.; Gu, Z.; Hong, S.; Lian, H. One-pot production of chitin with high purity from lobster shells using choline chloride–malonic acid deep eutectic solvent. *Carbohydr. Polym.* **2017**, *177*, 217–223. [CrossRef]
132. Hong, S.; Yuan, Y.; Yang, Q.; Zhu, P.; Lian, H. Versatile acid base sustainable solvent for fast extraction of various molecular weight chitin from lobster shell. *Carbohydr. Polym.* **2018**, *201*, 211–217. [CrossRef] [PubMed]
133. Einbu, A.; Vårum, K.M. Depolymerization and De-N-acetylation of Chitin Oligomers in Hydrochloric Acid. *Biomacromolecules* **2007**, *8*, 309–314. [CrossRef] [PubMed]
134. Einbu, A.; Vårum, K.M. Characterization of Chitin and Its Hydrolysis to GlcNAc and GlcN. *Biomacromolecules* **2008**, *9*, 1870–1875. [CrossRef] [PubMed]
135. Yamaguchi, R.; Arai, Y.; Itoh, T. A microfibril formation from depolymerized chitosan by N-acetylation. *Agric. Boil. Chem.* **1982**, *46*, 2379–2381.
136. Il'Ina, A.V.; Varlamov, V.P. Hydrolysis of chitosan in lactic acid. Прикладная биохимия и микробиология **2004**, *40*, 300–303. [CrossRef]
137. Tian, F.; Liu, Y.; Hu, K.; Zhao, B. Study of the depolymerization behavior of chitosan by hydrogen peroxide. *Carbohydr. Polym.* **2004**, *57*, 31–37. [CrossRef]
138. Prashanth, K.V.H.; Dharmesh, S.M.; Rao, K.S.J.; Tharanathan, R.N. Free radical-induced chitosan depolymerized products protect calf thymus DNA from oxidative damage. *Carbohydr. Res.* **2007**, *342*, 190–195. [CrossRef]
139. Trombotto, S.; Ladaviere, C.; Delolme, F.; Domard, A. Chemical Preparation and Structural Characterization of a Homogeneous Series of Chitin/Chitosan Oligomers. *Biomacromolecules* **2008**, *9*, 1731–1738. [CrossRef]
140. Mourya, V.K.; Inamdar, N.N.; Choudhari, Y.M. Chitooligosaccharides: Synthesis, characterization and applications. *Polym. Sci. Ser. A* **2011**, *53*, 583–612. [CrossRef]
141. Chylenski, P.; Petrović, D.M.; Müller, G.; Dahlström, M.; Bengtsson, O.; Lersch, M.; Siika-Aho, M.; Horn, S.J.; Eijsink, V.G.H. Enzymatic degradation of sulfite-pulped softwoods and the role of LPMOs. *Biotechnol. Biofuels* **2017**, *10*, 177. [CrossRef]
142. Müller, G.; Várnai, A.; Johansen, K.S.; Eijsink, V.G.H.; Horn, S.J. Harnessing the potential of LPMO-containing cellulase cocktails poses new demands on processing conditions. *Biotechnol. Biofuels* **2015**, *8*, 187. [CrossRef] [PubMed]
143. Wang, D.; Li, A.; Han, H.; Liu, T.; Yang, Q. A potent chitinase from Bacillus subtilis for the efficient bioconversion of chitin-containing wastes. *Int. J. Boil. Macromol.* **2018**, *116*, 863–868. [CrossRef] [PubMed]

144. Zhang, A.; Wei, G.; Mo, X.; Zhou, N.; Chen, K.; Ouyang, P. Enzymatic hydrolysis of chitin pretreated by bacterial fermentation to obtain pure N-acetyl-d-glucosamine. *Green Chem.* **2018**, *20*, 2320–2327. [CrossRef]
145. Naqvi, S.; Moerschbacher, B.M. The cell factory approach toward biotechnological production of high-value chitosan oligomers and their derivatives: An update. *Crit. Rev. Biotechnol.* **2017**, *37*, 11–25. [CrossRef]
146. Kadokawa, J.-I. Precision Polysaccharide Synthesis Catalyzed by Enzymes. *Chem. Rev.* **2011**, *111*, 4308–4345. [CrossRef]
147. Kobayashi, S.; Makino, A. Enzymatic Polymer Synthesis: An Opportunity for Green Polymer Chemistry. *Chem. Rev.* **2009**, *109*, 5288–5353. [CrossRef]
148. Samain, E.; Drouillard, S.; Heyraud, A.; Driguez, H.; Geremia, R.A. Gram-scale synthesis of recombinant chitooligosaccharides in Escherichia coli. *Carbohydr. Res.* **1997**, *302*, 35–42. [CrossRef]
149. Biely, P.; Kratky, Z.; Vrsanska, M. Substrate-Binding Site of Endo-1,4-P-Xylanase of the Yeast. *Eur. J. Biochem.* **1981**, *119*, 559–564. [CrossRef]
150. Pantaleone, D.; Yalpani, M.; Scollar, M. Unusual susceptibility of chitosan to enzymic hydrolysis. *Carbohydr. Res.* **1992**, *237*, 325–332. [CrossRef]
151. Zhang, H.; Neau, S.H. In vitro degradation of chitosan by a commercial enzyme preparation: Effect of molecular weight and degree of deacetylation. *Biomaterials* **2001**, *22*, 1653–1658. [CrossRef]
152. Kittur, F.S.; Kumar, A.B.V.; Varadaraj, M.C.; Tharanathan, R.N. Chitooligosaccharides—preparation with the aid of pectinase isozyme from Aspergillus niger and their antibacterial activity. *Carbohydr. Res.* **2005**, *340*, 1239–1245. [CrossRef] [PubMed]
153. Lee, D.-X.; Xia, W.-S.; Zhang, J.-L. Enzymatic preparation of chitooligosaccharides by commercial lipase. *Food Chem.* **2008**, *111*, 291–295. [CrossRef] [PubMed]
154. Kumar, A.V. Low molecular weight chitosans: preparation with the aid of papain and characterization. *Biochim. Biophys. Acta (BBA) Gen. Subj.* **2004**, *1670*, 137–146. [CrossRef] [PubMed]
155. Choi, W.-S.; Ahn, K.-J.; Lee, D.-W.; Byun, M.-W.; Park, H.-J. Preparation of chitosan oligomers by irradiation. *Polym. Degrad. Stab.* **2002**, *78*, 533–538. [CrossRef]
156. Lopatin, S.A.; Derbeneva, M.S.; Kulikov, S.N.; Varlamov, V.P.; Shpigun, O.A. Fractionation of chitosan by ultrafiltration. *J. Anal. Chem.* **2009**, *64*, 648–651. [CrossRef]
157. Hattori, T.; Anraku, N.; Kato, R. Capillary electrophoresis of chitooligosaccharides in acidic solution: Simple determination using a quaternary-ammonium-modified column and indirect photometric detection with Crystal Violet. *J. Chromatogr. B* **2010**, *878*, 477–480. [CrossRef] [PubMed]
158. Dong, H.; Wang, Y.; Zhao, L.; Zhou, J.; Xia, Q.; Jiang, L.; Fan, L. Purification of DP 6 to 8 chitooligosaccharides by nanofiltration from the prepared chitooligosaccharides syrup. *Bioresour. Bioprocess.* **2014**, *1*, 170. [CrossRef]
159. Le Dévédec, F.; Bazinet, L.; Furtos, A.; Venne, K.; Brunet, S.; Mateescu, M.A. Separation of chitosan oligomers by immobilized metal affinity chromatography. *J. Chromatogr. A* **2008**, *1194*, 165–171. [CrossRef]
160. Lv, M.; Hu, Y.; Gänzle, M.G.; Lin, J.; Wang, C.; Cai, J. Preparation of chitooligosaccharides from fungal waste mycelium by recombinant chitinase. *Carbohydr. Res.* **2016**, *430*, 1–7. [CrossRef]
161. Gao, X.A.; Jung, W.J.; Kuk, J.H.; Park, R.D. Reaction pattern of Bacillus cereus D-11 Chitosanase on chitooligosaccharide alchols. *J. Microbiol. Biotechnol.* **2009**, *19*, 358–361. [CrossRef]
162. Yi, L.; Sun, X.; Du, K.; Ouyang, Y.; Wu, C.; Xu, N.; Linhardt, R.J.; Zhang, Z. UP-HILIC-MS/MS to Determine the Action Pattern of Penicillium sp. Dextranase. *J. Am. Soc. Mass Spectrom.* **2015**, *26*, 1174–1185. [CrossRef] [PubMed]
163. Sørbotten, A.; Horn, S.J.; Eijsink, V.G.H.; Varum, K.M. Degradation of chitosans with chitinase B from Serratia marcescens: Production of chito-oligosaccharides and insight into enzyme processivity. *FEBS J.* **2005**, *272*, 538–549. [CrossRef] [PubMed]
164. Haebel, S.; Bahrke, S.; Peter, M.G. Quantitative Sequencing of Complex Mixtures of Heterochitooligosaccharides by vMALDI-Linear Ion Trap Mass Spectrometry. *Anal. Chem.* **2007**, *79*, 5557–5566. [CrossRef] [PubMed]
165. Dong, X.; Shen, A.; Gou, Z.; Chen, D.; Liang, X. Hydrophilic interaction/weak cation-exchange mixed-mode chromatography for chitooligosaccharides separation. *Carbohydr. Res.* **2012**, *361*, 195–199. [CrossRef] [PubMed]
166. Santos-Moriano, P.; Woodley, J.M.; Plou, F.J. Continuous production of chitooligosaccharides by an immobilized enzyme in a dual-reactor system. *J. Mol. Catal. B Enzym.* **2016**, *133*, 211–217. [CrossRef]

167. Sasaki, C.; Kristiansen, A.; Fukamizo, T.; Vårum, K.M. Biospecific Fractionation of Chitosan. *Biomacromolecules* **2003**, *4*, 1686–1690. [CrossRef]
168. Yoon, J.H. Enzymatic synthesis of chitooligosaccharides in organic cosolvents. *Enzym. Microb. Technol.* **2005**, *37*, 663–668. [CrossRef]
169. Lopatin, S.; Ilyin, M.; Pustobaev, V.; Bezchetnikova, Z.; Varlamov, V.; Davankov, V. Mass-Spectrometric Analysis of N-Acetylchitooligosaccharides Prepared through Enzymatic Hydrolysis of Chitosan. *Anal. Biochem.* **1995**, *227*, 285–288. [CrossRef]
170. Jung, W.-J.; Souleimanov, A.; Park, R.-D.; Smith, D.L. Enzymatic production of N-acetyl chitooligosaccharides by crude enzyme derived from Paenibacillus illioisensis KJA-424. *Carbohydr. Polym.* **2007**, *67*, 256–259. [CrossRef]
171. Cao, L.; Wu, J.; Li, X.; Zheng, L.; Wu, M.; Liu, P.; Huang, Q. Validated HPAEC-PAD Method for the Determination of Fully Deacetylated Chitooligosaccharides. *Int. J. Mol. Sci.* **2016**, *17*, 1699. [CrossRef]
172. Wu, H.; Yao, Z.; Bai, X.; Du, Y.; Lin, B. Anti-angiogenic activities of chitooligosaccharides. *Carbohydr. Polym.* **2008**, *73*, 105–110. [CrossRef]
173. Jiang, M.; Guo, Z.; Wang, C.; Yang, Y.; Liang, X.; Ding, F. Neural activity analysis of pure chito-oligomer components separated from a mixture of chitooligosaccharides. *Neurosci. Lett.* **2014**, *581*, 32–36. [CrossRef] [PubMed]
174. Hamer, S.N.; Cord-Landwehr, S.; Biarnés, X.; Planas, A.; Waegeman, H.; Moerschbacher, B.M.; Kolkenbrock, S. Enzymatic production of defined chitosan oligomers with a specific pattern of acetylation using a combination of chitin oligosaccharide deacetylases. *Sci. Rep.* **2015**, *5*, 8716. [CrossRef] [PubMed]
175. Paul, T.; Halder, S.K.; Das, A.; Ghosh, K.; Mandal, A.; Payra, P.; Barman, P.; Das Mohapatra, P.K.; Pati, B.R.; Mondal, K.C. Production of chitin and bioactive materials from Black tiger shrimp (Penaeus monodon) shell waste by the treatment of bacterial protease cocktail. *3 Biotech* **2015**, *5*, 483–493. [CrossRef] [PubMed]
176. Doan, C.T.; Tran, T.N.; Nguyen, V.B.; Nguyen, A.D.; Wang, S.-L. Reclamation of Marine Chitinous Materials for Chitosanase Production via Microbial Conversion by Paenibacillus macerans. *Mar. Drugs* **2018**, *16*, 429. [CrossRef]
177. Bosquez-Molina, E.; Zavaleta-Avejar, L. New Bioactive Biomaterials Based on Chitosan. In *Chitosan in the Preservation of Agricultural Commodities*; Elsevier: Amsterdam, The Netherlands, 2016; pp. 33–64.
178. Jiang, Y.; Fu, C.; Wu, S.; Liu, G.; Guo, J.; Su, Z. Determination of the Deacetylation Degree of Chitooligosaccharides. *Mar. Drugs* **2017**, *15*, 332. [CrossRef]
179. Limón, M.C.; Margolles-Clark, E.; Benítez, T.; Penttilä, M. Addition of substrate-binding domains increases substrate-binding capacity and specific activity of a chitinase from Trichoderma harzianum. *FEMS Microbiol. Lett.* **2001**, *198*, 57–63. [CrossRef]
180. Delgado-Jarana, J.; Limon, M.C.; Chacon, M.R.; Mejias, R.; Rincón, A.M.; Codón, A.C.; Benítez, T. Increased antifungal and chitinase specific activities of Trichoderma harzianum CECT 2413 by addition of a cellulose binding domain. *Appl. Microbiol. Biotechnol.* **2004**, *64*, 675–685.
181. Kowsari, M.; Motallebi, M.; Zamani, M. Protein engineering of chit42 towards improvement of chitinase and antifungal activities. *Curr. Microbiol.* **2014**, *68*, 495–502. [CrossRef]
182. Matroodi, S.; Motallebi, M.; Zamani, M.; Moradyar, M. Designing a new chitinase with more chitin binding and antifungal activity. *World J. Microbiol. Biotechnol.* **2013**, *29*, 1517–1523. [CrossRef]
183. Kurašin, M.; Kuusk, S.; Kuusk, P.; Sørlie, M.; Väljamäe, P. Slow Off-rates and Strong Product Binding Are Required for Processivity and Efficient Degradation of Recalcitrant Chitin by Family 18 Chitinases. *J. Boil. Chem.* **2015**, *290*, 29074–29085. [CrossRef] [PubMed]
184. Fan, Y.; Fang, W.; Xiao, Y.; Yang, X.; Zhang, Y.; Bidochka, M.J.; Pei, Y. Directed evolution for increased chitinase activity. *App. Microbiol. Biotechnol.* **2007**, *76*, 135–139. [CrossRef] [PubMed]
185. Songsiririthigul, C.; Pesatcha, P.; Eijsink, V.G.H.; Yamabhai, M. Directed evolution of a Bacillus chitinase. *Biotechnol. J.* **2009**, *4*, 501–509. [CrossRef] [PubMed]
186. Mekasha, S.; Byman, I.R.; Lynch, C.; Toupalová, H.; Anděra, L.; Næs, T.; Vaaje-Kolstad, G.; Eijsink, V.G. Development of enzyme cocktails for complete saccharification of chitin using mono-component enzymes from Serratia marcescens. *Process. Biochem.* **2017**, *56*, 132–138. [CrossRef]
187. Zhou, J.; Chen, J.; Xu, N.; Zhang, A.; Chen, K.; Xin, F.; Zhang, W.; Ma, J.; Fang, Y.; Jiang, M.; et al. The broad-specificity chitinases: their origin, characterization, and potential application. *Appl. Microbiol. Biotechnol.* **2019**, *103*, 3289–3295. [CrossRef]

188. Pérez-Martínez, A.S.; De León-Rodríguez, A.; Harris, L.J.; Herrera-Estrella, A.; De La Rosa, A.P.B. Overexpression, purification and characterization of the Trichoderma atroviride endochitinase, Ech42, in Pichia pastoris. *Protein Expr. Purif.* **2007**, *55*, 183–188. [CrossRef]
189. Dahiya, N.; Tewari, R.; Tiwari, R.P.; Hoondal, G.S. Chitinase Production in Solid-State Fermentation by Enterobacter sp. NRG4 Using Statistical Experimental Design. *Curr. Microbiol.* **2005**, *51*, 222–228. [CrossRef]
190. Nidheesh, T.; Pal, G.K.; Suresh, P. Chitooligomers preparation by chitosanase produced under solid state fermentation using shrimp by-products as substrate. *Carbohydr. Polym.* **2015**, *121*, 1–9. [CrossRef]
191. Orikoshi, H.; Nakayama, S.; Miyamoto, K.; Hanato, C.; Yasuda, M.; Inamori, Y.; Tsujibo, H. Roles of Four Chitinases (ChiA, ChiB, ChiC, and ChiD) in the Chitin Degradation System of Marine Bacterium Alteromonas sp. Strain O-7. *Appl. Environ. Microbiol.* **2005**, *71*, 1811–1815. [CrossRef]

marine drugs

MDPI

Review

Crab vs. Mushroom: A Review of Crustacean and Fungal Chitin in Wound Treatment

Mitchell Jones [1], Marina Kujundzic [2], Sabu John [1] and Alexander Bismarck [2,*]

[1] School of Engineering, RMIT University, Bundoora East Campus, P.O. Box 71, Bundoora VIC 3083, Australia
[2] Institute of Material Chemistry and Research, Polymer and Composite Engineering (PaCE) Group, Faculty of Chemistry, University of Vienna, Währinger Straße 42, 1090 Vienna, Austria
* Correspondence: alexander.bismarck@univie.ac.at

Received: 27 December 2019; Accepted: 15 January 2020; Published: 18 January 2020

Abstract: Chitin and its derivative chitosan are popular constituents in wound-treatment technologies due to their nanoscale fibrous morphology and attractive biomedical properties that accelerate healing and reduce scarring. These abundant natural polymers found in arthropod exoskeletons and fungal cell walls affect almost every phase of the healing process, acting as hemostatic and antibacterial agents that also support cell proliferation and attachment. However, key differences exist in the structure, properties, processing, and associated polymers of fungal and arthropod chitin, affecting their respective application to wound treatment. High purity crustacean-derived chitin and chitosan have been widely investigated for wound-treatment applications, with research incorporating chemically modified chitosan derivatives and advanced nanocomposite dressings utilizing biocompatible additives, such as natural polysaccharides, mineral clays, and metal nanoparticles used to achieve excellent mechanical and biomedical properties. Conversely, fungi-derived chitin is covalently decorated with β-glucan and has received less research interest despite its mass production potential, simple extraction process, variations in chitin and associated polymer content, and the established healing properties of fungal exopolysaccharides. This review investigates the proven biomedical properties of both fungal- and crustacean-derived chitin and chitosan, their healing mechanisms, and their potential to advance modern wound-treatment methods through further research and practical application.

Keywords: chitin; chitosan; wound treatment; derivatization; nanocomposites

1. Introduction

Accidents or diseases resulting in skin damage are a commonplace occurrence in everyday life, making wound dressings a critical element of modern healthcare [1]. Wound dressings are typically porous in nature, with good barrier properties and oxygen permeability, and assist healing by preventing bleeding, absorbing excess exudates, keeping wounds moist, and protecting them from the environment [2,3]. However, issues with conventional dressings, such as irritation after prolonged use, poor compatibility with wounds, and a lack of effectiveness in the treatment of chronic wounds, such as severe burns, diabetic wounds, and ulcers, necessitates improved wound-dressing technologies that are biocompatible, actively accelerate healing, and exhibit antibacterial and antifungal activity [4,5]. Use of nontoxic and antibacterial biological polymeric nanofibers, such as chitin and bacterial cellulose, in wound-dressing technologies has subsequently received significant attention. Nanofibers are particularly well suited to wound-dressing research due to their high surface-area-to-volume ratio, porosity, pore size distribution, and morphology, which mirror the skin's natural extracellular matrix, promoting cell adhesion and proliferation [3,6]. Chitin, a linear macromolecule composed of *N*-acetylglucosamine, and its derivative chitosan are among the most popular nanofibers used in wound-dressing research [1]. Naturally occurring in arthropod exoskeletons, mollusks, and fungi, chitin is one of the most abundant organic polymers on Earth and is easily extracted from these natural sources by using a mild alkaline treatment, the concentration of which can be increased if desired to produce chitosan, the deacetylated derivative of chitin [7]. Both chitin and chitosan exhibit properties beneficial to wound-dressing applications, including biocompatibility, biodegradability, hemostatic activity, healing acceleration, nontoxicity, adsorption, and anti-infection properties [1,3]. However, significant differences exist in the structure, properties, processing, and associated polymers of animal- and fungi-derived chitin, which have influenced their application in wound-dressing research, respectively. This review aims to investigate the key differences between animal and fungal chitin and the mechanisms through which chitin and chitosan assist wound healing, before examining the historical and current application of these chitin and chitosan variants to wound-dressing research. Advanced wound-dressing technologies utilizing chemically modified chitin and chitosan and nanocomposite architectures are also addressed, as well as the future potential of these chitin types in wound treatment.

2. Differences between Crustacean and Fungal Chitin

Chitin is one of the most abundant organic polymers on Earth, constituting the structural component of arthropod exoskeletons, mollusk radula, cephalopod endoskeletons, fungal cell walls, and fish and lissamphibian scales [8]. The largest source of chitin globally is suggested to be Zooplankton cuticles, with an estimated 379 million tons of Antarctic krill available worldwide [9,10]. However, fishing these tiny organisms is not commercially viable, and, subsequently, shellfish industry wastes, such as shrimp, crab, and lobster shells with chitin contents of 8–40%, are the main source of industrial chitin [11–13] (Table 1). Fungi provide an alternative source of chitin and, despite having lower chitin content than crustaceans (10–26% as a chitin-β-glucan complex), are experiencing increasing academic and commercial interest [14,15]. Unlike crustacean chitin, fungal chitin is not limited by seasonal and regional variation and does not require the aggressive acid treatment that crustacean chitin does for purification and demineralization, to remove calcium carbonate and other minerals [15,16]. It also supplements the rigid chitin structure with more pliable branched β-glucan, yielding a native nanocomposite architecture that can provide both strong and tough fiber networks when extracted [15,17].

Table 1. Polymorphs and examples of chitin sources with their respective chitinous constituent dry weight (d.wt.) compared to total source mass, chitin contents, and other major organic and inorganic constituents listed. Data from [14,18–30].

Polymorph	Sources	Chitin Content	Other Major Constituents
α	Crustacean shells		(chitinous shell up to 50% of crustacean d.wt.)
	Lobster Crab Krill	16–23% 25–30% 34–49%	20–60% calcium or magnesium carbonate, 20–40% protein
	Insect cuticles		(chitinous cuticle up to 50% of insect d.wt.)
	Cockroach Butterfly Silkworm	18–38% 22–64% 20–44%	20–50% protein, minerals, pigments and fat
	Fungal cell walls		(chitin–glucan nanofibers up to 26% of fungal biomass d.wt.)
	Mushrooms Mycelium Yeast Mold	8–43% 5–35% 1–3% 8–27%	50–60% β-glucan, protein
β	Squid pen Sea tube worms	31–49% 25–29%	Proteins and minerals

Both crustacean and fungal chitin have a similar molecular structure to cellulose, which is the structural component of the primary cell wall of all green plants, algae, and oomycetes. The main difference between cellulose and chitin is the replacement of the C2 hydroxyl group of cellulose with an acetamide group, which can be deacetylated to obtain chitosan (Figure 1). Two major polymorphic forms of chitin exist, α and β, with α-chitin the most common polymorph for both crustacean and fungal chitin and β-chitin occurring only in squid pen, sea tube worms, and some algae (centric diatom) [19].

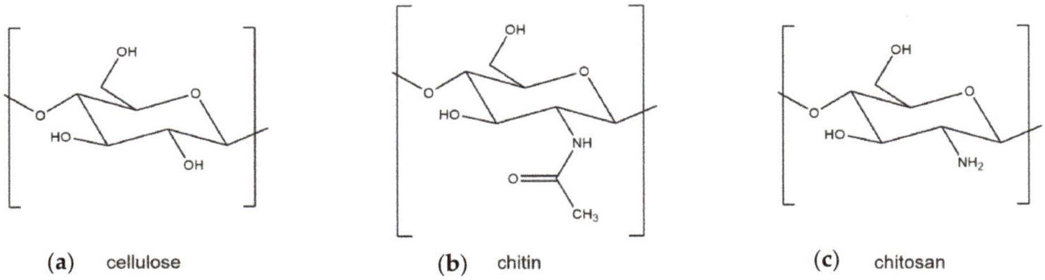

Figure 1. Molecular structures of (**a**) cellulose, (**b**) chitin, and (**c**) chitosan.

However, key differences exist between crustacean and fungal chitin. Crustacean chitin normally has minimal residual protein and binds with sclerotized proteins and minerals, whereas fungal chitin is associated with other polysaccharides, such as glucan, which can occur in quantities exceeding the chitin content itself [31]. Crosslinking between chitin and proteins is well established in both crustacean- and insect-derived chitin, although it is still unclear whether the bridging is partially covalent in nature, with the low quantity of residual protein present suggesting that there is little covalent bonding or that the bonds may be cleaved during the chitin extraction process [32–35]. On the other hand, the linkages between chitin and glucan in fungi have been proven to be covalent in nature [36–38]. Small differences exist between insoluble glucans in mushrooms, yeast, and hyphae. However, most commonly, β-glucan exhibiting a (1→3) backbone and (1→6) branching is associated with chitin [39]. The location of chitin also varies, being concentrated in the bud scar in yeast and in the cell wall of most other fungi. Notably, in some fungi, both chitin and chitosan are simultaneously co-synthesized, a feature unique to the fungal phylum Zygomycota [40,41].

The extraction processes for fungal and crustacean chitin are similar (Figure 2), with both processes initially requiring the raw material to be washed and homogenized. For fungi, the starting material is mycelial biomass or fruiting bodies, while for crustaceans, it is their shells.

Fungal chitin sources are generally easily homogenized using a kitchen blender [42], while the harder and more brittle crustacean shells must be crushed. The high mineral content of crustacean shells also requires an acidic demineralization step, typically completed by using 1–2 M hydrochloric acid (HCl) for up to 48 h, although concentrations ranging up to 11 M are possible [43]. This step is not required when processing fungal chitin. Deproteination is then completed for either fungal or crustacean chitin in mild alkaline conditions, typically 1 M sodium hydroxide (NaOH), before the final material is decolorized, using a bleaching step, if desired. Pure chitin is obtained from crustacean shells as a final product, whereas fungal chitin sources yield a chitin-β-glucan complex following extraction. Pure chitin can be derived from this complex, if desired, using acid treatments to degrade the glucan, yielding X-ray diffraction patterns resembling crustacean chitin [44].

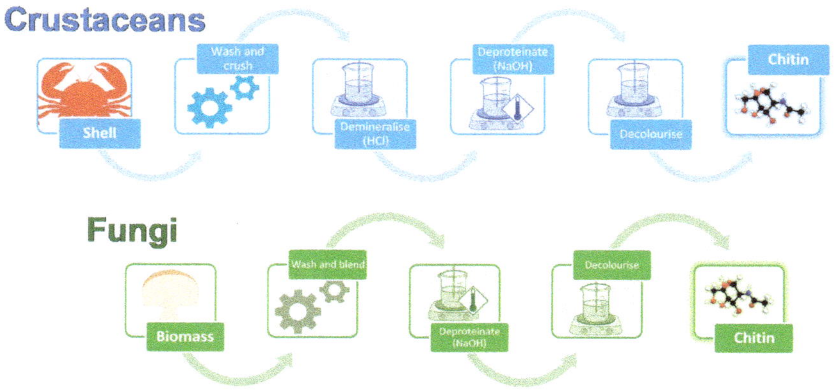

Figure 2. Chitin extraction process for crustacean- and fungi-derived chitin, comprising mechanical (crushing or blending) and chemical (demineralization, deproteination, and decolorization) treatments.

3. Generation and Properties of Chitosan

Chitosan can be generated from both fungal and crustacean chitin in a simple deacetylation process, whereby the acetyl group of chitin's acetamide group is cleaved off under strong alkaline conditions (Figure 3), typically sodium hydroxide (NaOH), with up to 98% yields possible [45]. Although chitin and chitosan both have useful biomedical properties, including biocompatibility, biodegradability, hemostatic activity, healing acceleration, nontoxicity, adsorption, and anti-infection potential [3], chitosan generally receives more scientific attention due to its more useful structure, which renders it soluble in aqueous acids. Chitosan's primary amine group can be protonated under mildly acidic conditions. Conversely, chitin is insoluble in all regular solvents, such as water, organic solvents, and mild acids or bases, due to the hydrogen bonding associated with the acetyl, amino, and hydroxyl groups in its polysaccharide chain [19]. Protonated chitosan's charge also makes it a bio adhesive, able to bond to negatively charged surfaces, such as mucous membranes, chelate heavy metal ions, and is biocompatible and biodegradable with superior antibacterial properties to chitin if hydrated or in the form of a hydrogel [30,46,47]. The primary and secondary hydroxyl groups on each repeating unit and the amine group of each deacetylated unit are also reactive and are readily chemically modified to alter the physical and mechanical properties of chitosan [48]. These advantages provide chitosan with greater processing and biomedical potential than chitin as a component for wound treatment materials. However, its use in biomedical materials is limited by its poor mechanical properties. Chitin is strong, with a nanofibril tensile strength of ~1.6–3.0 GPa [49], which results from hydrogen bonding between the chains of the macromolecules [50]. Conversely, the absence of the acetyl group, which contributes to hydrogen bond formation in chitin and stabilizes its crystalline structure, significantly compromises the mechanical properties of chitosan [51]. This makes chitosan alone mechanically unsuitable for applications that require durability, such as strong films or composites, despite its significant biomedical potential.

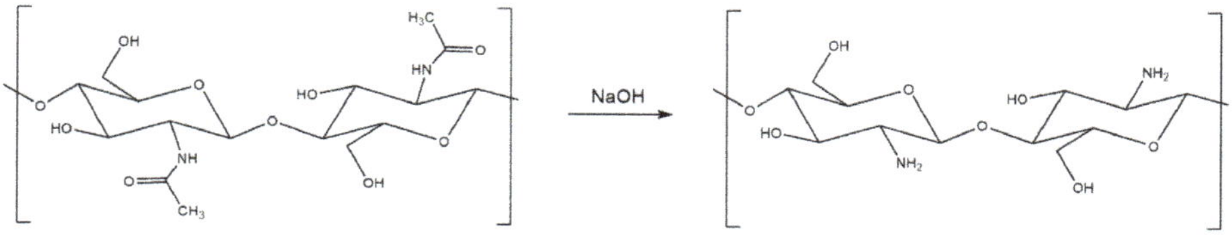

Figure 3. Reaction scheme for the deacetylation of chitin into chitosan, using sodium hydroxide (NaOH).

4. Healing Mechanisms of Chitin and Chitosan

Wound healing is a complex biological process comprising four stages: hemostasis, inflammation, proliferation, and remodeling [52] (Figure 4). These stages overlap in time [53] and follow a specific program, which is introduced and modulated by different cell types. Usually this mechanism works well enough to facilitate rapid repair of damaged skin. However, it does not regenerate the wounded skin completely, with scaring and loss of hair follicles or sweat glands common in healed skin [54]. Impaired wound healing function and chronic wounds in some patients is also common [52]. One of the major objectives of wound-healing technologies is to facilitate improved wound healing, tending toward wound regeneration [53,54]. Chitin and its derivates have been shown to be useful constituents in wound-dressing materials [55–57] and may potentially contribute to the development of skin substitutes facilitating skin regeneration since they appear to influence the wound-healing process on a molecular level.

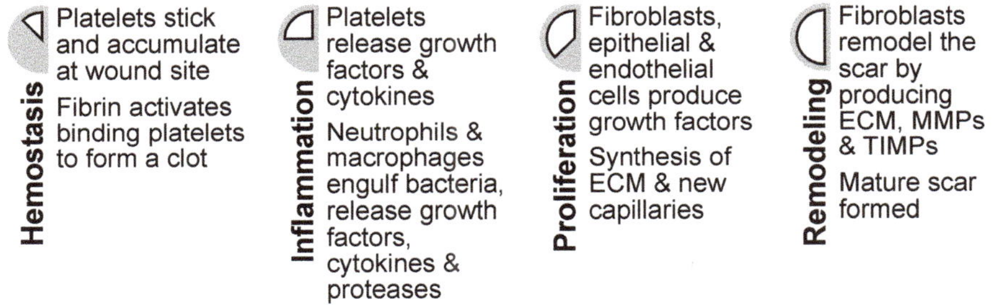

Figure 4. The four stages of wound healing (hemostasis, inflammation, proliferation, and remodeling) with descriptions of associated cellular activities.

The hemostasis phase starts immediately upon injury occurrence and is intended to stop hemorrhage by forming a fibrin clot [52] (Figure 5), a step which typically depends on platelets [54]. The formed clot re-establishes a barrier against the outside world and provides an improvised extracellular matrix, which is needed for cell migration [53]. Chitosan has hemostatic properties, reacting with red blood cells to form a coagulum [58] (Table 2), and acting independently from the regular coagulation mechanism, whereas, typically, red blood cells only have a supportive role in the formation of clots [59]. This improved hemostatic effect was also observed in whole blood, heparinized blood, and defibrinated blood [58], meaning that chitosan can potentially provide an improved clotting ability and aid hemostasis [60]. Studies have also been undertaken to assess the effectiveness of chitosan as a hemostatic in surgical settings, with wounds treated using chitosan exhibiting reduced bleeding compared to control wounds [61,62]. However, chitosan's hemostatic effectiveness has not been compared to other hemostatics, and chitin does not seem to have been investigated as a hemostatic.

Once the hemorrhage has been stopped, the degranulating fibrin clot and surrounding tissue cells trigger the next stages of healing by releasing cytokines and growth factors, which attract cells to the wound site [53]. Chitosan may induce a different clotting mechanism, meaning that the healing process may be altered. This potentially results in a modified healing response, facilitated by the release of fewer growth factors from the platelets [63]. One of the first cells to respond next are neutrophils, also called polymorphonuclear neutrophils or PMNs. PMNs clean foreign objects, like dirt and bacteria, from the wound and remove damaged cells and are one of the main cell types responsible for inflammation [53]. Both chitin and chitosan have been shown to have a positive chemotactic effect on canine PMNs [64,65], meaning that they attract PMNs. An in vitro study showed that chitin has a stronger effect than chitosan [65]. However, chitosan may potentially impact the wound to a greater extent, as it degrades more slowly than chitin [64]. A similar effect has been observed in bovine PMNs [66]. Studies undertaken in dogs also found increased infiltration of PMNs after 3 days in wounds treated with chitosan, compared to control wounds, and decreased inflammation after 28 days in wounds treated using chitin or chitosan [67,68]. This induced increase in PMNs may also improve wound cleansing and shorten the inflammation stage, potentially providing a positive impact on the wound healing process. PMNs have also been observed to release pro-inflammatory cytokines, which may activate surrounding fibroblasts and keratinocytes [54].

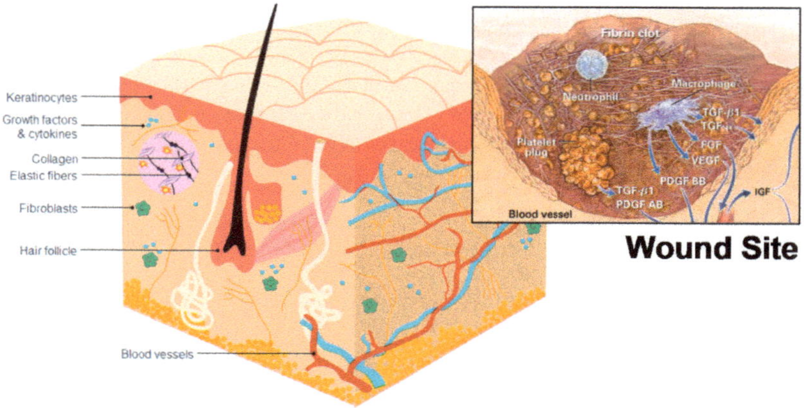

Figure 5. Skin structuring and locations of cells relevant to wound healing. Inset: a representation of a wound site and cells relating to the hemostasis and inflammation stages of wound healing. Reproduced with copyright permission from Singer and Clark [53].

Table 2. Cell types, their respective functions in wound healing, and the effect of chitin or chitosan upon these functions.

Cell Type	Function in Wound Healing	Effects of Chitin or Chitosan
Red blood cells	Supportive role in fibrin clot formation.	Chitosan forms a coagulum with red blood cells.
Polymorphonuclear neutrophils (PMN)	Clean wound site of foreign particles and cell debris.	Chitin and chitosan attract PMNs to wound site.
Macrophages	Consume dead cells, attract fibroblasts, support skin and blood vessel replacement and synthesis of the extracellular matrix.	Chitin and chitosan attract macrophages. Chitosan stimulates cytokine production (TGF-β1, PDGF, IL-1).
Fibroblasts	Reformation of the dermis and synthesis of extracellular matrix.	Indirect effect through macrophage cytokines and stimulates IL-8 production.
Keratinocytes	Reformation of epidermis.	Indirect effect through macrophage cytokines.

Macrophages, which consume PMNs [69], become the next dominant leukocyte in the inflammation stage. Macrophages have been shown to be essential for wound healing, as they have a key role in transitioning the wound from the inflammation stage to the cell proliferation stage [52,53]. They have many functions, such as phagocytosis of dead or infected cells, attraction of many cells to the wound site, and they also support the formation of granulation tissue, blood vessels, and the extracellular matrix [53]. Defective wound repair has been observed in animals depleted of macrophages [53]. The same study, which showed increased PMN infiltration, also showed macrophages increasingly infiltrating wounds treated with chitosan in comparison to control wounds [67]. A potential reason for this may be chitosan-induced activation of a complement called C5, which attracts macrophages and PMNs [67]. Chitosan has also been shown to increase the mRNA expression and synthesis of TGF-β1 (transforming growth factor-beta 1) and PDGF (platelet-derived growth factor) in macrophages in vitro [70]. Both TGF-β1 and PDGF are chemotactic for macrophages and fibroblasts, with TGF-β1 also affecting keratinocytes, which make up the outermost layer of skin, [54] and PDGF, inducing fibroblast proliferation and collagen production [70]. It has also been observed that 70% deacylated chitin increases in vitro [71] and in vivo [72] secretion of IL-1 in macrophages, which affects fibroblast proliferation [73] and collagen production [67]. Chitosan (over 95% deacylated) on the other hand shows no effect in vitro [71] and lesser effects than the 70% deacylated chitin in vivo [72].

Fibroblasts, which lay a new skin fundament in the wound, are also a key cell type for wound healing. They produce the extracellular cell matrix [53], the structure between cells, which consists mainly of collagen [74]. Collagen plays a key role in scar formation, as excessive collagen deposition can lead to scars [53]. Insufficient collagen deposition has also been linked to chronic wounds [63]. Therefore, a balance of collagen production and degradation is necessary to ensure full regeneration. As described above, chitin and chitosan affect the secretion of different cytokines in macrophages, which in turn affect the proliferation of fibroblasts and collagen production. However, the effect of chitin and chitosan on fibroblasts is not only indirect in nature, with chitosan inducing increased IL-8 production in fibroblasts [66], a strong chemotactic for PMNs and regulator of keratinocyte migration and proliferation [73]. Another important role of fibroblasts is the production of the extracellular cell matrix. In vitro studies have shown no direct effects of chitosan on the fibroblasts producing the extracellular matrix [66]. However, indirect effects through microphage stimulation, and therefore fibroblast stimulation, may affect this stage. It has also been hypothesized that chitin and chitosan could be incorporated into the extracellular matrix, through the use of lysozyme [60], an enzyme capable of degrading chitin and chitosan.

The effects of molecular weight and degree of deacetylation on the wound-healing potential of chitin and chitosan have also been studied, albeit to a lesser extent. An in vivo study on incisions in rats investigated the effect of chitin (300 kDa, <10% deacetylation), chitosan (80 kDa, >80% deacetylation), and their oligomers and monomers on wound break strength and collagenase activity [75]. The results showed that wounds treated using chitosan (chitosan, oligomer, and monomer) were stronger than those treated using chitin. In both cases, treatments using oligomers were associated with the highest wound break strength, although chitosan had comparable performance, and chitosan monomers were associated with the highest collagenase activity. A further in vitro study on fibroblasts investigated differences in healing based on the molecular weight and degree of deacetylation of chitin and chitosan [76], utilizing chitin with a degree of deacetylation of 37% and molecular weights of 37 and 197 kDa, and chitosan with degrees of deacetylation of 58% and 89% and molecular weights of 12 kDa/194 kDa and 13 kDa/263 kDa, respectively. The results showed that chitosan with a higher degree of deacetylation had a greater effect on fibroblast proliferation, which was further enhanced at lower molecular weights.

The molecular weights of the chitin and chitosan used in these studies falls in the low-molecular-weight range, as both chitin and chitosan can have molecular weights >1000 kDa [77]. However, another in vivo study investigating surgical burns in rats used a broader range of molecular weights, ranging from 70 to 750 kDa and peaking at 2000 kDa [78]. However, the degree of deacetylation of each sample was not varied, with a fixed value of 63%, 75%, and 92%, for each respective molecular weight. The results showed that the 2000 kDa chitosan performed significantly better than the other molecular weights both in wound contraction and collagenase activity, a result that the author attributed to its high molecular weight [78]. However, since the degree of deacetylation has a greater effect on wound healing than the molecular weight in the low-molecular-weight range [75,76], the effects of different degrees of deacetylation at high molecular weights should also be examined.

It is however clear that chitosan with a higher degree of deacetylation exhibits higher biological activity than that with a lower degree of deacetylation [75,76]. The effect of molecular weight on wound healing in the low-molecular-weight range studied (<300 kDa) also seems to be enhanced at lower molecular weights (<100 kDa). However, since chitin and chitosan can exhibit molecular weights that fall well outside this range, further studies for higher molecular weights (>300 kDa) are required, especially when considering the correlation between the hemostatic activity of chitosan and higher molecular weights [79].

5. Fungi-Derived Chitin and Chitosan Wound Dressings

Medical applications of fungi date back to ancient times, where it was used as a styptic to stop bleeding and as a crude precursor to modern antibiotics in the treatment of infections [80–83]. However, true academic interest in medical materials derived from fungi did not begin until the 1970s, when the mycelia of several fungal species were investigated as wound-healing accelerants. Prudden et al. [84] studied the topical application of powdered mycelium from *Phycomycetes mucor*, *Penicillium notatum*, and *Aspergillus niger* on rat wounds to confirm the healing properties of glucosamine (polymer units of chitosan), which was thought to be responsible for the healing potential of the cartilage material historically used in wound treatment [84]. Wounded rat skin treated with powdered mycelium was found to have a higher tensile strength than untreated or cartilage powder treated wounds as they healed, with *P. mucor* associated with the highest skin tensile strengths (Figure 6). In further investigations, a chitin-β-glucan powder was also produced through NaOH and HCl treatment of the same mycelium and compared to purified crustacean chitin, again as a topically applied healing accelerant on rat wounds. Lobster and king crab chitin outperformed the purified mycelium powder; however, all fungal species except *A. niger* provided higher skin tensile strength than the cartilage and shrimp chitin healing agents [85].

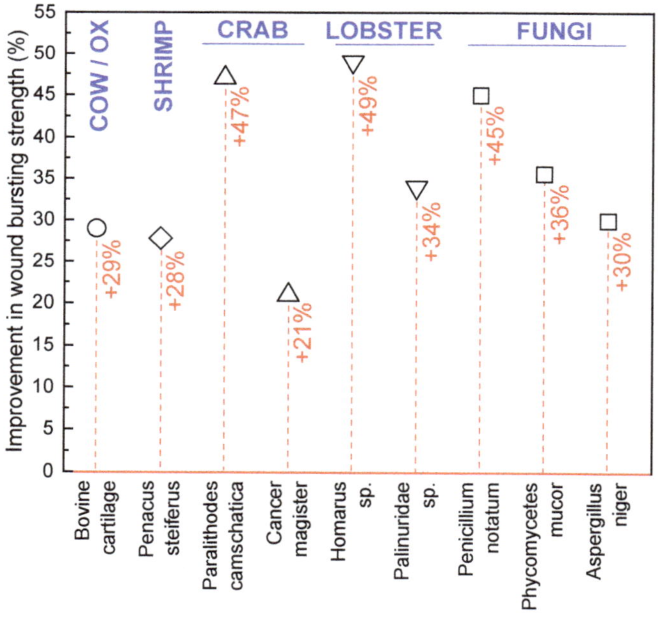

Figure 6. Improvement in the bursting strength (%) of wounds treated using bovine cartilage and shrimp, crab, lobster, and fungal chitin, compared to an untreated control wound. Data from Balassa and Prudden [85].

Following these successes, chitin quickly gained popularity academically as a wound-healing accelerant, with most subsequent work focusing on the healing potential of crustacean chitin. However, the lower costs and simpler purification of fungal chitin did attract research interest, with further studies utilizing NaOH and acetic acid purified *Aspergillus oryzae*, *Mucor mucedo*, and *Phycomyces blakesleeanus* mycelium demonstrating increased cell proliferation in fibroblasts at low concentrations.

This cell-proliferating effect facilitated through the use of the fungal material was found to correlate with the chitin or chitosan content of the material, with *P. blakesleeanus* showing the highest proliferation at 0.01% and 0.5% w/v. Additionally cell attractant properties were found in *P. blakesleeanus* and *M. mucedo*, which were suggested to assist in wound healing [86].

Commercialization of fungi-derived wound treatment materials occurred in 1997, with a research group from Taiwan extracting a chitin-polysaccharide mixture from *Ganoderma tsugae*, comprising β-1-3-glucan (~60%) and *N*-acetylglucosamine (~40%), and creating a weavable skin substitute called Sacchachitin (Figure 7). This novel wound dressing was tested on rats [56] and Guinea pigs [87], before being tested in a preliminary clinical trial on two human patients with chronic wounds, in 2005 [55]. Animal studies showed that Sacchachitin improved wound healing significantly compared to conventional gauze and had comparable performance to Beschitin, a commercially available wound dressing from crustacean chitin, developed in 1988 [87]. Improvements in healing were also observed in human trials for chronic wounds open for seven months or longer, with the underlying healing mechanisms being fibroblast and keratinocyte proliferation and the activity of matrix metalloproteinases (MMPs) (human cells) [55]. A Sacchachitin nanogel derivative was also produced for the treatment of corneal burns in rabbits, demonstrating promise with significant increases in cornea cell proliferation and wound closure stimulation, in addition to enhanced corneal wound healing due to the inhibition of protein breakdown [88].

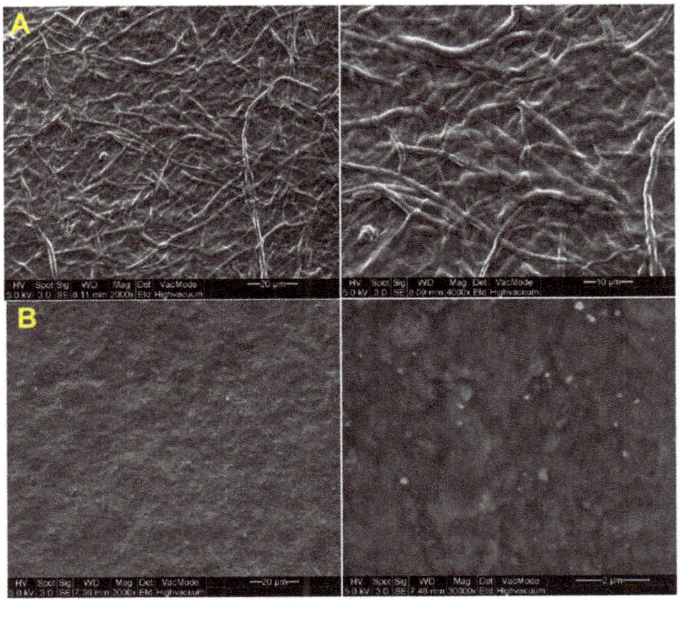

Figure 7. SE (scanning electron) micrographs of (**A**) fibrous and (**B**) micronized Sacchachitin. Reproduced from Chen, Lee, Chen, Ho, Lui, Sheu, and Su [88] (open access).

More recently, with the rise of research interest into the wound-treatment potential of purer crustacean chitin derivatives, academic interest in the medical applications of fungal material has shifted to the investigation of fungal exopolysaccharides (EPS). EPS are not components of the fungal intercellular matrix or cell wall, where chitin is typically found, but rather occur on the cell surface or in the extracellular matrix [89]. Compared to other fungal polysaccharides, they are mass producible in a short time and easily isolated and purified [89]. Thai studies investigating the EPS of 16 different native fungal strains identified three strains that were biocompatible with Vero cells, which are primate cells resembling fibroblasts, and increased interleukin-8 (IL-8) production in fibroblasts, improving wound healing [90]. EPS have also been combined with traditional antibacterial agents, such as ciprofloxacin, to create active-agent-loaded fungi-derived wound dressings [91]. Fungal β-glucans, such as lentinan from *L. edodes* (shiitake), schizophyllan from *S. commune* (split gill), zymosan from *S. cereviase* (baker's yeast), pleuran from *P. ostreatus* (oyster), and ganoderan from *G. lucidum* (reishii), have also been extensively studied due to the human immune system's ability to recognize them, promoting immune stimulation, antibacterial, antitumor, anticancer, and antioxidant properties [92–95]. These findings, coupled with the varying chitin, chitosan, and polysaccharide profiles of the over 5.1 million species of fungi in existence [96] and recent advances in fungal material technology [7,14,17,97–101], suggest that fungi-derived wound treatments warrant further investigation. In particular, the native chitin-β-glucan composite architecture of fungal chitin could be utilized to achieve scaffolds exceeding the mechanical performance of crustacean chitin [17] and novel antibacterial properties resulting from composite dressings incorporating naturally generated complexes of fungal chitin, chitosan, β-glucans, and exopolysaccharides could pave the way for new low-cost, natural, and mass-producible dressing technologies.

6. Crustacean-Derived Chitin and Chitosan Wound Dressings

6.1. Derivatization of Chitin and Chitosan to Improve Solubility and Biomedical Properties

Most research concerning the application of crustacean-derived chitin and chitosan in wound dressings focuses on either chemical modification (derivatization) or material engineering practices, such as hybridization or incorporation of chitin or chitosan into nanocomposites, to address the physical, biomedical, or mechanical shortcomings of each respective polymer. Derivatization often deals with improving the solubility of chitin and chitosan [102], which typically have low solubility in common solvents, with chitin being insoluble in water and most organic solvents, and chitosan being insoluble in most organic solvents and aqueous solutions above pH 6.5. This hinders the processing of chitin and chitosan and limits their applications. Other goals of derivatization include the addition or enhancement of existing biomedical properties of chitin or chitosan, such as antibacterial activity [103], hydrogel formation [104,105], and wound-healing acceleration. The most common derivatizations are carboxymethylation, which introduces the carboxymethyl functional group, and quaternation, which converts a tertiary amine to a quaternary ammonium compound; however, other derivatizations are also possible.

Carboxymethylation of chitin and chitosan is commonly regarded as one of the most useful derivatizations. Through the addition of the carboxymethyl group to chitin or chitosan, an anionic functional group (carboxyl) is introduced. This addition makes chitin or chitosan more hydrophilic and improves solubility, both in water and some organic solvents [106]. Carboxymethylation of chitin and chitosan is also known to improve biocompatibility and antibacterial properties and can be used to create hydrogels more effectively [106,107]. The specific properties of a carboxymethylated chitosan depend on the degree of carboxymethylation and the substituent position of the carboxymethyl group [108]. Four different substituent patterns for chitosan have been reported: *O*-carboxymethyl chitosan, *N*-carboxymethyl chitosan, *N,O*-carboxymethyl chitosan, and *N,N*-dicarboxymethyl chitosan [107] (Figure 8).

Although all of these variants are water-soluble, *N,O*-carboxymethyl chitosan has better antibacterial properties than *O*-carboxymethyl chitosan and unmodified chitosan [109,110]. These improved antibacterial properties are most likely the reason for the heightened research interest in *N,O*-carboxymethyl chitosan. *N*-carboxymethyl chitosan has been shown to improve wound healing in mice by inducing production of inflammatory cytokines [108] and *N,N*-dicarboxymethyl chitosan has been shown to be associated with bone regeneration by chelating calcium and magnesium [111,112]; however, both substrates have received less attention from the research community.

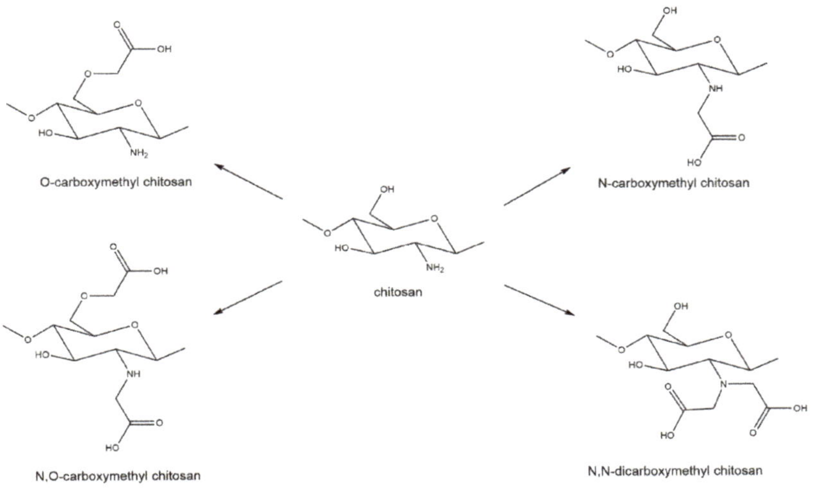

Figure 8. Carboxymethylation derivatizations of chitosan generating O-carboxymethyl chitosan, *N*-carboxymethyl chitosan, *N,O*-carboxymethyl chitosan, and *N,N*-dicarboxymethyl chitosan.

Notably, carboxymethylated chitin or chitosan can be further functionalized through the introduction of additional substituents to the backbone of the chitin or chitosan structure or the carboxyl group of the carboxymethyl. Some examples of further functionalization include the addition of acrylic groups, like 2-hydroxy-3-methacryloyloxypropylate, to the backbone, resulting in a tissue adhesive utilizable in wound-closure applications [113]. Ethylenediamine can also be introduced at both 3-OH and 6-OH positions in chitin or chitosan to create 3,6-*O*-*N*-acetylethylenediamine modified chitosan (AEDMCS), which has improved solubility in water over a wide pH range (3–11, compared to 3–6) and exhibits improved antibacterial properties, against both Gram-negative and Gram-positive bacteria [114]. Further functionalization of carboxymethyl chitin at the carboxyl group also provides the opportunity to produce improved hydrogels, such as those incorporating tyramine groups. The phenolic group of tyramine can be enzymatically crosslinked by using horseradish peroxides (HRP), which can be used to tune hydrogel properties [115].

Quaternization is another popular chitin- and chitosan-derivatization process, which converts a tertiary amine to a quaternary ammonium compound, enhancing solubility in water and organic solvents, as well as increasing antibacterial activity [109,116,117]. These improved properties are associated with the addition of the permanent cationic group $RN(CH_3)_3^+$, with the increased charge generating a higher polar character in chitin or chitosan and enhancing solubility in polar solvents, like water and some organic solvents. The leading hypothesis regarding the improved antibacterial properties of these derivatives is that increases in cationic groups result in interaction with the negative surface of bacteria, which inhibits bacterial growth [109,116,118,119]. Various substituent patterns are achievable depending on how chitin or chitosan are derivatized. Chitin's accessible position for derivatization is the 6-OH group [120,121]. However, simultaneous quaternization of the 6-OH and 3-OH positions also seems to be possible and may provide superior antifungal activity than 6-OH quaternization alone [118]. Conversely, derivatization of chitosan is most readily achieved through *N*-quaternization, as the amine group simply needs to be methylated, resulting in *N,N,N*-trimethylchitosan (TMC), which exhibits improved solubility and antibacterial properties. However, the unintended methylation of the OH-groups of chitosan can also accrue under the classical synthesis route, which may reduce the solubility of the product. Such potential methylation has led to the creation of *O*-methylation free TMC synthesis procedures [116]. Other quaternization positions in chitosan include the 6-OH group and the diquaternization of both N and O positions [119].

The mechanical properties of chitosan-based wound dressings are also sometimes the focus of derivatizations utilizing crosslinking. Despite the unsuitability of polyvinyl alcohol (PVA) and polyvinylpyrrolidone (PVP) hydrogels themselves as wound-dressing materials due to their insufficient elasticity and limited hydrophilicity [122], they are popular crosslinkers for chitosan-based hydrogels, to improve their tensile properties [123–126]. Crosslinking with genipin, a chemical compound found in gardenia fruit extract, is also popular [3,127].

Many other derivatizations of chitin and chitosan are also possible, including sulfonation, which leads to properties resembling heparin, a blood thinner [128], and phosphorylation, which increases solubility and antibacterial properties [129]. Introduction of ether groups is also possible, creating derivatives like hydroxypropyl chitosan, which has antifungal properties against fruit fungi [130], or hydroxyethyl β-chitin (HEC) and hydroxybutyl β-chitin, which are antibacterial chitin derivatives that can be turned into gels through heating [131].

6.2. Chitin and Chitosan Nanocomposite Architectures as Wound Dressings

Recent advances in chitin- and chitosan-based wound dressings include polymer, mineral, and metal additives, rather than utilizing pure chitin or chitosan. These additives are typically included to improve the mechanical properties, such as tensile strength and modulus, and biomedical properties, such as antibacterial and antifungal activity of the dressings [1]. However, improvements in these properties must be achieved without compromising dressing biocompatibility, such as blood compatibility and cytocompatibility, physical properties, such as porosity and surface area, which affect cell and fibroblast attachment, and wetting and barrier properties, such as hydrophilicity, water uptake capacity, oxygen, carbon dioxide, and water vapor transmission rates [124,132]. This is important since chitin and chitosan themselves are biocompatible and able to be degraded by several enzymes [133], such as lysozyme in vivo [134]. The degradation rate is governed by the molecular weight and degree of deacetylation [133,134] of the chitosan with further manipulation based on fiber diameter and mesh porosity also possible in chitosan fiber-mesh scaffolds [135].

Biocompatible additives include natural polysaccharides, such as cellulose, and mineral clays, such as the aluminum phyllosilicate clays bentonite and halloysite. These additives are primarily used as reinforcements to improve the mechanical properties of wound dressings [1], which is especially important in chitosan-based wound dressings, which suffer from poor tensile strength and elasticity [132]. Cellulose nanocrystals [127,136] increase the tensile properties of chitosan-based wound dressings, with the additional possibility of utilizing bacterial cellulose to facilitate amine coupling, to increase strength rather than conventional impregnation or physical blending methods [137]. Alternatively, chitin itself, which has a high tensile strength and modulus, can be used to reinforce chitosan, with both chitin nanofibers [132] and nanocrystals [3] improving the tensile strength of chitosan-based wound dressings. Combinations of chitin and silk fibroin are also popular in wound-dressing research [138–140], as are combinations of chitosan and sodium alginate, which has hemostatic and gel-forming properties, keeping the wound moist and preventing fiber entrapment during removal [141,142]. Use of these fibrous nanomaterials in wound dressings not only improves tensile strength, but also typically increases surface area, improving fibroblast attachment and spreading [143], without significantly affecting biocompatibility or barrier properties [3,124].

Minerals, such the aluminum phyllosilicate clays bentonite and halloysite, can alternatively provide increases in tensile strength [144,145], while additionally increasing glass transition temperature and enhancing some biomedical wound dressing properties. For example, bentonite clays are nontoxic, have a high cation-exchange capacity, and provide some degree of antimicrobial activity, while also being low in cost and abundant [146,147]. Bentonite is very hydrophilic and is subsequently able to absorb large amounts of wound fluid, increasing the water uptake capacity of dressings and maintaining the moist environment necessary for wound healing [148]. Halloysite nanotubes are also popular nanofillers to improve the mechanical properties of wound dressings due to their unique rod-like structure and hydrophilicity, meaning that they are easily solution-mixed with chitosan in aqueous solution, facilitating easy nanocomposite preparation [149–151]. Graphene oxide is also sometimes included due to its amphiphilicity, high intrinsic strength, and ample oxygen-bearing groups, in addition to its high surface area, which, like nanofibers, was found to improve fibroblast attachment and spreading [143].

However, while many additives are included in wound dressings as reinforcement, others serve purely to enhance the antibacterial properties of the dressing. Metal nanoparticles are popular additives to chitosan-based wound dressings due to their ability to alter the metabolic activity of bacteria they encounter, crossing the bacterial membrane and affecting the shape and function of the cell membrane [143,152] (Figure 9). The presence of these nanoparticles in the metabolic pathway causes oxidative stress, enzyme inhibition, protein deactivation and altered membrane permeability, electrolyte balance, and gene expression, which results in microbial death [153]. Most commonly, silver (Ag), gold (Au), copper (Cu) zinc oxide (ZnO), and titanium dioxide (TiO_2) nanoparticles were incorporated into chitosan-based wound dressings, to enhance antibacterial activity [5,126,154–159]. Ag and Au nanoparticles reduce oxygen molecules, to form reactive intermediates with strong positive redox potential, such as superoxide and hydroxyl radicals (Ag nanoparticles), and singlet oxygen (Au nanoparticles). Metal oxides, such as ZnO and TiO_2, behave similarly, interacting with water or hydroxide ions to form hydroxyl radicals, which can be reduced to superoxide. These radicals then degrade active components governing normal bacterial morphological and physiological function, providing an antibacterial effect [153]. Similar antibiotic activity has also been investigated by using honey and antibiotic-loaded chitosan-based wound dressings, but has received less attention than wound dressings utilizing metal nanoparticles [4,152,160,161].

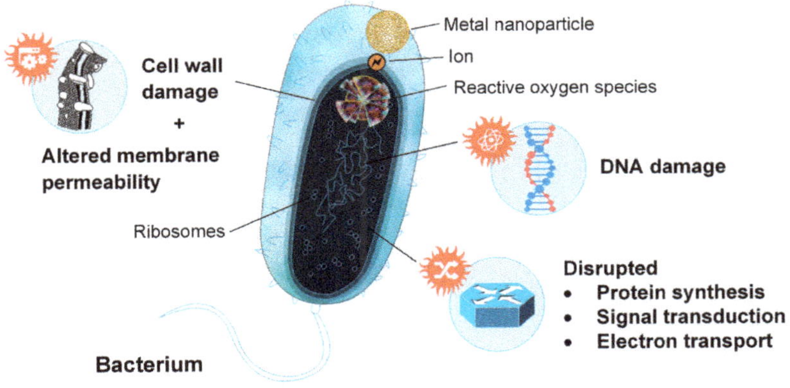

Figure 9. Metal nanoparticle interfacing with bacterium and representations of the mechanisms facilitating microbial death.

7. Human Clinical Trials Utilizing Chitin and Chitosan for Wound Treatment

Commercialization of chitin and chitosan-based wound treatment products, such as Axiostat®, Beschitin® W, Bexident® Post, Celox®, Chitohem®, HemCon®, Medisorb® R, Surgi shield®, and SEQUA® San Chitosan, in addition to custom-prepared treatments, have prompted several human clinical trials of chitin and chitosan for wound-healing applications. These studies predominantly focus on chitosan and chitosan derivatives for use as wound dressings, gels, powders, films, membranes, and even mouthwash for oral, nasal, ear, and skin applications, in addition to treatment of ulcers and serious hemorrhages (Table 3).

Table 3. Human clinical trials utilizing commercially available and custom-made chitin and chitosan wound treatments, resulting in significant improvements in the healing of ear, nasal, oral, and skin wounds, in addition to treatment of ulcers and serious hemorrhages. Data from [162–177].

Application	Wound Type	Treatment Utilized	Treatment Constituents	Ref.
Ear	Membrane perforation	Beschitin® W (membrane)	Chitin, unknown	[162]
Hemorrhage	Obstetric hemorrhage	Celox® (powder/gauze)	Chitosan, unknown	[163]
Nasal	Postoperative	Surgi shield® (gel)	8% carboxymethyl chitosan, unknown	[164]
Oral	Aphthous stomatitis	Mouthwash	0.5% chitosan powder, polyacrylic acid, methyl-/propylparaben, glycerin	[165]
		Adhesive film	Chitosan powder, sesame oil	[166]
	Postoperative	HemCon® (dressing)	Chitosan, unknown	[167]
	Tooth extraction	Bexident® Post (gel)	Chitosan, chlorhexidine, allantoin, dexpanthenol	[168]
		Chitohem® (powder)	Chitosan, unknown	[169]
Skin	Diabetic	Medisorb® R (membrane/powder)	Butyric-acetic chitin copolyesters, unknown	[170]
	Postoperative	Membrane	Chitosan only	[171]
		Dressing	Carboxymethyl chitosan, unknown	[172]
	Puncture	HemCon® (dressing)	Chitosan, unknown	[173]
	Superficial	Axiostat® (dressing)	Chitosan, unknown	[174]
		Film	Oligochitosan, glycerol	[175]
Ulcers	Pressure, vascular, diabetic ulcers	Topical gel	2% chitosan powder, acetic acid, regenerated cellulose	[176]
		SEQUA® San Chitosan (dressing)	Chitosan, unknown	[177]

These wound treatments have experienced significant success in oral clinical trials where they have been used to treat aphthous stomatitis (mouth ulcers), postoperative and tooth extraction wounds. Chitosan mouthwash (0.5%) reduced aphthous stomatitis pain and ulcer size, exhibiting comparable performance to Triamcinolone, a corticosteroid product [165]. Similar results could also be achieved by using a mucoadhesive film [166]. Dental surgery clinical trials also found chitosan-based wound treatments to significantly shorten bleeding time and improve wound healing for patients undergoing minor surgery and tooth extractions [167,168]. Clinical trials examining the effect of chitosan on a range of other wounds also exhibited very promising results, with improved cell adherence, hemostasis and re-epithelialization [164,171], less itching and sensitivity [171], less exudate and odor [175], and reductions in wound healing time [170,173], post-hemodialysis puncture site bleeding [173], and rebleeding [174] in diabetic, puncture, superficial, skin graft, and sinus postoperative wounds. Chitosan has also been utilized in clinical trials for treatment of ulcers with notable reductions in exudate, pain on dressing removal, wound area and depth when compared to traditional Vaseline gauze dressings [176,177]. Additionally, military-grade chitosan-based wound-treatment products, such as Celox®, have been used as lower-cost alternatives to oxytocin, prostaglandin, and uterine balloons in the treatment of life-threatening obstetric hemorrhages, completely stopping uncontrolled bleeding within seconds to minutes. Although chitosan was used in most clinical trials, it should also be noted that chitin membranes have been used to assist in the closure of chronic tympanic membrane perforations in the ear [162].

8. Conclusions

Chitin and its chitosan derivative have experienced significant research interest for wound-dressing applications since the 1970s due to their ability to accelerate healing and reduce scarring. While chitin historically received academic attention due to its biomedical properties, its deacetylated derivative chitosan has been the focus of more recent scientific research due to its superior healing properties. These beneficial properties of chitin and chitosan include nontoxicity, biocompatibility, biodegradability, and antimicrobial activity and are achieved through numerous mechanisms, such as hemostatic activity and support in cellular proliferation and attachment. Crustacean-derived chitosan has been widely investigated and used in wound-healing research due to its high yields and purity, with significant advances in wound dressings incorporating chemically modified chitosan derivatives to improve solubility and antimicrobial activity. Chitosan blends incorporating biocompatible additives, such as natural polysaccharides, synthetic polymers, mineral clays, and metal nanoparticles, have also been utilized to generate advanced wound dressings with excellent mechanical and biomedical properties. Fungi, on the other hand, have received significantly less scientific interest due to their lower chitin content. Moreover, the chitin present in fungi is covalently linked to β-glucan. However, the mass production potential and simple extraction processes associated with fungal chitin, coupled with variations in the chitin content of fungal species, recent advances in fungal materials technologies, and the discovery of healing properties in fungal exopolysaccharides suggest that further investigation of the healing potential of fungal polysaccharide constituents is warranted. With proven biomedical properties, both fungi- and crustacean-derived chitin and chitosan constitute powerful natural medicinal agents, with the potential to advance modern medicine and wound treatment through further research and practical application.

Author Contributions: M.J. and M.K. conceptualized the manuscript, performed all data review and analysis, designed the figures, and wrote the manuscript; A.B. and S.J. supervised the work and contributed to manuscript review and proofing. All authors have read and agreed to the published version of the manuscript.

Funding: M.J. was sponsored by an Australian Government Research Training Program Scholarship at RMIT. Open Access Funding by the University of Vienna.

Conflicts of Interest: The authors declare no conflicts of interest.

References

1. Morganti, P.; Morganti, G.; Coltelli, M.B. Chitin Nanomaterials and Nanocomposites for Tissue Repair. In *Marine-Derived Biomaterials for Tissue Engineering Applications*; Springer: Berlin, Germany, 2019; pp. 523–544.
2. Khil, M.S.; Cha, D.I.; Kim, H.Y.; Kim, I.S.; Bhattarai, N. Electrospun nanofibrous polyurethane membrane as wound dressing. *J. Biomed. Mater. Res. Part B Appl. Biomater.* **2003**, *67*, 675–679. [CrossRef] [PubMed]
3. Naseri, N.; Algan, C.; Jacobs, V.; John, M.; Oksman, K.; Mathew, A.P. Electrospun chitosan-based nanocomposite mats reinforced with chitin nanocrystals for wound dressing. *Carbohydr. Polym.* **2014**, *109*, 7–15. [CrossRef] [PubMed]
4. Shah, A.; Buabeid, M.A.; Arafa, E.-S.A.; Hussain, I.; Li, L.; Murtaza, G. The wound healing and antibacterial potential of triple-component nanocomposite (chitosan-silver-sericin) films loaded with moxifloxacin. *Int. J. Pharm.* **2019**, *564*, 22–38. [CrossRef] [PubMed]
5. Murali, S.; Kumar, S.; Koh, J.; Seena, S.; Singh, P.; Ramalho, A.; Sobral, A.J. Bio-based chitosan/gelatin/Ag@ ZnO bionanocomposites: Synthesis and mechanical and antibacterial properties. *Cellulose* **2019**, *26*, 1–15. [CrossRef]
6. Li, W.J.; Laurencin, C.T.; Caterson, E.J.; Tuan, R.S.; Ko, F.K. Electrospun nanofibrous structure: A novel scaffold for tissue engineering. *J. Biomed. Mater. Res.* **2002**, *60*, 613–621. [CrossRef]
7. Nawawi, W.; Jones, M.; Murphy, R.J.; Lee, K.-Y.; Kontturi, E.; Bismarck, A. Nanomaterials derived from fungal sources—Is it the new hype? *Biomacromolecules* **2019**, *21*, 30–55. [CrossRef]
8. Morin-Crini, N.; Lichtfouse, E.; Torri, G.; Crini, G. Applications of chitosan in food, pharmaceuticals, medicine, cosmetics, agriculture, textiles, pulp and paper, biotechnology, and environmental chemistry. *Environ. Chem. Lett.* **2019**, *17*, 1667–1692. [CrossRef]
9. Atkinson, A.; Siegel, V.; Pakhomov, E.; Jessopp, M.; Loeb, V. A re-appraisal of the total biomass and annual production of Antarctic krill. *Deep Sea Res. Part I Oceanogr. Res. Pap.* **2009**, *56*, 727–740. [CrossRef]
10. Jeuniaux, C.; Voss-Foucart, M.F. Chitin biomass and production in the marine environment. *Biochem. Syst. Ecol.* **1991**, *19*, 347–356. [CrossRef]
11. Kurita, K. Chitin and chitosan: Functional biopolymers from marine crustaceans. *Mar. Biotechnol.* **2006**, *8*, 203. [CrossRef]
12. Charoenvuttitham, P.; Shi, J.; Mittal, G.S. Chitin extraction from black tiger shrimp (*Penaeus monodon*) waste using organic acids. *Sep. Sci. Technol.* **2006**, *41*, 1135–1153. [CrossRef]
13. Gopalan Nair, K.; Dufresne, A. Crab shell chitin whisker reinforced natural rubber nanocomposites. 1. Processing and swelling behavior. *Biomacromolecules* **2003**, *4*, 657–665. [CrossRef] [PubMed]
14. Jones, M.; Weiland, K.; Kujundzic, M.; Theiner, J.; Kahlig, H.; Kontturi, E.; John, S.; Bismarck, A.; Mautner, A. Waste-Derived Low-Cost Mycelium Nanopapers with Tunable Mechanical and Surface Properties. *Biomacromolecules* **2019**, *20*, 3513–3523. [CrossRef] [PubMed]
15. Di Mario, F.; Rapana, P.; Tomati, U.; Galli, E. Chitin and chitosan from Basidiomycetes. *Int. J. Biol. Macromol.* **2008**, *43*, 8–12. [CrossRef]
16. Hassainia, A.; Satha, H.; Boufi, S. Chitin from Agaricus bisporus: Extraction and characterization. *Int. J. Biol. Macromol.* **2018**, *117*, 1334–1342. [CrossRef]
17. Nawawi, W.; Lee, K.-Y.; Kontturi, E.; Murphy, R.; Bismarck, A. Chitin nanopaper from mushroom extract: Natural composite of nanofibres and glucan from a single bio-based source. *ACS Sustain. Chem. Eng.* **2019**, *7*, 6492–6496. [CrossRef]
18. Nguyen, T.T.; Barber, A.R.; Corbin, K.; Zhang, W. Lobster processing by-products as valuable bioresource of marine functional ingredients, nutraceuticals, and pharmaceuticals. *Bioresour. Bioprocess.* **2017**, *4*, 27. [CrossRef]
19. Rinaudo, M. Chitin and chitosan: Properties and applications. *Prog. Polym. Sci.* **2006**, *31*, 603–632. [CrossRef]
20. Abo Elsoud, M.M.; El Kady, E.M. Current trends in fungal biosynthesis of chitin and chitosan. *Bull. Natl. Res. Cent.* **2019**, *43*, 59. [CrossRef]
21. Arbia, W.; Arbia, L.; Adour, L.; Amrane, A. Chitin extraction from crustacean shells using biological methods—A review. *Food Technol. Biotechnol.* **2013**, *51*, 12–25.
22. Cuong, H.N.; Minh, N.C.; Van Hoa, N.; Trung, T.S. Preparation and characterization of high purity β-chitin from squid pens (*Loligo chenisis*). *Int. J. Biol. Macromol.* **2016**, *93*, 442–447. [CrossRef] [PubMed]

23. Fesel, P.H.; Zuccaro, A. β-glucan: Crucial component of the fungal cell wall and elusive MAMP in plants. *Fungal Genet. Biol.* **2016**, *90*, 53–60. [CrossRef] [PubMed]
24. Gaill, F.; Shillito, B.; Menard, F.; Goffinet, G.; Childress, J.J. Rate and process of tube production by the deep-sea hydrothermal vent tubeworm *Riftia pachyptila*. *Mar. Ecol. Prog. Ser.* **1997**, *148*, 135–143. [CrossRef]
25. Kaya, M.; Bitim, B.; Mujtaba, M.; Koyuncu, T. Surface morphology of chitin highly related with the isolated body part of butterfly (*Argynnis pandora*). *Int. J. Biol. Macromol.* **2015**, *81*, 443–449. [CrossRef]
26. Naczk, M.; Synowiecki, J.; Sikorski, Z.E. The gross chemical composition of Antarctic krill shell waste. *Food Chem.* **1981**, *7*, 175–179. [CrossRef]
27. Pandharipande, S.; Bhagat, P.H. Synthesis of chitin from crab shells and its utilization in preparation of nanostructured film. *Synthesis* **2016**, *5*, 1378–1383.
28. Paulino, A.T.; Simionato, J.I.; Garcia, J.C.; Nozaki, J. Characterization of chitosan and chitin produced from silkworm crysalides. *Carbohydr. Polym.* **2006**, *64*, 98–103. [CrossRef]
29. Tauber, O.E. The distribution of chitin in an insect. *J. Morphol.* **1934**, *56*, 51–58. [CrossRef]
30. Janesch, J.; Jones, M.; Bacher, M.; Kontturi, E.; Bismarck, A.; Mautner, A. Mushroom-derived chitosan-glucan nanopaper filters for the treatment of water. *React. Funct. Polym.* **2019**, *146*, 104428. [CrossRef]
31. Muzzarelli, R.A. Chitin nanostructures in living organisms. In *Chitin*; Springer: Berlin, Germany, 2011; pp. 1–34.
32. Hackman, R. Studies on chitin IV. The occurrence of complexes in which chitin and protein are covalently linked. *Aust. J. Biol. Sci.* **1960**, *13*, 568–577. [CrossRef]
33. Attwood, M.M.; Zola, H. The association between chitin and protein in some chitinous tissues. *Comp. Biochem. Physiol.* **1967**, *20*, 993–998. [CrossRef]
34. Kramer, K.J.; Hopkins, T.L.; Schaefer, J. Applications of solids NMR to the analysis of insect sclerotized structures. *Insect Biochem. Mol. Biol.* **1995**, *25*, 1067–1080. [CrossRef]
35. Percot, A.; Viton, C.; Domard, A. Characterization of shrimp shell deproteinization. *Biomacromolecules* **2003**, *4*, 1380–1385. [CrossRef] [PubMed]
36. Sietsma, J.; Wessels, J. Evidence for covalent linkages between chitin and β-glucan in a fungal wall. *Microbiology* **1979**, *114*, 99–108. [CrossRef]
37. Kollár, R.; Reinhold, B.B.; Petráková, E.; Yeh, H.J.; Ashwell, G.; Drgonová, J.; Kapteyn, J.C.; Klis, F.M.; Cabib, E. Architecture of the yeast cell wall β (1→6)-glucan interconnects mannoprotein, β (1→3)-glucan, and chitin. *J. Biol. Chem.* **1997**, *272*, 17762–17775. [CrossRef] [PubMed]
38. Heux, L.; Brugnerotto, J.; Desbrieres, J.; Versali, M.-F.; Rinaudo, M. Solid state NMR for determination of degree of acetylation of chitin and chitosan. *Biomacromolecules* **2000**, *1*, 746–751. [CrossRef] [PubMed]
39. Latge, J.P. The cell wall: A carbohydrate armour for the fungal cell. *Mol. Microbiol.* **2007**, *66*, 279–290. [CrossRef]
40. Bartnicki-Garcia, S.; Nickerson, W.J. Isolation, composition, and structure of cell walls of filamentous and yeast-like forms of Mucor rouxii. *Biochim. Biophys. Acta* **1962**, *58*, 102–119. [CrossRef]
41. Karimi, K.; Zamani, A. Mucor indicus: Biology and industrial application perspectives: A review. *Biotechnol. Adv.* **2013**, *31*, 466–481. [CrossRef]
42. Rice, M. Get an Old Blender and Make Your Own Deckle and Mould. *Mushroom J. Wild Mushrooming* **1992**, *10*, 22–26.
43. Younes, I.; Rinaudo, M. Chitin and chitosan preparation from marine sources. Structure, properties and applications. *Mar. Drugs* **2015**, *13*, 1133–1174. [CrossRef] [PubMed]
44. Sietsma, J.; Wessels, J. Chemical analysis of the hyphal walls of Schizophyllum commune. *Biochim. Biophys. Acta Gen. Subj.* **1977**, *496*, 225–239. [CrossRef]
45. Peniston, Q.P.; Johnson, E.L. Process for the Manufacture of Chitosan. U.S. Patent No. 4,195,175, 25 March 1980.
46. Thanou, M.; Verhoef, J.; Junginger, H. Oral drug absorption enhancement by chitosan and its derivatives. *Adv. Drug Deliv. Rev.* **2001**, *52*, 117–126. [CrossRef]
47. No, H.K.; Park, N.Y.; Lee, S.H.; Meyers, S.P. Antibacterial activity of chitosans and chitosan oligomers with different molecular weights. *Int. J. Food Microbiol.* **2002**, *74*, 65–72. [CrossRef]
48. Islam, S.; Bhuiyan, M.R.; Islam, M. Chitin and chitosan: Structure, properties and applications in biomedical engineering. *J. Polym. Environ.* **2017**, *25*, 854–866. [CrossRef]

49. Bamba, Y.; Ogawa, Y.; Saito, T.; Berglund, L.A.; Isogai, A. Estimating the Strength of Single Chitin Nanofibrils via Sonication-Induced Fragmentation. *Biomacromolecules* **2017**, *18*, 4405–4410. [CrossRef]
50. Webster, J.; Weber, R. *Introduction to Fungi*; Cambridge University Press: Cambrige, UK, 2007.
51. Cui, J.; Yu, Z.; Lau, D. Effect of Acetyl Group on Mechanical Properties of Chitin/Chitosan Nanocrystal: A Molecular Dynamics Study. *Int. J. Mol. Sci.* **2016**, *17*, 61. [CrossRef]
52. Guo, S.A.; DiPietro, L.A. Factors affecting wound healing. *J. Dent. Res.* **2010**, *89*, 219–229. [CrossRef]
53. Singer, A.J.; Clark, R.A. Cutaneous wound healing. *N. Engl. J. Med.* **1999**, *341*, 738–746. [CrossRef]
54. Martin, P. Wound healing-aiming for perfect skin regeneration. *Science* **1997**, *276*, 75–81. [CrossRef]
55. Su, C.-H.; Liu, S.-H.; Yu, S.-Y.; Hsieh, Y.-L.; Ho, H.-O.; Hu, C.-H.; Sheu, M.-T. Development of fungal mycelia as a skin substitute: Characterization of keratinocyte proliferation and matrix metalloproteinase expression during improvement in the wound-healing process. *J. Biomed. Mater. Res. Part A* **2005**, *72*, 220–227. [CrossRef] [PubMed]
56. Su, C.-H.; Sun, C.-S.; Juan, S.-W.; Hu, C.-H.; Ke, W.-T.; Sheu, M.-T. Fungal mycelia as the source of chitin and polysaccharides and their applications as skin substitutes. *Biomaterials* **1997**, *18*, 1169–1174. [CrossRef]
57. Ohshima, Y.; Nishino, K.; Yonekura, Y.; Kishimoto, S.; Wakabayashi, S. Clinical application of chitin non-woven fabric as wound dressing. *Eur. J. Plast. Surg.* **1987**, *10*, 66–69. [CrossRef]
58. Malette, W.; Quigley, H.; Adickes, E. Chitosan effect in vascular surgery, tissue culture and tissue regeneration. In *Nature and Technology*; Springer: Berlin, Germany, 1986; pp. 435–442.
59. Andrews, D.A.; Low, P.S. Role of red blood cells in thrombosis. *Curr. Opin. Hematol.* **1999**, *6*, 76. [CrossRef] [PubMed]
60. Muzzarelli, R.A. Biochemical significance of exogenous chitins and chitosans in animals and patients. *Carbohydr. Polym.* **1993**, *20*, 7–16. [CrossRef]
61. Klokkevold, P.R.; Lew, D.S.; Ellis, D.G.; Bertolami, C.N. Effect of chitosan on lingual hemostasis in rabbits. *J. Oral Maxillofac. Surg.* **1991**, *49*, 858–863. [CrossRef]
62. Brandenberg, G.; Leibrock, L.G.; Shuman, R.; Malette, W.G.; Quigley, H. Chitosan: A New Topical Hemostatic Agent for Diffuse Capillary Bleeding in Brain Tissue. *Neurosurgery* **1984**, *15*, 9–13. [CrossRef]
63. Diegelmann, R.F.; Dunn, J.D.; Lindblad, W.J.; Cohen, I.K. Analysis of the effects of chitosan on inflammation, angiogenesis, fibroplasia, and collagen deposition in polyvinyl alcohol sponge implants in rat wounds. *Wound Repair Regen.* **1996**, *4*, 48–52. [CrossRef]
64. Usami, Y.; Minami, S.; Okamoto, Y.; Matsuhashi, A.; Shigemasa, Y. Influence of chain length of N-acetyl-D-glucosamine and D-glucosamine residues on direct and complement-mediated chemotactic activities for canine polymorphonuclear cells. *Carbohydr. Polym.* **1997**, *32*, 115–122. [CrossRef]
65. Usami, Y.; Okamoto, Y.; Minami, S.; Matsuhashi, A.; Kumazawa, N.H.; Tanioka, S.-I.; Shigemasa, Y. Migration of canine neutrophils to chitin and chitosan. *J. Vet. Med. Sci.* **1994**, *56*, 1215–1216. [CrossRef]
66. Ueno, H.; Mori, T.; Fujinaga, T. Topical formulations and wound healing applications of chitosan. *Adv. Drug Deliv. Rev.* **2001**, *52*, 105–115. [CrossRef]
67. Ueno, H.; Yamada, H.; Tanaka, I.; Kaba, N.; Matsuura, M.; Okumura, M.; Kadosawa, T.; Fujinaga, T. Accelerating effects of chitosan for healing at early phase of experimental open wound in dogs. *Biomaterials* **1999**, *20*, 1407–1414. [CrossRef]
68. Okamoto, Y.; Shibazaki, K.; Minami, S.; Matsuhashi, A.; Tanioka, S.-I.; Shigemasa, Y. Evaluation of chitin and chitosan on open wound healing in dogs. *J. Vet. Med. Sci.* **1995**, *57*, 851–854. [CrossRef] [PubMed]
69. Martin, P.; Leibovich, S.J. Inflammatory cells during wound repair: The good, the bad and the ugly. *Trends Cell Biol.* **2005**, *15*, 599–607. [CrossRef] [PubMed]
70. Ueno, H.; Nakamura, F.; Murakami, M.; Okumura, M.; Kadosawa, T.; Fujinaga, T. Evaluation effects of chitosan for the extracellular matrix production by fibroblasts and the growth factors production by macrophages. *Biomaterials* **2001**, *22*, 2125–2130. [CrossRef]
71. Nishimura, K.; Ishihara, C.; Ukei, S.; Tokura, S.; Azuma, I. Stimulation of cytokine production in mice using deacetylated chitin. *Vaccine* **1986**, *4*, 151–156. [CrossRef]
72. Nishimura, K.; Nishimura, S.; Nishi, N.; Saiki, I.; Tokura, S.; Azuma, I. Immunological activity of chitin and its derivatives. *Vaccine* **1984**, *2*, 93–99. [CrossRef]
73. Barrientos, S.; Stojadinovic, O.; Golinko, M.S.; Brem, H.; Tomic-Canic, M. Growth factors and cytokines in wound healing. *Wound Repair Regen.* **2008**, *16*, 585–601. [CrossRef]

74. Theocharis, A.D.; Skandalis, S.S.; Gialeli, C.; Karamanos, N.K. Extracellular matrix structure. *Adv. Drug Deliv. Rev.* **2016**, *97*, 4–27. [CrossRef]
75. Minagawa, T.; Okamura, Y.; Shigemasa, Y.; Minami, S.; Okamoto, Y. Effects of molecular weight and deacetylation degree of chitin/chitosan on wound healing. *Carbohydr. Polym.* **2007**, *67*, 640–644. [CrossRef]
76. Howling, G.I.; Dettmar, P.W.; Goddard, P.A.; Hampson, F.C.; Dornish, M.; Wood, E.J. The effect of chitin and chitosan on the proliferation of human skin fibroblasts and keratinocytes in vitro. *Biomaterials* **2001**, *22*, 2959–2966. [CrossRef]
77. Pillai, C.; Paul, W.; Sharma, C.P. Chitin and chitosan polymers: Chemistry, solubility and fiber formation. *Prog. Polym. Sci.* **2009**, *34*, 641–678. [CrossRef]
78. Alsarra, I.A. Chitosan topical gel formulation in the management of burn wounds. *Int. J. Biol. Macromol.* **2009**, *45*, 16–21. [CrossRef] [PubMed]
79. Yang, J.; Tian, F.; Wang, Z.; Wang, Q.; Zeng, Y.J.; Chen, S.Q. Effect of chitosan molecular weight and deacetylation degree on hemostasis. *J. Biomed. Mater. Res. Part B Appl. Biomater.* **2008**, *84*, 131–137. [CrossRef]
80. Wainwright, M.; Rally, L.; Ali, T.A. The scientific basis of mould therapy. *Mycologist* **1992**, *6*, 108–110. [CrossRef]
81. Wainwright, M. Moulds in folk medicine. *Folklore* **1989**, *100*, 162–166. [CrossRef]
82. Baker, T. Fungal styptics. *Mycologist* **1989**, *3*, 19–20. [CrossRef]
83. Wainwright, M. Moulds in ancient and more recent medicine. *Mycologist* **1989**, *3*, 21–23. [CrossRef]
84. Prudden, J.F.; Migel, P.; Hanson, P.; Friedrich, L.; Balassa, L. The discovery of a potent pure chemical wound-healing accelerator. *Am. J. Surg.* **1970**, *119*, 560–564. [CrossRef]
85. Balassa, L.; Prudden, J. In Applications of chitin and chitosan in wound-healing acceleration. In Proceedings of the 1st International Conference on Chitin/Chitosan, Springfield, VA, USA, 11–13 April 1977; National Technical Information. pp. 296–305.
86. Chung, L.Y.; Schmidt, R.J.; Hamlyn, P.F.; Sagar, B.F.; Andrew, A.M.; Turner, T.D. Biocompatibility of potential wound management products: Fungal mycelia as a source of chitin/chitosan and their effect on the proliferation of human F1000 fibroblasts in culture. *J. Biomed. Mater. Res.* **1994**, *28*, 463–469. [CrossRef]
87. Chung, L.Y.; Schmidt, R.; Hamlyn, P.; Sagar, B.F.; Andrews, A.; Turner, T. Biocompatibility of potential wound management products: Hydrogen peroxide generation by fungal chitin/chitosans and their effects on the proliferation of murine L929 fibroblasts in culture. *J. Biomed. Mater. Res.* **1998**, *39*, 300–307. [CrossRef]
88. Chen, R.-N.; Lee, L.-W.; Chen, L.-C.; Ho, H.-O.; Lui, S.-C.; Sheu, M.-T.; Su, C.-H. Wound-healing effect of micronized sacchachitin (mSC) nanogel on corneal epithelium. *Int. J. Nanomed.* **2012**, *7*, 4697.
89. Mahapatra, S.; Banerjee, D. Fungal exopolysaccharide: Production, composition and applications. *Microbiol. Insights* **2013**, *6*, 1–16. [CrossRef] [PubMed]
90. Madla, S.; Methacanon, P.; Prasitsil, M.; Kirtikara, K. Characterization of biocompatible fungi-derived polymers that induce IL-8 production. *Carbohydr. Polym.* **2005**, *59*, 275–280. [CrossRef]
91. Üzere, Y.Ö.M.O.K.; Polimer, A.A.Y.F. Antibacterial agent loaded fungal polymer for use as a wound dressing. *J. Biol. Chem.* **2011**, *39*, 297–303.
92. Stalhberger, T.; Simenel, C.; Clavaud, C.; Eijsink, V.G.; Jourdain, R.; Delepierre, M.; Latgé, J.-P.; Breton, L.; Fontaine, T. Chemical organization of the cell wall polysaccharide core of Malassezia restricta. *J. Biol. Chem.* **2014**, *289*, 12647–12656. [CrossRef] [PubMed]
93. Synytsya, A.; Novák, M. Structural diversity of fungal glucans. *Carbohydr. Polym.* **2013**, *92*, 792–809. [CrossRef]
94. Goodridge, H.S.; Wolf, A.J.; Underhill, D.M. β-glucan recognition by the innate immune system. *Immunol. Rev.* **2009**, *230*, 38–50. [CrossRef]
95. Wasser, S. Medicinal mushroom science: Current perspectives, advances, evidences, and challenges. *Biomed. J.* **2014**, *37*, 345–356. [CrossRef]
96. Blackwell, M. The Fungi: 1, 2, 3 … 5.1 million species? *Am. J. Bot.* **2011**, *98*, 426–438. [CrossRef]
97. Jones, M.; Huynh, T.; Dekiwadia, C.; Daver, F.; John, S. Mycelium Composites: A Review of Engineering Characteristics and Growth Kinetics. *J. Bionanoscience* **2017**, *11*, 241–257. [CrossRef]
98. Wösten, H.; Krijgsheld, P.; Montalti, M.; Läkk, H.; Summerer, L. Growing Fungi Structures in Space. Available online: http://www.esa.int/gsp/ACT/doc/ARI/ARI%20Study%20Report/ACT-RPT-HAB-ARI-16-6101-Fungi_structures.pdf (accessed on 26 November 2019).

99. Wösten, H.A. Filamentous fungi for the production of enzymes, chemicals and materials. *Curr. Opin. Biotechnol.* **2019**, *59*, 65–70. [CrossRef] [PubMed]
100. Camere, S.; Karana, E. Fabricating materials from living organisms: An emerging design practice. *J. Clean. Prod.* **2018**, *186*, 570–584. [CrossRef]
101. Jones, M.; Mautner, A.; Luenco, S.; Bismarck, A.; John, S. Engineered mycelium composite construction materials from fungal biorefineries: A critical review. *Mater. Des.* **2019**, *187*, 108397. [CrossRef]
102. Oh, B.H.L.; Bismarck, A.; Chan-Park, M.B. High Internal Phase Emulsion Templating with Self-Emulsifying and Thermoresponsive Chitosan-graft-PNIPAM-graft-Oligoproline. *Biomacromolecules* **2014**, *15*, 1777–1787. [CrossRef]
103. Benhabiles, M.; Salah, R.; Lounici, H.; Drouiche, N.; Goosen, M.; Mameri, N. Antibacterial activity of chitin, chitosan and its oligomers prepared from shrimp shell waste. *Food Hydrocoll.* **2012**, *29*, 48–56. [CrossRef]
104. Ribeiro, M.P.; Espiga, A.; Silva, D.; Baptista, P.; Henriques, J.; Ferreira, C.; Silva, J.C.; Borges, J.P.; Pires, E.; Chaves, P. Development of a new chitosan hydrogel for wound dressing. *Wound Repair Regen.* **2009**, *17*, 817–824. [CrossRef]
105. Bhattarai, N.; Gunn, J.; Zhang, M. Chitosan-based hydrogels for controlled, localized drug delivery. *Adv. Drug Deliv. Rev.* **2010**, *62*, 83–99. [CrossRef]
106. Upadhyaya, L.; Singh, J.; Agarwal, V.; Tewari, R.P. Biomedical applications of carboxymethyl chitosans. *Carbohydr. Polym.* **2013**, *91*, 452–466. [CrossRef]
107. Liu, H.; Liu, J.; Qi, C.; Fang, Y.; Zhang, L.; Zhuo, R.; Jiang, X. Thermosensitive injectable in-situ forming carboxymethyl chitin hydrogel for three-dimensional cell culture. *Acta Biomater.* **2016**, *35*, 228–237. [CrossRef]
108. Chang, J.; Liu, W.; Han, B.; Peng, S.; He, B.; Gu, Z. Investigation of the skin repair and healing mechanism of N-carboxymethyl chitosan in second-degree burn wounds. *Wound Repair Regen.* **2013**, *21*, 113–121. [CrossRef] [PubMed]
109. Xiao, F.L.; Yun, L.G.; Dong, Z.Y.; Zhi, L.; Kang, D.Y. Antibacterial action of chitosan and carboxymethylated chitosan. *J. Appl. Polym. Sci.* **2001**, *79*, 1324–1335.
110. Anitha, A.; Rani, V.D.; Krishna, R.; Sreeja, V.; Selvamurugan, N.; Nair, S.; Tamura, H.; Jayakumar, R. Synthesis, characterization, cytotoxicity and antibacterial studies of chitosan, O-carboxymethyl and N, O-carboxymethyl chitosan nanoparticles. *Carbohydr. Polym.* **2009**, *78*, 672–677. [CrossRef]
111. Mattioli-Belmonte, M.; Nicoli-Aldini, N.; De Benedittis, A.; Sgarbi, G.; Amati, S.; Fini, M.; Biagini, G.; Muzzarelli, R. Morphological study of bone regeneration in the presence of 6-oxychitin. *Carbohydr. Polym.* **1999**, *40*, 23–27. [CrossRef]
112. Muzzarelli, R.A.; Ramos, V.; Stanic, V.; Dubini, B.; Mattioli-Belmonte, M.; Tosi, G.; Giardino, R. Osteogenesis promoted by calcium phosphate N, N-dicarboxymethyl chitosan. *Carbohydr. Polym.* **1998**, *36*, 267–276. [CrossRef]
113. Azuma, K.; Nishihara, M.; Shimizu, H.; Itoh, Y.; Takashima, O.; Osaki, T.; Itoh, N.; Imagawa, T.; Murahata, Y.; Tsuka, T. Biological adhesive based on carboxymethyl chitin derivatives and chitin nanofibers. *Biomaterials* **2015**, *42*, 20–29. [CrossRef]
114. Dang, Q.; Liu, K.; Liu, C.; Xu, T.; Yan, J.; Yan, F.; Cha, D.; Zhang, Q.; Cao, Y. Preparation, characterization, and evaluation of 3, 6-ON-acetylethylenediamine modified chitosan as potential antimicrobial wound dressing material. *Carbohydr. Polym.* **2018**, *180*, 1–12. [CrossRef]
115. Bi, B.; Liu, H.; Kang, W.; Zhuo, R.; Jiang, X. An injectable enzymatically crosslinked tyramine-modified carboxymethyl chitin hydrogel for biomedical applications. *Colloids Surf. B Biointerfaces* **2019**, *175*, 614–624. [CrossRef]
116. Xu, T.; Xin, M.; Li, M.; Huang, H.; Zhou, S. Synthesis, characteristic and antibacterial activity of N, N, N-trimethyl chitosan and its carboxymethyl derivatives. *Carbohydr. Polym.* **2010**, *81*, 931–936. [CrossRef]
117. Cheah, W.Y.; Show, P.-L.; Ng, I.-S.; Lin, G.-Y.; Chiu, C.-Y.; Chang, Y.-K. Antibacterial activity of quaternized chitosan modified nanofiber membrane. *Int. J. Biol. Macromol.* **2019**, *126*, 569–577. [CrossRef]
118. Luan, F.; Wei, L.; Zhang, J.; Tan, W.; Chen, Y.; Wang, P.; Dong, F.; Li, Q.; Guo, Z. Synthesis, Characterization, and Antifungal Activity of N-Quaternized and N-Diquaternized Chitin Derivatives. *Starch Stärke* **2018**, *70*, 1800026. [CrossRef]
119. Khattak, S.; Wahid, F.; Liu, L.-P.; Jia, S.-R.; Chu, L.-Q.; Xie, Y.-Y.; Li, Z.-X.; Zhong, C. Applications of cellulose and chitin/chitosan derivatives and composites as antibacterial materials: Current state and perspectives. *Appl. Microbiol. Biotechnol.* **2019**, *103*, 1989–2006. [CrossRef] [PubMed]

120. Ding, F.; Shi, X.; Li, X.; Cai, J.; Duan, B.; Du, Y. Homogeneous synthesis and characterization of quaternized chitin in NaOH/urea aqueous solution. *Carbohydr. Polym.* **2012**, *87*, 422–426. [CrossRef]
121. Xu, H.; Fang, Z.; Tian, W.; Wang, Y.; Ye, Q.; Zhang, L.; Cai, J. Green Fabrication of Amphiphilic Quaternized β-Chitin Derivatives with Excellent Biocompatibility and Antibacterial Activities for Wound Healing. *Adv. Mater.* **2018**, *30*, 1801100. [CrossRef] [PubMed]
122. Kamoun, E.A.; Chen, X.; Mohy Eldin, M.S.; Kenawy, E.-R.S. Crosslinked poly (vinyl alcohol) hydrogels for wound dressing applications: A review of remarkably blended polymers. *Arab. J. Chem.* **2015**, *8*, 1–14. [CrossRef]
123. Yang, X.; Zhu, Z.; Liu, Q.; Chen, X.; Ma, M. Effects of PVA, agar contents, and irradiation doses on properties of PVA/ws-chitosan/glycerol hydrogels made by γ-irradiation followed by freeze-thawing. *Radiat. Phys. Chem.* **2008**, *77*, 954–960. [CrossRef]
124. Poonguzhali, R.; Basha, S.K.; Kumari, V.S. Synthesis and characterization of chitosan-PVP-nanocellulose composites for in-vitro wound dressing application. *Int. J. Biol. Macromol.* **2017**, *105*, 111–120. [CrossRef]
125. Hasan, A.; Waibhaw, G.; Tiwari, S.; Dharmalingam, K.; Shukla, I.; Pandey, L.M. Fabrication and characterization of chitosan, polyvinylpyrrolidone, and cellulose nanowhiskers nanocomposite films for wound healing drug delivery application. *J. Biomed. Mater. Res. Part A* **2017**, *105*, 2391–2404. [CrossRef]
126. Khorasani, M.T.; Joorabloo, A.; Adeli, H.; Mansoori-Moghadam, Z.; Moghaddam, A. Design and optimization of process parameters of polyvinyl (alcohol)/chitosan/nano zinc oxide hydrogels as wound healing materials. *Carbohydr. Polym.* **2019**, *207*, 542–554. [CrossRef]
127. Naseri, N.; Mathew, A.P.; Girandon, L.; Fröhlich, M.; Oksman, K. Porous electrospun nanocomposite mats based on chitosan–cellulose nanocrystals for wound dressing: Effect of surface characteristics of nanocrystals. *Cellulose* **2015**, *22*, 521–534. [CrossRef]
128. Vongchan, P.; Sajomsang, W.; Subyen, D.; Kongtawelert, P. Anticoagulant activity of a sulfated chitosan. *Carbohydr. Res.* **2002**, *337*, 1239–1242. [CrossRef]
129. Shanmugam, A.; Kathiresan, K.; Nayak, L. Preparation, characterization and antibacterial activity of chitosan and phosphorylated chitosan from cuttlebone of Sepia kobiensis (Hoyle, 1885). *Biotechnol. Rep.* **2016**, *9*, 25–30. [CrossRef] [PubMed]
130. Peng, Y.; Han, B.; Liu, W.; Xu, X. Preparation and antimicrobial activity of hydroxypropyl chitosan. *Carbohydr. Res.* **2005**, *340*, 1846–1851. [CrossRef] [PubMed]
131. Xu, H.; Wu, S.; Wei, P.; Xie, F.; Xu, X.; Cai, J.; Liu, Y. Versatile synthesis, characterization and properties of β-chitin derivatives from aqueous KOH/urea solution. *Carbohydr. Polym.* **2020**, *227*, 115345. [CrossRef]
132. Shelma, R.; Paul, W.; Sharma, C.P. Chitin nanofibre reinforced thin chitosan films for wound healing application. *Trends Biomater. Artif. Organs* **2008**, *22*, 111–115.
133. Zhang, H.; Neau, S.H. In Vitro degradation of chitosan by a commercial enzyme preparation: Effect of molecular weight and degree of deacetylation. *Biomaterials* **2001**, *22*, 1653–1658. [CrossRef]
134. Vårum, K.M.; Myhr, M.M.; Hjerde, R.J.; Smidsrød, O. In Vitro degradation rates of partially N-acetylated chitosans in human serum. *Carbohydr. Res.* **1997**, *299*, 99–101. [CrossRef]
135. Cunha-Reis, C.; TuzlaKoglu, K.; Baas, E.; Yang, Y.; El Haj, A.; Reis, R. Influence of porosity and fibre diameter on the degradation of chitosan fibre-mesh scaffolds and cell adhesion. *J. Mater. Sci. Mater. Med.* **2007**, *18*, 195–200. [CrossRef]
136. Li, Q.; Zhou, J.; Zhang, L. Structure and properties of the nanocomposite films of chitosan reinforced with cellulose whiskers. *J. Polym. Sci. Part B Polym. Phys.* **2009**, *47*, 1069–1077. [CrossRef]
137. Lai, C.; Zhang, S.; Chen, X.; Sheng, L. Nanocomposite films based on TEMPO-mediated oxidized bacterial cellulose and chitosan. *Cellulose* **2014**, *21*, 2757–2772. [CrossRef]
138. Mehrabani, M.G.; Karimian, R.; Rakhshaei, R.; Pakdel, F.; Eslami, H.; Fakhrzadeh, V.; Rahimi, M.; Salehi, R.; Kafil, H.S. Chitin/silk fibroin/TiO2 bio-nanocomposite as a biocompatible wound dressing bandage with strong antimicrobial activity. *Int. J. Biol. Macromol.* **2018**, *116*, 966–976. [CrossRef] [PubMed]
139. Mehrabani, M.G.; Karimian, R.; Mehramouz, B.; Rahimi, M.; Kafil, H.S. Preparation of biocompatible and biodegradable silk fibroin/chitin/silver nanoparticles 3D scaffolds as a bandage for antimicrobial wound dressing. *Int. J. Biol. Macromol.* **2018**, *114*, 961–971. [CrossRef] [PubMed]
140. Niamsa, N.; Srisuwan, Y.; Baimark, Y.; Phinyocheep, P.; Kittipoom, S. Preparation of nanocomposite chitosan/silk fibroin blend films containing nanopore structures. *Carbohydr. Polym.* **2009**, *78*, 60–65. [CrossRef]

141. Devi, M.P.; Sekar, M.; Chamundeswari, M.; Moorthy, A.; Krithiga, G.; Murugan, N.S.; Sastry, T. A novel wound dressing material-fibrin-chitosan-sodium alginate composite sheet. *Bull. Mater. Sci.* **2012**, *35*, 1157–1163. [CrossRef]
142. Knill, C.; Kennedy, J.; Mistry, J.; Miraftab, M.; Smart, G.; Groocock, M.; Williams, H. Alginate fibres modified with unhydrolysed and hydrolysed chitosans for wound dressings. *Carbohydr. Polym.* **2004**, *55*, 65–76. [CrossRef]
143. Dubey, P.; Gopinath, P. PEGylated graphene oxide-based nanocomposite-grafted chitosan/polyvinyl alcohol nanofiber as an advanced antibacterial wound dressing. *RSC Adv.* **2016**, *6*, 69103–69116. [CrossRef]
144. Koosha, M.; Mirzadeh, H.; Shokrgozar, M.A.; Farokhi, M. Nanoclay-reinforced electrospun chitosan/PVA nanocomposite nanofibers for biomedical applications. *RSC Adv.* **2015**, *5*, 10479–10487. [CrossRef]
145. Xu, Y.; Ren, X.; Hanna, M.A. Chitosan/clay nanocomposite film preparation and characterization. *J. Appl. Polym. Sci.* **2006**, *99*, 1684–1691. [CrossRef]
146. Sothornvit, R.; Rhim, J.-W.; Hong, S.-I. Effect of nano-clay type on the physical and antimicrobial properties of whey protein isolate/clay composite films. *J. Food Eng.* **2009**, *91*, 468–473. [CrossRef]
147. Gupta, S.S.; Bhattacharyya, K.G. Adsorption of heavy metals on kaolinite and montmorillonite: A review. *Phys. Chem. Chem. Phys.* **2012**, *14*, 6698–6723. [CrossRef]
148. Devi, N.; Dutta, J. Preparation and characterization of chitosan-bentonite nanocomposite films for wound healing application. *Int. J. Biol. Macromol.* **2017**, *104*, 1897–1904. [CrossRef] [PubMed]
149. Liu, M.; Zhang, Y.; Wu, C.; Xiong, S.; Zhou, C. Chitosan/halloysite nanotubes bionanocomposites: Structure, mechanical properties and biocompatibility. *Int. J. Biol. Macromol.* **2012**, *51*, 566–575. [CrossRef] [PubMed]
150. Sandri, G.; Aguzzi, C.; Rossi, S.; Bonferoni, M.C.; Bruni, G.; Boselli, C.; Cornaglia, A.I.; Riva, F.; Viseras, C.; Caramella, C. Halloysite and chitosan oligosaccharide nanocomposite for wound healing. *Acta Biomater.* **2017**, *57*, 216–224. [CrossRef] [PubMed]
151. Devi, N.; Dutta, J. Development and in vitro characterization of chitosan/starch/halloysite nanotubes ternary nanocomposite films. *Int. J. Biol. Macromol.* **2019**, *127*, 222–231. [CrossRef] [PubMed]
152. Noori, S.; Kokabi, M.; Hassan, Z. Poly (vinyl alcohol)/chitosan/honey/clay responsive nanocomposite hydrogel wound dressing. *J. Appl. Polym. Sci.* **2018**, *135*, 46311. [CrossRef]
153. Wang, L.; Hu, C.; Shao, L. The antimicrobial activity of nanoparticles: Present situation and prospects for the future. *Int. J. Nanomed.* **2017**, *12*, 1227–1249. [CrossRef]
154. Archana, D.; Singh, B.K.; Dutta, J.; Dutta, P. In Vivo evaluation of chitosan–PVP–titanium dioxide nanocomposite as wound dressing material. *Carbohydr. Polym.* **2013**, *95*, 530–539. [CrossRef]
155. Khorasani, M.T.; Joorabloo, A.; Moghaddam, A.; Shamsi, H.; MansooriMoghadam, Z. Incorporation of ZnO nanoparticles into heparinised polyvinyl alcohol/chitosan hydrogels for wound dressing application. *Int. J. Biol. Macromol.* **2018**, *114*, 1203–1215. [CrossRef]
156. Lu, Z.; Gao, J.; He, Q.; Wu, J.; Liang, D.; Yang, H.; Chen, R. Enhanced antibacterial and wound healing activities of microporous chitosan-Ag/ZnO composite dressing. *Carbohydr. Polym.* **2017**, *156*, 460–469. [CrossRef]
157. Zhai, M.; Xu, Y.; Zhou, B.; Jing, W. Keratin-chitosan/n-ZnO nanocomposite hydrogel for antimicrobial treatment of burn wound healing: Characterization and biomedical application. *J. Photochem. Photobiol. B Biol.* **2018**, *180*, 253–258. [CrossRef]
158. Jayaramudu, T.; Varaprasad, K.; Pyarasani, R.D.; Reddy, K.K.; Kumar, K.D.; Akbari-Fakhrabadi, A.; Mangalaraja, R.; Amalraj, J. Chitosan capped copper oxide/copper nanoparticles encapsulated microbial resistant nanocomposite films. *Int. J. Biol. Macromol.* **2019**, *128*, 499–508. [CrossRef] [PubMed]
159. Liang, D.; Lu, Z.; Yang, H.; Gao, J.; Chen, R. Novel asymmetric wettable AgNPs/chitosan wound dressing: In vitro and in vivo evaluation. *ACS Appl. Mater. Interfaces* **2016**, *8*, 3958–3968. [CrossRef] [PubMed]
160. Sarhan, W.A.; Azzazy, H.M.; El-Sherbiny, I.M. Honey/chitosan nanofiber wound dressing enriched with Allium sativum and Cleome droserifolia: Enhanced antimicrobial and wound healing activity. *ACS Appl. Mater. Interfaces* **2016**, *8*, 6379–6390. [CrossRef] [PubMed]
161. Pulat, M.; Kahraman, A.S.; Tan, N.; Gümüşderelioğlu, M. Sequential antibiotic and growth factor releasing chitosan-PAAm semi-IPN hydrogel as a novel wound dressing. *J. Biomater. Sci. Polym. Ed.* **2013**, *24*, 807–819. [CrossRef] [PubMed]

162. Kakehata, S.; Hirose, Y.; Kitani, R.; Futai, K.; Maruya, S.-I.; Ishii, K.; Shinkawa, H. Autologous serum eardrops therapy with a chitin membrane for closing tympanic membrane perforations. *Otol. Neurotol.* **2008**, *29*, 791–795. [CrossRef]
163. Carles, G.; Dabiri, C.; Mchirgui, A. Different uses of chitosan for treating serious obstetric hemorrhages. *J. Gynecol. Obstet. Hum. Reprod.* **2016**, *46*, 693–695. [CrossRef]
164. Chung, Y.-J.; An, S.-Y.; Yeon, J.-Y.; Shim, W.S.; Mo, J.-H. Effect of a chitosan gel on hemostasis and prevention of adhesion after endoscopic sinus surgery. *Clin. Exp. Otorhinolaryngol.* **2016**, *9*, 143. [CrossRef]
165. Rahmani, F.; Moghadamnia, A.A.; Kazemi, S.; Shirzad, A.; Motallebnejad, M. Effect of 0.5% Chitosan mouthwash on recurrent aphthous stomatitis: A randomized double-blind crossover clinical trial. *Electron. Physician* **2018**, *10*, 6912. [CrossRef]
166. Shao, Y.; Zhou, H. Clinical evaluation of an oral mucoadhesive film containing chitosan for the treatment of recurrent aphthous stomatitis: A randomized, double-blind study. *J. Dermatol. Treat.* **2019**, 1–5. [CrossRef]
167. Kumar, K.A.; Kumar, J.; Sarvagna, J.; Gadde, P.; Chikkaboriah, S. Hemostasis and post-operative care of oral surgical wounds by hemcon dental dressing in patients on oral anticoagulant therapy: A split mouth randomized controlled clinical trial. *J. Clin. Diagn. Res.* **2016**, *10*, ZC37. [CrossRef]
168. Madrazo-Jiménez, M.; Rodríguez-Caballero, Á.; Serrera-Figallo, M.-Á.; Garrido-Serrano, R.; Gutiérrez-Corrales, A.; Gutiérrez-Pérez, J.-L.; Torres-Lagares, D. The effects of a topical gel containing chitosan, 0, 2% chlorhexidine, allantoin and despanthenol on the wound healing process subsequent to impacted lower third molar extraction. *Med. Oral Patol. Oral Y Cir. Bucal* **2016**, *21*, e696. [CrossRef] [PubMed]
169. Shafaeifard, S.; Sarkarat, F.; Pahlevan, R.; Ezati, A.; Keyhanlou, F. Investigating the effect of Chitohem powder on coagulation time and the complications following tooth extraction. *J. Res. Dent. Sci.* **2017**, *14*, 138–143.
170. Latańska, I.; Kozera-Żywczyk, A.; Paluchowska, E.B.; Owczarek, W.; Kaszuba, A.; Noweta, M.; Tazbir, J.; Kolesińska, B.; Draczyński, Z.; Sujka, W. Characteristic Features of Wound Dressings Based on Butyric-Acetic Chitin Copolyesters—Results of Clinical Trials. *Materials* **2019**, *12*, 4170. [CrossRef] [PubMed]
171. Azad, A.K.; Sermsintham, N.; Chandrkrachang, S.; Stevens, W.F. Chitosan membrane as a wound-healing dressing: Characterization and clinical application. *J. Biomed. Mater. Res. Part B Appl. Biomater.* **2004**, *69*, 216–222. [CrossRef]
172. Angspatt, A.; Taweerattanasil, B.; Janvikul, W.; Chokrungvaranont, P.; Sirimaharaj, W. Carboxymethylchitosan, alginate and tulle gauze wound dressings: A comparative study in the treatment of partial-thickness wounds. *Asian Biomed.* **2011**, *5*, 413–416.
173. Bachtell, N.; Goodell, T.; Grunkemeier, G.; Jin, R.; Gregory, K. Treatment of dialysis access puncture wound bleeding with chitosan dressings. *Dial. Transplant.* **2006**, *35*, 672–681. [CrossRef]
174. Ketan, P.; Anjali, P.; Rignesh, P.; Bhavika, P.; Priyank, P.; Dev, P. Assessing the Efficacy of Haemostatic Dressing Axiostat® In Trauma Care at a Tertiary Care Hospital in India: A Comparison with Conventional Cotton Gauze. *Indian J. Emerg. Med.* **2016**, *2*, 93–99. [CrossRef]
175. Halim, A.S.; Nor, F.M.; Mat Saad, A.Z.; Mohd Nasir, N.A.; Norsa'adah, B.; Ujang, Z. Efficacy of chitosan derivative films versus hydrocolloid dressing on superficial wounds. *J. Taibah Univ. Med. Sci.* **2018**, *13*, 512–520. [CrossRef]
176. Campani, V.; Pagnozzi, E.; Mataro, I.; Mayol, L.; Perna, A.; D'Urso, F.; Carillo, A.; Cammarota, M.; Maiuri, M.; De Rosa, G. Chitosan Gel to Treat Pressure Ulcers: A Clinical Pilot Study. *Pharmaceutics* **2018**, *10*, 15. [CrossRef]
177. Mo, X.; Cen, J.; Gibson, E.; Wang, R.; Percival, S.L. An open multicenter comparative randomized clinical study on chitosan. *Wound Repair Regen.* **2015**, *23*, 518–524. [CrossRef]

MDPI
St. Alban-Anlage 66
4052 Basel
Switzerland
Tel. +41 61 683 77 34
Fax +41 61 302 89 18
www.mdpi.com

Marine Drugs Editorial Office
E-mail: marinedrugs@mdpi.com
www.mdpi.com/journal/marinedrugs

www.ingramcontent.com/pod-product-compliance
Lightning Source LLC
LaVergne TN
LVHW070144100526
838202LV00015B/1888
* 9 7 8 3 0 3 9 3 6 0 7 2 7 *